D0623002

Brain and the Gaze

On the Active Boundaries of Vision

Jan Lauwereyns

The MIT Press
Cambridge, Massachusetts
London, England

O PTO

MIT Press books may be purchased at special quantity discounts for business or sales promotional use. For information, please email special_sales@mitpress.mit.edu or write to Special Sales Department, The MIT Press, 55 Hayward Street, Cambridge, MA 02142.

This book was set in Syntax and Times Roman by Toppan Best-set Premedia Limited, Hong Kong. Printed and bound in the United States of America.

Library of Congress Cataloging-in-Publication Data

Lauwereyns, Jan, 1969–
Brain and the gaze : on the active boundaries of vision / Jan Lauwereyns.
    p.   cm.
Includes bibliographical references and index.
ISBN 978-0-262-01791-6 (hardcover : alk. paper)
1. Vision—Popular works.   I. Title.
QP475.5.L38   2012
612.8'4—dc23
2012004935

10 9 8 7 6 5 4 3 2 1

Contents

Prelude: Output for Input

How do we gain access to things as they are? The question requires no defense—it is about as basic and important as it gets. How can we tell what is true from what is false? How does perception work? Questions such as these arise naturally, frequently, with slight variations, at different times and in different circumstances, in the minds of mothers, children, judges, journalists, scientists, artists, philosophers, police officers, politicians, bankers, insurance agents, managers, and most other human beings. In my head, these questions also resonate with the voices of thinkers and poets like William James (1890|1950b) and Wallace Stevens (1951). Says William James in volume 2 of his *Principles of Psychology*, at the beginning of chapter XXI on "The Perception of Reality" (1890|1950b, p. 283):

Everyone knows the difference between imagining a thing and believing in its existence, between supposing a proposition and acquiescing in its truth. In the case of acquiescence or belief, the object is not only apprehended by the mind, but it is held to have reality. Belief is thus the mental state or function of cognizing reality. As used in the following pages, "Belief" will mean every degree of assurance, including the highest possible certainty and conviction.

Everyone has experienced the difference between truly perceiving an object and merely imagining it. But do we *know* the difference? When and how can we be certain that we are "cognizing reality"? Gigerenzer (2002) assures us that in this life nothing is certain but death and taxes. Even William James appears to start stuttering in the quoted passage, struggling with a peculiar definition of "belief." The definition is valid only within the context of his text ("the following pages"), James implies. Outside it, the tricky word "belief" may often be associated with conviction, but not necessarily as a function of reality. In *The Necessary Angel: Essays on Reality and the Imagination*, Wallace Stevens (1951, p. 33) offers a suggestion I would like to read as a reply to James:

We have been a little insane about the truth. We have had an obsession. In its ultimate extension, the truth about which we have been insane will lead us to look beyond the truth to something in which the imagination will be the dominant complement. It is not only that the imagination adheres to reality, but, also, that reality adheres to the imagination and the interdependence is essential.

To gain access to things as they are, Stevens seems to argue, we need both imagination and reality. Without imagination, we have no way of cognizing reality. Perception revolves around the interplay between reality and the imagination. Without the active, creative component of "imagination"—a covert, internal process that projects virtual information and generates expectations and biases—there would be no perception—no opportunity to tune into real data, or to let actual signals rise above noise.

How do we gain access to things as they are? In the search for potential, partial answers to this question, we need to focus on the essential interdependence of reality and the imagination. We need to investigate the active nature of perception.

This Inspired and Careless Decision

What are the basic principles that govern the interaction between the world, the brain, and the praxis of perception? As a point of departure, I would like to take one of the most famous eye movements in world history (or rather mythology): that of Orpheus, the legendary Greek poet whose heart-wrenching laments convinced the gods to let him take his beloved Eurydice back to the world of the living on the condition that he not look back. Tragically, he did.

Why did Orpheus look back? Was it out of curiosity for the underworld or, more specifically, the shape of Eurydice as a ghost? Or was it out of impatience or anxiety, wishing to check, unsure whether Eurydice was actually following him back to life? Orpheus's terrible deed—an attempt at gathering visual information—has fascinated not only poets such as Rainer Maria Rilke (1995, p. 55, lines written in 1904: "his sight would race ahead of him like a dog, / stop, come back, then rushing off again,") and Jean Cocteau (director of the stunningly beautiful 1950 movie *Orphée*). It also received special attention in Maurice Blanchot's (1955|1989) classic essay on *The Space of Literature*, which opens, on an unnumbered page, with this straightforward admission: "A book, even a fragmentary one, has a center which attracts it. (…) [H]ere, toward the pages entitled 'Orpheus's Gaze.'"

Blanchot recognized in Orpheus's unfortunate act of perception an emblem of what poetry (and literature in general) is all about. The last paragraph of the pages in question is titled *The Leap* (p. 176). There we read this:

Writing begins with Orpheus's Gaze. And this gaze is the movement of desire that shatters the song's destiny, that disrupts concern for it, and in this inspired and careless decision reaches the origin, consecrates the song.

I am not entirely sure I understand this statement, or whether it is in fact comprehensible in a practical, neatly definable sense. But I like its curious sound (especially in the French original) and its beautiful word combinations ("the movement of desire," "the song's destiny," and "this inspired and careless decision"). The paradoxes keep reverberating: Action at the end, "that shatters destiny," brings us back to the beginning, "reaches the origin"; the loss of "the song's destiny" actually "consecrates the song." Everything happens autonomously or involuntarily, perhaps unconsciously, "inspired and careless." However, what really intrigues me here is the idea of connecting gaze dynamics with the imagination, with the creative dimension in literature—a quintessentially human enterprise, aimed at forging new thoughts and ideas, devoted to reading and writing meaningfulness into the world.

I read Blanchot's statement as an intuitive description of active perception. Active perception works paradoxically, with output for input, motor processes for sensory processes, eye movements for visual information. These paradoxical processes occur largely autonomously and involuntarily—we are seldom aware of the eye movements we make. We tend to forget that we actually, unwittingly, but nonneutrally, choose (or "construct") what we see, even though we routinely take our self-made pictures to be veridical representations of reality. Through these processes we create meaning—we recognize things to be things (objects or events) that carry semantic information. Meaning would be the target of the movement of desire. With our eye movements, we attempt to gain access to things as they are—a product of the interdependence of reality and the imagination, to paraphrase Wallace Stevens.

Exactly how does the interdependence work? How can we translate imagination into something tractable for the science of perception? Repeatedly rereading James, Stevens, and Blanchot, I realized I kept coming back to the topic of active perception, recognizing important roles for bias and sensitivity—concepts that I have explored previously (Lauwereyns, 2010)—in the interplay between imagination and reality.

Thus, the inspired and careless decision forced itself upon me, to write this book. The gaze would be my paradigm, the brain my cosubject and co-object.

For the structure of my title, *Brain and the Gaze*, I borrowed that of *Death and the Maiden*, thinking of the conventional English translation of the (unofficial) title of Franz Schubert's String Quartet No. 14 in D minor. (I did not know Keith Jarrett's *Death and the Flower* until after I had already decided on my title.) Brain stood for death (Thanatos, negation, discrimination, language), the gaze for the maiden (Eros, positive energy, connection, life).

I needed a subtitle to emphasize that the writing would be about visual perception and active processes—*On the Active Boundaries of Vision*. The last word serves as a tribute to the scientific genius of David Marr (1982|2010). The "Active Boundaries" are borrowed from the title of a collection of essays by the great American poet Michael Palmer (2008), in which he explores the "fugitive perceptions and resistant meanings" of poetry, "an art that is in many respects essentially unknowable, its silences articulate, its freedoms perversely demanding" (p. viii). Palmer stubbornly, wonderfully closely, pursued the elusive, what is "essentially unknowable." My topic will be more mundane even if I will occasionally visit poetry along the way to sharpen or soften a point or to start a discussion. My focus is on perception, a basic function, a natural question for any study of psychological principles—something I *believe* (in James's sense of the word) to be essentially knowable. The learning is possible and is being achieved, more or less, to an ever greater degree. With *Brain and the Gaze: On the Active Boundaries of Vision*, it is my objective to learn and to share the learning.

My Promises

Between writing the book and having written it, I needs must have my outline, my compass. The following preview offers what lies behind the author, before the reader. Prospective exercises of this kind, which generate expectations and create context, are crucial players in perception. In the act of pointing to future events, I am inviting your semantic system to read in particular ways—such a deictic gesture must be the most non-neutral (*biased!*) activity in a book on brain and the gaze. We (always both readers and writers) are warned. Every book makes its promises. Here are mine.

This is a book about active perception and its brain mechanisms. Every single chapter will focus on the gaze as the principal paradigm for active perception. The book is written first and foremost for neuroscientists, both students and experts. It is designed as a critical and engaging account, written by a single author, targeting maximal internal consistency in style and tone. The work, then, also wishes to be an attractive point of entry to the study of perception, its neural underpinnings and its broader psychological and philosophical implications. My home turf is neuroscience and, more specifically, cognitive neuroscience. Always returning to this vantage point, I aim to bring "other perspectives" (from Continental philosophy, phenomenology, and ecological psychology) to bear on the topics and issues that interest neuroscientists. The critical examinations via philosophical and psychological texts will always endeavor to produce relevant thoughts and ideas for neuroscientists.

At the same time, the book will not be overly technical. It will extend a helping hand to relatively inexperienced students as well as readers from different fields who encounter the various concepts about perception and the brain for the first time. Though libraries and shops should classify the book under "neuroscience," I do believe that these sections are visited not only by neuroscientists but also by readers who are interested in specific topics such as perception—readers from neighboring academic fields (e.g., literary theory, social studies, economics, linguistics) and readers outside academia (e.g., those with a vested interest in art) who are keen to understand how we are able to see the things we see.

I will avoid mixing jargons. With cognitive neuroscientists as my primary audience, my speech will include Plain English and Neuroscience English. But even when using Neuroscience English, I will endeavor to give nonneuroscientists enough cues to acquire the necessary bit of Neuroscience English on the spot.

Yet, also for neuroscientists the book's approach will look unfamiliar. I will take the novelty as both a wonderful challenge and an undeniable risk. This is not a standard monograph but a book that demands freedom of thought, to rethink the cognitive neuroscience of perception by engaging in a frank and open-minded discussion with critics of neuroscience from phenomenology to psychoanalysis. The goal is not to build a defense but to look ahead toward ways in which alternate views may help us reinterpret the available data and devise promising new lines of investigation.

Research on perception has been transformed over the past two decades with the development of, and easy access to, powerful tools for imaging and computation. Aroused, or even a little annoyed, by the high-powered enterprise of cognitive neuroscience, thinkers such as the psychoanalyst Žižek (2006|2009), or the empirically oriented philosopher Noë (2004) and other proponents of "embodied cognition," have formulated critical responses, which have echoed or updated complaints from previous generations, such as those raised by Merleau-Ponty (1945|2008) and Gibson (1979|1986). Several issues recur in these criticisms: the active, or even constructive, nature of perception; the implications of perspective and subjectivity; the content and depth of representation; and the appropriate criteria for truth and relevance. However, the insights from ecological perception, phenomenology, and embodied cognition have as yet not been translated to neuroscience. There could be at least two reasons for this. On the one hand, these insights occasionally sounded like divisive "attacks" rather than constructive criticisms and so may have elicited (if anything at all) a withdrawal response from the neuroscience community. On the other hand, these insights have in many cases failed to give concrete pointers to how they might be incorporated for new empirical efforts in neuroscience research, and so the criticisms may have baffled rather than inspired neuroscientists.

The present book will rise to the challenge of incorporating the dynamic and constructive aspects into an account of the neural underpinnings that underlie perception. The agenda, then, is to read closely the criticisms from ecological perception, phenomenology, and embodied cognition in order to take home what may be useful for neuroscience. The emphasis will naturally be on visual perception since gaze dynamics represent arguably the clearest case of "action in perception." However, the book will compare visual perception with other modalities to understand what is unique about gaze and visual perception versus what is true for perception in general.

As I am a bit of a numerological fetishist, I will have seven plus (not minus) two chapters (giving me the holy number of nine, the number of books Sappho wrote): seven proper chapters, accompanied by the important ritual events of opening (with the present "prelude") and closing (with the "coda"). Before introducing the seven chapters, I would like to take a little detour (if you are in a rush, please jump to the next paragraph). I am writing, and wrote, the first draft of the following outline when I started the linear writing phase of this book (on February 23,

2011, with an inescapable, if rather dark, sense of occasion, on the day that New Zealand Prime Minister John Key declared a national emergency, following the terrible earthquake in Christchurch; it was also the hundred-and-ninetieth anniversary of the death of the great poet John Keats and, infinitely more trivially, the thirteenth anniversary of my Ph.D. defense on "the intentionality of visual selective attention"). Thus, there was a particular moment in time that counts as the beginning. However, I will be adjusting this outline throughout my work on the book, retrospectively tweaking the promises so that I might hope to deliver. This is how active perception works: with the interplay between imagination and reality, expectation and confirmation, refined sensitivity and improved bias. As mentioned above, the act of pointing remains the most nonneutral activity, especially in a book on brain and the gaze. We (always both readers and writers) are warned. I will continually be checking my promises.

Looking Forward to the Past

Chapter 1, "Free Viewing," starts from the observation that perception takes time and makes trajectories. The world does not come to us all at once. Arguably the first and most fundamental principle to note about perception is the dynamic and constrained nature of the process. Any observer must integrate little bits and pieces of information across time and space in order to understand what is happening in a given situation. The book opens with an exploration of the *active boundaries* within which the interaction between the world, the brain, and the praxis of perception takes place. The point of departure is the special nature of eye movements as a type of observer behavior that is intrinsically devoted to the acquisition of real-world information. Yet, our eye movements perform the task of information gathering in a decidedly biased fashion: not random, not systematic or machine-like, but chaotic, exhibiting a form of "bounded unpredictability." Here, the concept of *informativeness* will be introduced as a key player in the attractor dynamics of perception. Information may have intrinsic value and act as a proximate form of reinforcement, promoting exploration and "perception for perception." Research, it will be argued, often stands to benefit from an economic analysis of perception, using information value as the critical, observer-dependent currency. The discussion also raises the implicit denial of agency in perception, or why we trust our self-made perceptions to be veridical.

In chapter 2, "A Sensorimotor System," I will introduce the anatomical constraints that help shape the active boundaries of vision. The focus is on the actual implications of our biology. Aiming to give the body its due place in embodied cognition, in fact, requires more than merely acknowledging that functions such as perception are situated and limited in scope. While proposals such as those of Merleau-Ponty (1945|2008) have rightfully pulled the role of the body to the foreground, the task of characterizing and investigating the particularities of anatomically grounded biases and tendencies remains largely before us. The chapter sketches the contours of this task by focusing on the intrinsically dialectical nature of the brain's visual system, with a basic introduction of the neural circuits for eye movement control. The brain, it turns out, is organized in such a way as to facilitate negotiation. This pervasive interaction occurs between various polarities in perception, including center and surround, figure and ground, object and context, fovea and parafovea, and ventral and dorsal processing. The interaction is orchestrated strategically over space and over time by using context as a cue to generate specific expectations. The process implies integration of views, which raises important theoretical issues about the underlying algorithms and representations. In this chapter, I offer an initial exploration of these issues via a discussion of Noë's (2004) enactive view of perception.

Chapter 3, "The Moving Retina," takes a closer look at the notion of a visual *system*. What are, properly speaking, the systematic features of the brain's visual system? I will investigate this topic by reconsidering the mechanisms of active perception that are at work at the level of the retina—the first, most machine-like stage of visual processing. The retina does not receive feedback signals from downstream brain areas and so would appear to function in a strictly "bottom-up" fashion. However, newly emerging research has emphasized the complexity of information processing at the level of the retina, going beyond what has classically been determined as "sensory." Moreover, with eye movements, the retina is continually moving as a function of higher-order control, which can be regarded as an indirect form of feedback. These two observations warrant a new look at the function of the retina from the perspective of active perception. In the final analysis, the anatomical constraints imply possible directions of information processing, but actual perception revolves around how these options are translated into real or virtual phenomena of things around us. How and when does perception begin? Is the "machine" turned on automatically by certain stimuli? How do these processes relate to consciousness? Important topics here include the extent of automaticity and autonomy in vision, the effects of training and expertise, and the existence of modules devoted to specific categories of information such as faces or snakes. Recurrent in these discussions will be the theme of purpose and intentionality, which can be rephrased as a general bias toward meaning.

For chapter 4, "Seeing and Grasping," I will begin with perhaps the least controversial statement about vision, saying that it performs a function in service of cognition. Seeking a common ground among all theories and intuitions about perception, we may note that seeing is universally understood as a way of (metaphorically) grasping the visual presence of objects and events. Chapter 4 explores the merits and demerits of taking the cognitive stance to the extreme, with the hypothesis that vision does not merely detect or discriminate physical objects and events passively but in a very proactive sense defines and delineates (virtual) objects and events. That is to say, objects only become objects by virtue of how they emerge as graspable units in vision. The focus on the active role of the observer in this process is sharpened through close readings of Gaston Bachelard's *The Poetics of Space* (1958|1994) and Žižek's (2006|2009) *The Parallax View*. The proposed mechanisms and characteristics are compared with available empirical data on, among other things, the internal monitoring of eye movements, predictive remapping, ego- versus allocentric coding, and the coordination between visual selection and purposeful action. Selective processing and dynamic sensitivity imply tractable costs and benefits in the effort, speed, and accuracy of information processing. This proposal develops with a discussion of Gibson's (1979|1986) ecological perception. Here I will argue that biases and sensitivities determine the economy of perception in the critical currency of information value, or meaning.

In chapter 5, "The Intensive Approach," the core cognitive function of vision is explored further by highlighting the implicit assumptions of causality and meaningfulness. The tending toward meaning in perception works via complex, parallel, and divergent projections of information. Every step along the way changes the information and modulates the neural activity, thus chasing away Cartesian ghosts and observers-within-observers. The notion of echo variations is emphasized with the functions of the thalamus, or the brain's inner chamber, which proves to be anything but a simple relay station. The varying echoes of information attest to the existence of representations of objects and features at different levels of abstraction. I will emphasize the *intensive* nature of representations: selective, amplified, shaped by purpose, and reliant on virtual information. Magnitude and duration turn out to be critical properties of neural representations, often neglected by theorists. The neural and cognitive mechanisms of intensive processing are discussed with examples of afterimages, filling in, and visual working memory. Reading Dennett (1991) allows me to sharpen my thoughts about these phenomena. I will characterize active vision as an intensive form of traveling back and forth between memory, sensation, and imagination. This portrayal benefits from concepts and ideas in the works of Kant (1781|2007) and other masters of philosophical investigation. A few words are devoted to subjective experiments, Goethe (1810|2006), and the ever-fascinating topic of colors.

Chapter 6 is titled "The Gaze of Others." In it, I will explore the role of the gaze as object for perception (i.e., the gaze of others as a visual stimulus). This introduces yet another crossover between perception and action. I will argue that there exists a natural connection between our own ability of gaze control and our reading of other people's gaze. Eye movements allow the observer to receive different portions of visual information from one moment to the next and are perfectly in accord with the theory of intromission, which states that light enters the eye, and not the other way around—a truth carved in stone since the days of Alhazen (a thousand years ago). However, eye movements also constitute, or produce, visual information in at least two different ways, both of which warrant a reappraisal of the much-maligned emission theory. First, eye movements can have a formative influence on the observer's preference: What we happen to see is, more often than not, what we end up liking; that is, vision modulates affect. Second, eye movements communicate the observer's "focus of attention" to other observers and are intuitively read as signals that index *informativeness*, with important emotional and social implications. Chapter 6 examines both strains of "emission effects" pertaining to the gaze by exploring the connection between fixation (choice) and association (inclusion). Relevant topics to be addressed here are the mirror system, shared attention, and the theory of mind, as well as the counterparts of these concepts in cultural studies and psychoanalysis.

"Out of sight, out of mind," the saying goes. Chapter 7, "Seeing and Nothingness," reflects on the truth of this prescientific wisdom by translating the role of indexing in vision to a more general proposal on the intrinsic *intentionality* of vision and consciousness. The concept of intentionality, here, implies that the act of seeing necessarily takes an object. There is no vision, unless we see *something*. There is no consciousness, unless we are conscious of *something*. Yet, the "mind's eye" can be directed, via imagination and memory, to things that are not there. Thus, if perception (as will have been argued in previous chapters) is primarily a cognitive act on the basis of virtual information, then how can it be distinguished from other cognitive acts on the basis of virtual information, such as dreaming, imagining, and remembering? The clue must reside in the critical interaction with the immediate world, the physical presence of things as they are. The world offers a level of detail and a physical stability matched by no internal process. Perception, unlike all other cognitive acts, works directly and intensively with sensory information that is as close as we can ever get to the actual physical processes before us. This interaction with the immediate world—or the interplay between hypothesis and test, between imagination and reality—ultimately provides us with the necessary platform to distinguish fact from fiction, truths from falsehoods, and "what is" from "what is not"—both highly practical and deeply philosophical questions. The book, then, converges on an intensive view of perception, combining intent (purpose, meaning) with effortful processing of a limited real-world field (typically centered on objects). Active perception combines motor and sensory processes to create and receive meaningful objects—always only a few, and always preferably important ones, useful or dangerous, beautiful or strange.

Laboratory of Sensorimotor Research

So it is my intention to bridge the gap between "the motor side" and "the sensory side" in neuroscience. The book title and subtitle emphasize this already, with "the gaze" and "vision" in close proximity of one another. The motor and sensory sides are even closer together in the Laboratory of Sensorimotor Research, one of the places I would like to think of as my true home in science—a thought that takes me to my acknowledgments.

My interest in brain and the gaze was cultivated in several of such true homes: the Laboratory of Experimental Psychology, led by Géry d'Ydewalle, when I was an undergraduate, and then a graduate, student from 1991 to 1998 at the University of Leuven, Belgium; the Eyelab of John Henderson and Fernanda Ferreira, during an intense year in 1996–1997 when I was a visiting student at Michigan State University; and the research unit led by Okihide Hikosaka, during my days as a postdoc, first at Juntendo University in Tokyo, Japan, and then at the National

Institutes of Health (NIH), in Bethesda, Maryland. Eye tracking was the favorite method in the first two labs, populated by the dying breed of hardcore cognitive psychologists. The third was a neurophysiology lab, specialized in single-unit studies with monkeys performing eye movement tasks.

When Okihide Hikosaka was offered the opportunity to set up his lab at the NIH, it came as an invitation to join the Laboratory of Sensorimotor Research, the house for science built by Robert H. Wurtz—Bob. If anyone has the appropriate expertise to write a book on brain and the gaze, it would have to be Bob Wurtz. Until he does finally write that book, I will merely stand in and write the present book in honor of the man who should have written it.

Of course, me being me, I cannot write the book Bob would have written. Not only do I lack his massive expertise but, for better or worse, my mind has been shaped by other influences—literary. Blanchot was there already from the beginning, but I have been, and continue to be, amazed by the works of many writers, poets, friends, teachers, and colleagues, not less numerous or brilliant than the beautiful minds I have met, and continue to meet, in science. Working on the present book, I tell neuroscientists I am writing the book "that Bob should write," but to my literary friends I say I am writing the book "that Heidi would write if she were a neuroscientist"—Heidi Thomson, my former colleague at Victoria University of Wellington, New Zealand, who unlocked the English Romantic poets for me (particularly Keats and Coleridge), pointing to the omnipresent gaze dynamics in their work. This book is a work written in dialogue with the virtual voice of Heidi Thomson—an excellent model of "the literary scholar"—almost as much as it is a tribute to Bob Wurtz—the perfect exemplar of "the neuroscientist."

Refusing, in a Coleridgean vein, the easy dialectics and writing in threes, the third major source of inspiration for this book is Minoru Tsukada, whose greatness resides first and foremost in his amazing ability to integrate his personae as neuroscientist, painter, and lover of life. The man is one of the main reasons why I am still in science—he provides existence proof that the integration of the three Kantian domains is more than merely possible. In very concrete ways my sensei has also been a crucial source of support at critical moments. With his keen aesthetic eye and fascination for dynamics in the brain, Minoru Tsukada also embodied several intentional undercurrents that wrote themselves into the fabric of this book.

I do not have enough space here to thank all the many people who inspired me to write this book, or in the writing of this book. If they know me, they know my thoughts are structured (anatomized for bias) so as to be with them always. Nevertheless, and conscious of the risk of naming names, I would like to give explicit thanks to Bob Prior and Susan Buckley, my lifeline at the MIT Press; Johan Velter and Arnoud van Adrichem, my partners in literary crime; Matt Weaver, my former and very talented Ph.D. student; and Muneyoshi Takahashi, my current postdoc, who more than anyone provided and protected the literary space that I needed for writing this book.

I would also like to acknowledge institutional support: from the International Education Center and the Graduate School of Systems Life Sciences at Kyushu University, Japan; the Brain Science Center at Tamagawa University, Japan; and the School of Psychology at Victoria University of Wellington, New Zealand. This work was made possible in part thanks to project grant RGP0039|2010 from the Human Frontier Science Program.

Last and never less than most important, I would be unable to accomplish anything if it were not for my home base, Nanami ("Seven Seas"), Shinsei ("Pure Star"), and the quiet cherry blossom well, Shizuka ("Peaceful").

1 Free Viewing

Yet did I never breathe its pure serene
Till I heard Chapman speak out loud and bold:
Then felt I like some watcher of the skies
When a new planet swims into his ken

These lines were written by John Keats, in his 1816 sonnet "On First Looking into Chapman's Homer" (1978|2003, p. 34). They form lines seven to ten, right around the spot where we may expect, according to Italian tradition, the so-called *volta*, or sudden turn in perspective, tone, or theme. Through the ages and in English hands—notably William Shakespeare's and Edmund Spenser's—the character and techniques of the sonnet did change somewhat. And John Keats, the youngest and arguably the most talented of the British Romantic poets, was never one for shrinking back from inventing his own forms. But here, in this sonnet, the *volta* operates in prototypical fashion. In the critical ninth line Keats connects his discovery of Homer's "pure serene" in Chapman's translation with a great vertical leap, an upward shift of gaze, "Then felt I like some watcher of the skies."

The tenth line makes the poem sublime—not with a new *volta*, but by elaborating on the image of the stargazer. We know the watcher of the skies will be elated, mystified and overawed, "When a new planet swims into his ken." Through this image, we understand better than through any more direct admission how Keats must have felt when first looking into Chapman's Homer. The new knowledge, the previously unidentified object in the sky, is sure to paint more than merely a smile on the face of the observer. Perhaps the sound of Keats's line of verse, with the slightly archaic "ken," works particularly (almost nostalgically) well on ears attuned to German, Scottish, or Dutch, where the verb "to ken" (in Middle English: *kennen*) means "to know" or "to understand." In the sonnet, the range of knowing converges on the field of vision. Now within his ken, the stargazer is able both visually to process and mentally to cognize the new planet. Mind and the visual sense perfectly agree in this wonderful instance of perception.

Yet, the instance appears not to be a point in time, not in the sense of a precise instant that we might try to clock the way we would the next world record in the hundred-meter sprint, with at least two digits behind the dot after the nine (unless Usain Bolt, or the next breed of sprinter, manages to take it down to eight). The perception of the new planet seems to be drawn out over time, not reducible to one exact moment, but living in a vague momentariness, spanning several seconds and probably requiring more than one eye movement. John Keats might have had the discovery of the planet Uranus in mind, by the astronomer William Herschel, an event that unfolded over several nights in the months of March and April 1781. (Herschel first thought he had charted an unknown comet but later realized it was the first new planet to be discovered in over a thousand years; Holmes, 2008.) We imagine the stargazer a little unsure at first, briefly noticing something out of the corner of his eye, then losing track of the object when he aims his focal vision at the place where he thought he saw something, only to then gradually convince himself that there is really something out there, millions of years old perhaps, but new for him—out of the darkness, a new planet, sluggishly *swimming* into his ken.

The Dynamics of Gaze

To see things as they are, we need time. The new planet must be given the opportunity to swim. In the quoted lines it may seem as if Keats portrays the perception to be a passive one, something that happens to, and remains beyond the control of, the observer. Such may be the feeling we ultimately have when perceiving things. We grasp what is there, we believe in its truth, to repeat William James's phrase—we accept what is given. However, the data require the act of collection. We must *create* the opportunity for the new planet to come swimming into our ken. John Keats emphasized this as well in his sonnet "On First Looking into Chapman's Homer" (1978|2003, p. 34). The poem opened with the words "Much have I travell'd" and abstracted the long journey to the point where the "I" finally gets to breathe the "pure serene" when Chapman speaks "out loud and bold."

We must look here, look there. The stargazer will employ his or her telescopes, she or he will check the weather, wait for clear skies. Effort comes into it. We have no choice but to make trajectories, to compare. We must travel over time and over space. The whole of the world at once is too large to be graspable or even meaningful in its undifferentiated massiveness. We can only work with little bits and pieces, in which we recognize structures, patterns with predictable outcomes, statistical regularities, semantic values, and important implications. Let this be our most basic truth about perception—axiom the first: Perception is a limited process. It is a happening, dynamic and constrained, situated at particular coordinates in time and space.

Here is a similar thought, wonderfully expressed by Alva Noë, author of the inspiring monograph *Action in Perception* (2004, p. 164):

Perceiving how things are is a mode of exploring how things appear. How they appear is, however, an aspect of how they are. To explore appearance is thus to explore the environment, the world. To discover how things are, from how they appear, is to discover an order or pattern in their appearances. The process of perceiving, of finding out how things are, is a process of meeting the world; it is an activity of skillful exploration.

It is one of the most lucid and agreeable statements in Noë's wonderful book, which, in good philosophic (and neuroscientific) tradition, I will proceed to disagree with on almost everything else. Even in the quoted excerpt I feel perhaps a little queasy about equating perception with an activity of skillful exploration. Such activity surely contributes to perception, but does it necessarily have to be "skillful," and, to ask a Clinton-esque question, what is the meaning of "is" here? I might also have preferred the word "function" over "mode" in the first sentence. But still, I find Noë's words very appealing here, with their emphasis on perception as a process that involves exploration and discovery, that is, action bound to time and space.

Noë (2004) rightfully puts his foot down firmly on the role of action in perception. On the second page of *Action in Perception*, he exposes a common tendency of ours: "We tend, when thinking about perception, to make vision, not touch, our paradigm, and we tend to think of vision on a photographic model," the implication being that the two tendencies are fallacious. Surely, to think of vision on a photographic model must be wrong. In fact, Noë's complaint is hardly a new one. On the first actual page of text in Richard L. Gregory's classic *Eye and Brain: The Psychology of Seeing*, we read what was written long ago (as measured in neuroscience time): "The eye is often described as like a camera, but it is the quite uncamera-like features of perception which are most interesting"

(1966, p.7). We know we should not rely on the photographic model, but somehow it keeps returning, implicitly, in hidden assumptions. Perhaps we should try to understand the parameters and conditions of its intrinsic attraction before simply rejecting the photographic model as misleading. After all, if perception is about finding out how things are, then we should be able to test the quality of perception—its accuracy and "objectivity"—against other reports, traces, or reflections of how things are. The photographic model has dominated as the most convincing method to capture visual traces. Could it be that the photographic model works metaphorically to reinforce our conviction? With it, we reassert that what we perceive is really out there, just like photos reflect the patterns of light that enter the camera.

Cognitive neuroscience would do well to keep the photographic model closer, the way the famous fictitious Mafioso Michael Corleone (according to Vito in *The Godfather Part II*) would keep his friends close but his enemies closer (a wisdom whose first dawning is variously attributed to Chinese or Italian philosophers of war or scheming). The photographic model can be our null hypothesis. The task of cognitive neuroscience is to show *how* human perception works differently, with emphasis on the action, on the doing. Noë (2004, p. 1) would have us think of perception as a process of groping and grasping, preferring the paradigm of touch:

Perception is not something that happens to us, or in us. It is something we do. Think of a blind person tap-tapping his or her way around a cluttered space, perceiving that space by touch, not all at once, but through time, by skillful probing and movement. This is, or at least ought to be, our paradigm of what perceiving is.

It is the core tenet of Noë's "enactive approach to perception." Still on the first page, he states that "we *enact* our perceptual experience, we act it out." In these expressions the "acting" may almost seem to rhyme with the Hollywood profession, where the doing involves pretense and the action is a matter of playing, not how things are, but how they can be imagined—an intriguing idea, with an important role for the imagination, but this does not match with the rest of Noë's text. The enacting, here, I think, is meant only in the sense of *executing*, of *carrying out*.

I dare not assume to understand, or to be able to imagine, the experience of a blind person, skillfully probing and moving around, mapping space by touch. Indeed, it is my very lack of such skills that prevents me from being able to imagine what it would be like. I cannot understand the layout of objects by touch. When I close my eyes, my most salient experience is the lack of visual input. If I walk across the room with eyes closed, I feel uneasy, uncertain, my balance is off, and I expect every second to trip over an undefined *this*, to stumble upon a mysterious *that*.

The appropriate paradigm to study perception *is* vision. It is no accident that we think about it first. Vision is the sense we rely on most frequently and extensively to obtain and to exchange information. Seeing is so naturally dominant a form of perception that it has worked itself into our idioms for understanding, even when other senses are involved, as in "I see what you're saying" (a title with a fine double entendre in Andersson et al., 2011). Moreover, even from the perspective of action in perception, vision rightfully comes to mind as a sense fundamentally shaped by our movements—our eye movements, our head movements, the dynamics of gaze when we look here, and there, and here again.

To see things as they are, we need to move our eyes constantly. The most urgent reason for this is that our eyes are particularly choosy cameras, to speak with the (erroneous!) photographic model. Our eyes do not give us a full view of things before us—far from it. They fail to "photograph" everything in front of us, in our field of vision. At any one moment in time, we see only a small fraction in sharp detail, as in the middle panel of figure 1.1 (the "Foveal" view), not the left panel (the view enjoyed by "Eternity"). The rest is a blur, as in the right panel

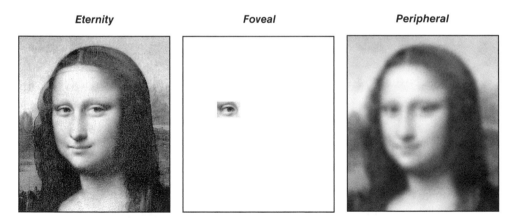

Eternity   *Foveal*   *Peripheral*

Figure 1.1
Three views of Leonardo da Vinci's *Mona Lisa*, or *La Gioconda*, painted between 1503 and 1519, quite possibly the most famous portrait in world history. The left panel shows the face in full detail, as we might recognize it truly to be for all eternity. The middle panel picks a small detail of the face, about as much as we can effectively process with our sharpest powers of vision at any particular moment in time. The right panel shows the low-frequency information contained in the picture, (very) roughly corresponding to the amount of detail we can process in our peripheral vision.

(the "Peripheral" view). The small fraction that we see in sharp detail corresponds to the center of the eye, the *fovea*. It covers no more than two degrees of visual angle, that is, roughly one percent of our visual field. To get detailed visual information, then, we need to aim and re-aim the fovea all the time, moving our eyes, shifting our gaze, focusing on this, that, and the other thing, until we have covered enough of the visual field to "get the picture," at which point we probably have to start moving our eyes again because things might have changed in the meantime.

For the full explanation of foveal versus peripheral vision, I will gladly refer to textbooks (e.g., Kandel, Schwartz, & Jessell, 2000; Palmer, 1999) and even more gladly to the delightful *Vision and Art: The Biology of Seeing* by Margaret Livingstone (2002|2008), from which I borrowed a few ideas for figure 1.1. But the story in brief is this. In the back of the eye we have the *retina*, which consists of several layers of cells, including the photoreceptor cells. Speaking in Neuroscience English, the photoreceptor cells transduce the energy of light, or translate the electromagnetic waves to changes of the membrane potential. In Plain English: The photoreceptor cells bleach in response to light, and this chemical process affects other cells. The photoreceptors come in two large families: rods, which do not need much light, respond slowly, and convey no color information, and their counterparts, the cones, which have the opposite characteristics. The fovea is at the center of the retina; it is populated almost exclusively by cones. As we move away from the fovea, the ratio of cones over rods changes. Close to the fovea, there are still quite a lot of cones, but the rods gain in strength. Further away from the fovea, there are very few cones; the rods rule.

Foveal vision, the center of our gaze, serviced by cones, gives us color and sharp detail for a tiny portion of the visual field. Peripheral vision, fed by information from rods, provides us with a general, roughish outline of the background. When cued to take note of it, people are often surprised to observe just how narrow their range of sharp (foveal) vision really is. Two degrees of visual angle corresponds to about the width of your thumb at arm's length—or the word "degrees" at the beginning of this sentence if you hold the book at a reasonable distance (say, 30 centimeters). Try it. Stretch your right arm out before you. Stick your thumb up. Fixate it. How much can you see left and right of your thumb without moving your eyes? Or go back to the sentence that began with "Two degrees." Focus on the word "degrees." Make sure not to move your eyes. How many words can you recognize left, right, above, below?

Literally speaking, my instructions in the previous sentences are nonsensical, filled with paradoxes. First, I ask you to focus on something. Then, in the next sentence, which you should not be able to read if you have indeed fixed your gaze as I asked, I give you further instructions. You can only carry out something structurally similar to what I asked if you hold the instructions in memory and then control your gaze as directed while attempting to concentrate "mentally" on peripheral information. Much of what you do, then, takes place *inside your head*: the maintenance in memory of the instructions, the mental concentration on peripheral visual information, and the attempts at linking up visual patterns with words or things that you know, that you have with you somehow, always—in your memory, your lexicon, your hidden archives. "Perception," said Noë (2004, p. 1), "is not something that happens (…) in us." But many of its aspects *do* happen inside us. The inside/outside will be a crucial dimension throughout the study of perception.

Covert versus Overt Processing

One particularly fascinating aspect about perception-inside-the-head is that we are indeed able to focus selectively on visual information in a way that does not follow from our eye, head, or body movements. We *can* look strategically out of the corner of our eyes—stalkers and private eyes are presumably expert at it, pretending not to be staring at you but at the beautiful tree in blossom. Posner (1980) was the first in a long line of researchers (including, e.g., Weaver, Phillips, & Lauwereyns, 2010) to study this kind of concentration on peripheral information systematically in the laboratory, providing elegant evidence of spatial orienting independent of gaze fixation. Cued to process one side of the screen, participants were able to "see" the targets there faster and with fewer errors than on the opposite side while the eyes remained fixed on a marker in the middle of the screen. Posner (1980) proposed that this form of orienting reflects a *covert attention* system. The word "attention" might be a bit problematic (more on this in the final section of this chapter). For now I would rather replace it by the slightly more neutral sound of "selective visual processing." However, the interesting distinction is between covert versus overt processing: "Covert" refers to mechanisms of selection that pertain to information processing inside the head, independent of body, head, or eye position; "overt" stands for mechanisms of orienting that are accompanied—or enacted—by movements of the body, head, or eye.

Alva Noë will agree that this is a crucial dimension that should always be in the foreground of our theoretical and empirical investigations of perception.

Does the existence of covert visual processing prove the enactive view of perception wrong? It certainly puts boundaries on the role of overt movement, which occasionally sounds a bit overstated in Noë (2004). But more will need to be learned, particularly with respect to the underlying neural mechanisms, and the "premotor theory" of covert selective visual processing. A brief flash forward: It could be that the covert processing involves *virtual* movement planning—a thought that Noë will undoubtedly appreciate yet also a thought that becomes compelling only by scrutinizing what happens inside the head during perception. As I said, the inside/outside will be a crucial dimension throughout. The enactive view of perception should inspire neuroscientists not only to consider what happens outside our heads but also to look with renewed precision and slightly different questions inside our heads.

The dialectics of overt and covert visual processing, of foveal and peripheral processing, also plays a prominent role in the Keats quote at the start of this chapter. When the stargazer found a new planet swimming into his ken, I suggested it was a process that took several seconds and probably a few eye movements. I imagine that the new planet would be incredibly distant, its light very faint in the night sky, such that it can only be picked up by rods, in peripheral vision. The stargazer might have accidentally caught a glance of it at first. Then, when he looked straight at the new planet, with foveal vision, it would vanish into the darkness, invisible via cones (or as the contemporary poet Keith Waldrop [2009, p. 100] writes: "In the spectral twilight, my dark-adapted eyes find stars— lost again if I try to look at them"). However, looking deliberately out of the corner of his eyes, aiming his foveal vision on purpose slightly away from his target, the stargazer would notice the new planet gradually, swimmingly, returning, as the rods start picking up the faint light again. This "return" would be an essential component for the experience in the ken; upon the return, the new planet is understood to be an object that can be re-cognized.

The smile of the Mona Lisa may be another case that thrives on the dialectics between overt and covert visual processing. Livingstone (2002|2008) discovered that the smile of *La Gioconda* is clearly there as a shadow round the mouth in peripheral vision, where things look blurry (i.e., information of low spatial frequency). On the other hand, the information of high spatial frequency, the fine detail, available to foveal vision, would show lips, more or less neutrally closed. Thus, if we aim the center of our gaze at the mouth, we see no smile. If we focus on the eyes or the hair, a smiley face emerges.

These two phenomenological examples suggest that the dialectics of overt versus covert processing can be quite subtle and complex—elusive or difficult to track in laboratory settings. Yet they have a strong impact on our experience. We will have to confront these dialectics with full force, along with the questions of what happens inside versus outside the head. We need the enactive view of perception to challenge us. So we read again.

"Perception," said Noë (2004, p. 1), "is not something that happens (…) in us." The statement keeps biting me. The negative is tricky, for it invites the slightly mystified question "Where does it happen, if not *in* us?" Can it be outside, *Out of Our Heads?* The latter phrase is the provocative title of Noë's 2009 book, to which I will return. For now, I will leave my answer open, feeling the need to explore a bit further, looking at various types of data and ideas. I grant that perception is not something that depends *only* on what happens inside our heads; all kinds of movements and interaction with the world are crucial, as we sit down, turn on the lamp, open the book, and make eye movements to be able to see the words I have written here. We will need to take extreme care to consider both what happens inside our heads and what happens elsewhere, in and with our entire bodies, and around us, in the spaces that provide the external situation of our perception. I will harp many times on the need for this extreme care—it is advice that has not sufficiently been heeded or heard in neuroscience.

Often, and for good reason in terms of data processing, we work with very constrained experimental settings. We look at neural correlates of visual processing when extremely simple stimuli are presented on a particular portion of the retina under conditions without any movement (as in the classic experiments by Hubel and Wiesel, 1959). Or we study only certain reinforced types of eye movement (trained, and performed on command) while the position of the head is fixed and the movement range of the rest of the body is limited (as in the very successful paradigm introduced by Wurtz, 1969). Such carefully controlled experiments have been, and continue to be, vital to the enterprise of cognitive neuroscience and to our understanding of what *does* happen inside our heads during perception. At the same time, though, we must—through convergent operations—learn the limits of the simple processes by comparing with the complex, by collecting other data, say, under free viewing conditions when any kind of eye movement is allowed but the head is fixed (e.g., Gibboni, Zimmerman, & Gothard, 2009; Mazer & Gallant, 2003) or under head-unrestrained conditions when particular gaze shifts are performed on command (e.g., Cecala & Freedman, 2009). Someday soon it should be possible to study neural correlates under head- and body-unrestrained free viewing conditions (but on March 9, 2011, PubMed returned zero items for "unrestrained free viewing").

Much of this research on neural correlates of visual perception, particularly at the level of single neurons, is carried out with monkeys (by lowering electrodes into the brain, near but not inside individual neurons, close enough to be able to record their action potentials). These so-called "single-unit studies" give unique electrophysiological data in terms of temporal and spatial precision, as yet unmatched by other, noninvasive techniques that can be applied with humans. The situation is unfortunate from any perspective, including the ethical and scientific. Nevertheless, many scientists believe that the information gained from such experiments warrants their existence. I do not always agree. Sometimes I do. For research specifically targeting eye movements and visual perception, monkeys are the appropriate (nonhuman) animal model, because rats (the main alternative for this kind of electrophysiology) show limited visual processing abilities.

Curiously, with respect to recording under unrestrained conditions, the work with monkeys seems to lag behind studies on spatial cognition with rats. We (I must plead guilty for a tiny bit of this rat work) are able to obtain compelling data about covert spatial coding with freely moving animals. Some of the activity reflects future paths (Johnson & Redish, 2007; Van der Meer et al., 2010) or impending spatial choices (Takahashi et al., 2009), independent of the rat's motor processes and current spatial position (in terms of body and head orientation as well as in terms of physical location in the maze or in the Skinner box). I will say more about the implications of these studies later when discussing the contents of internal coding. But here I would like to note that present technology allows researchers to collect sufficient data about various aspects of body position and motor activity, so that restraining during single- or multi-unit recording may not always be as necessary as researchers tend to think, perhaps out of habit rather than with their full powers of rational reasoning.

Speaking of movements of the body, head, and eye, perhaps this is a good place for a linguistic clarification. In the neuroscience literature, the word "gaze" is often used specifically for the combination of eye and head position. This will be the definition I adopt. What I gaze at is what appears in my foveal vision, in consequence of whichever movements I make, of eye, head, or any body part. In much of the empirical literature, experiments are conducted with the head fixed or stable so that shifts of gaze are produced by eye movements alone. Often the underlying or implicit assumption is that all other kinds of muscle activity are thereby controlled. Corneil and colleagues (2008) showed this to be a false assumption in the case of reflexive covert orienting, with evidence of neck muscle activity that appeared to match neural activity in the superior colliculus. It is a stern warning that we should watch out with, and be as explicit as we can about, any assumptions we make. With the head fixed, the observer is put in an unusual, if not unnatural, situation. If we see no other way to control factors such as retinal eccentricity of stimulation (i.e., where light falls on the retina), or noise and instability during neurophysiological recording, then we may still prefer head-fixed recording conditions. However, we had better be wary of overgeneralizing the implications of the results we obtain in those conditions.

The data by Corneil and colleagues (2008) suggest that we are effectively producing gaze shifts, even under so-called covert orienting conditions—perhaps the monkey's neck muscles were enacting a movement, which was blocked in the experimental setup with restrained head. To put it more strongly, the covert orienting condition was not covert at all; it went accompanied by body movement (muscle contraction in the neck). Worse, the observation that the muscle contraction correlated to some extent with superior colliculus activity points to a likely confounding factor in previous research on "covert" orienting (e.g., Robinson & Kertzman, 1995): Thinking they saw a neural mechanism relating to covert orienting, the researchers might actually have recorded signals that corresponded to the control of neck muscles. From this, I believe, we can learn three things. First, we prefer unrestrained conditions, recording (and accounting for) as much as possible of the various aspects of body movement (via video, motion sensors, electromyography). Second, the task of disentangling covert and overt processing is extremely difficult and extremely important; it should always be in the foreground of the minds of perception researchers. Third, we do well to study the paradigms and techniques of cognitive psychology, a field that *specializes* in the art of deducing hidden cognitive processes from measurable behavior.

I admit, the third message is a bit of a wildcard, not a conclusion based on the study by Corneil and colleagues (2008) but a need felt in the face of a difficult issue. To talk about covert cognitive processing, about perception, we have to move beyond first-order correlations between sensory input and neural activity, or between motor output and neural activity. It *is* possible to move beyond the first-order correlations, with nice and elegant, and relatively simple, experiments. These are found in cognitive psychology, the science derived from, and developed with, the groundbreaking ideas of researchers and thinkers like Franciscus Donders (1869, 1969) and then, a century later, Donald E. Broadbent (1958|1961), Ulric Neisser (1967), the already mentioned Michael I. Posner (Posner & Keele, 1968; Posner & Mitchell, 1967), Saul Sternberg (1969a, 1969b), and Anne Treisman (Treisman, 1969; Treisman & Gelade, 1980; Treisman & Sato, 1990), to name a few icons—with a remarkable flurry of activity around the year 1969 (a personal favorite in the twentieth century).

Cognitive psychologists like to compare task situations with different computational requirements—different types of decision making, with simple versus complex information, few versus many items, composed of these versus those features, and so on. Through these comparisons, we can try to isolate hidden components. Using nothing fancier than reaction time data (or how long it takes for an observer to make a correct response to a stimulus), Donders (1869, 1969) invented the subtraction method, still a popular and very efficient conceptual tool in cognitive neuroscience, particularly in neuroimaging studies using functional magnetic resonance imaging (fMRI). Let me very briefly give the gist of how the subtraction method works. (If you know the method by heart, you can skip the next three paragraphs—or read them anyway because the logic of Donders is a thing of beauty and therefore a joy forever, to misquote John Keats.)

Imagine you are sitting in front of a computer screen (figure 1.2 provides a visual aid); there are two response buttons, one for your left index finger, one for your right index finger. Sometimes the word "RED" appears in the middle of the screen. Sometimes the word is "GREEN." The computer generates the words and clocks your response times (the time between the word appearing and you pressing the correct button). Now, there will be three tasks. *Task 1*: If you see a word, any color, press the left button. *Task 2*: If you see "RED," not "GREEN," press the left button ("GREEN" requires no response). *Task 3*: If you see "RED," press the left button; if you see "GREEN," press the right button.

Let us analyze your responses to "RED" in the three cases (cf. the lower right part of figure 1.2). If you are not blind, if your hands are not broken or missing, if your mind is generally healthy, if you can read, if you follow the instructions (many ifs, I must admit), then your responses will probably be the fastest for task 1 and the slowest for task 3. Yet, in

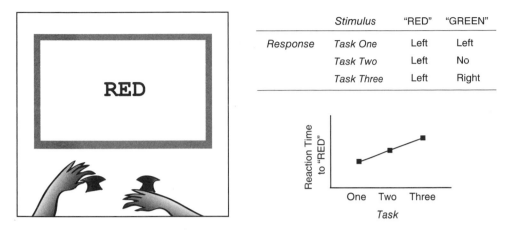

Stimulus	"RED"	"GREEN"
Response	Task One	Left	Left
	Task Two	Left	No
	Task Three	Left	Right

Figure 1.2
Schematic illustration of the subtraction method, as invented by Franciscus Donders (1869, 1969). The left panel shows the experimental setup, with a computer screen, two response buttons, and the hands of the subject (you). The table (upper right) represents the three different tasks, indicating which button to press in response to the two possible stimuli, "RED" or "GREEN." The graph (lower right) abstracts typical data for the given tasks. The ordinate has reaction time in response to "RED." The three tasks are situated next to each other on the abscissa. Reaction time is the shortest for task 1 and the longest for task 3.

all three cases, the sensory input and the motor output stay the same. There is the word "RED" in the middle of the screen, and you are pressing the left button with your left index finger. Why can you do that faster in task 1 than in task 2 or task 3? In task 1, you need only to detect a word on the screen, and you know what to do. Task 2 requires all of the same processes as task 1 *plus* word discrimination. Task 3 requires still more; now you need motor selection as well. The logic of Donders proposes that through the comparison across conditions we are able to track mental processes, such as word discrimination and motor selection. The extra time required for your response reflects different covert processes.

The method is not foolproof. Even in my example with the three tasks, some overt processes might slip in and covary with reaction time. The tension in your left hand will probably be higher in task 1 and task 2 than in task 3—this would be preparatory motor activity, be it not yet a full-blown button press. It would likely show up in the electromyogram of the muscles in your left hand. We will be wise to treat the proposal by Donders (1869, 1969) as a *hypothesis* about the source of reaction time variation. The need for cognitive psychology was, after all, only the third message taken home from the study by Corneil and colleagues (2008);

we should not forget the previous two and aim to measure all relevant body parameters while we devise experiments *à la* cognitive psychology to examine the dialectics of overt and covert processing.

Biased Viewing

I would like to be impartial, or better yet, equally partial to overt and covert processing—not just neutral, but fond of both. With Posner (1980), I am intrigued by our ability to separate the gaze from our current focus of visual information processing. More generally speaking, there are, of course, many other instances in which the visual input at the center of our gaze hardly impacts on our thinking. Today, the 14th of March, 2011, I am having more than my usual share of trouble on a Monday morning concentrating on the computer monitor and this evolving text. My mind is prone to wandering, after a nerve-racking weekend in the aftermath of the massive earthquake and tsunami in northeastern Japan (the region where most of my extended family *lives*, with great emphasis on the present tense). Eight point nine or even nine point zero on the moment magnitude scale… The awestruck gaze, fixed on the view of a place in ruins, may be controlled less by the details of the scenery than by the more abstract metaphoric and metonymic movements that occur in our minds. The gaze may stay inert, with eyes open yet mind unresponsive, as we daydream. We may even close our eyes and ruminate on remembered traces of things as they were (the magical pine tree islets of Matsushima) or imagined traces of things as they might be (my parents-in-law standing in line to receive a jerrican of water). These cases, with gaze and mind seemingly disconnected, will require further exploration. However, let us begin with the default situation.

Usually, naturally, our gaze *does* link up with the visual information that enters our minds. Given the constraints of foveal and peripheral processing, perception requires a very active gaze. We make frequent head and eye movements as we aim to absorb the visual information before us. Head and eye movements presumably are coordinated jointly to direct the gaze at particular portions of the scene (Einhäuser et al., 2009). The amount of work done by the head versus the eye depends on the species, as it is influenced by factors such as the layout of the retina and the relative ease of different types of movement. In rats, most of the work is done by the head rather than the eyes (Hikosaka & Sakamoto, 1987). Primates, especially humans, do relatively much of the gaze control via eye movements.

In the laboratory, with head-restrained conditions, the subjects are often forced to control their gaze solely via eye movements—they are by far the most extensively studied type of overt orienting behavior in vision research. For simplicity, I will take the data about eye movements to provide valid information about gaze control in general. This may be an unwarranted assumption particularly with respect to issues of spatial mapping—or the question whether the coordinates used for movement control are head centered ("craniotopic"), eye centered ("retinotopic"), world or object centered, and so forth. I will highlight the risk of overgeneralization when it is most salient but offer it here as a caveat that applies to any eye movement research that wishes to discuss gaze dynamics.

Not only should we consider head versus eye movements. There are also different types of eye movement. With "eye movement" I mean movement of the eyeballs, as controlled by the eye muscles (the "extra-ocular muscles"), not eye blinks or other movements of the eyelids. The eyelids do, of course, play an important role as well: The opening versus closing of our eyes has very obvious and very dramatic influences on perception. I will come back to this thought when discussing the topic of blocking out visual information in concert with other forms of "not-seeing," such as the ones already briefly alluded to in relation to day-dreaming, remembering, and imagining. Talking about eye movements, however, there is one important—simple and effective—distinction to make, by the nature of the displacement. Smooth eye movement occurs when we track a moving target, say, a bird flying overhead. It is a kind of gaze fixation in motion when we manage to keep the target in our foveal vision. This type of eye movement is called "smooth pursuit" but is not the most common. Much more frequent are the shifts of gaze produced by a "jump" of the eyes, a very quick displacement with abrupt onset. This type of eye movement is called a "saccade" and features prominently, if not exclusively, in most eye movement research.

Saccades typically last about thirty to forty milliseconds, depending on the size of the displacement as measured in visual angle. We may occasionally make relatively large saccades, of twenty degrees of visual angle or even more, but the distances covered by the majority of saccades are much smaller, averaging around two degrees of visual angle when reading English, four degrees when processing faces, and five degrees when looking at natural scenes, with some individual and cultural variation (Rayner et al., 2007). With saccades, we can aim our foveal vision at particular details in the scene before us. The actual visual processing, however, is accomplished during the periods of fixation in between the eye movements when the gaze remains stable. Like saccade size, fixation duration varies depending on the task and on individual and cultural factors. Very roughly, fixation durations tend to average somewhere between 200 and 300 milliseconds. Put differently, to give a not entirely nonsensical number, in many visual processing situations we make about three eye movements every second (see also Henderson, 2003, for a succinct review of a very large literature).

We are normally not aware of making so many eye movements when exploring a visual scene. We do not consciously aim our eyes as we read a text or look at a photograph. If urged to do so, cued to look at a particular detail in a photograph, or following the instructions of an experimenter in a laboratory setting, we can, of course, voluntarily control our eyes in a particular direction. But usually, rather than thinking about where or how to move our eyes, we reflect on the content of what we see. We just look around, oblivious to the fact that we have to make eye movements to see what we see. Active visual perception, then, is driven by an implicit behavior, remarkable in many ways. Eye movements *are* behavioral responses, even hailed as the preferred paradigm for carefully controlled studies of decision making (Glimcher, 2003; Platt, 2002; Platt & Glimcher, 1999). Yet, in natural, free viewing conditions, these behavioral responses operate as a perceptual mechanism that cuts across, or through, the artificial input–output structure of stimulus and response. This input–output structure has dominated for many decades in various schools of psychology as well as neuroscience, providing neat but inherently flawed chapters of sensory versus motor processes (see Hurley, 1998, for a vigorous indictment). Eye movements, by default, are output for input. They are response *and* stimulus. Their primary function is not to elicit a change in the environment—no displacement of any object or body—but to provide us with access to visual information about our current environment.

Eye movements play around, and influence, the active boundaries of vision; they help shape the interaction between the world, the brain, and the praxis of perception. The study of visual perception, therefore, finds a suitable point of departure in the analysis of this intrinsic observer behavior. How do we acquire information about things as they are? Guy T. Buswell (1920, 1935) was perhaps the most energetic pioneer to analyze the patterns of eye movement systematically in various tasks, including, first of all, reading. Buswell made use of a device developed by C. T. Gray and colleagues at the University of Chicago. The device captured beams of light that bounced off the cornea of the subject onto a moving film. It would be only one of many different techniques developed over the years to track eye movements (see Hansen and Ji, 2010, for an update). Buswell's interest was sparked by a very specific question: "In oral reading the eye always moves at a greater or less distance in advance of the voice" (1920, p. 1, the first sentence). He wanted a technique to measure the "eye–voice span," so he could characterize skilled versus "immature" readers. Gradually Buswell came to realize the full breadth of the role of eye movements in perception.

Another notable pioneer, the Russian Alfred L. Yarbus (1965|1967) convincingly demonstrated, through a series of experiments conducted in the 1950s and early 1960s, the specifically information-oriented nature of eye movements. Figure 1.3 illustrates his point with the Mona Lisa. If our eyes have to move for us to acquire visual details, then there are, in principle, at least three qualitatively different strategies we might apply to peruse a visual scene. We might follow an algorithm that would ensure complete coverage of the visual image (left panel). This would be similar to how a scanner — a machine — processes visual images, strictly from left to right and from top to bottom, for instance. An algorithm like this would guarantee an equal distribution of processing resources to every detail in the image. We can apply this strategy, if we force ourselves. In

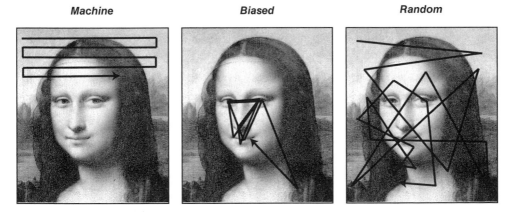

Machine   *Biased*   *Random*

Figure 1.3
Three possible scan paths for the eyes, looking at Leonardo da Vinci's *Mona Lisa*. The left panel shows a systematic, machine-like scan path, moving from left to right and from top to bottom. The middle panel shows a chaotic scan path, which appears to be biased toward specific regions of the portrait, particularly the eyes and mouth. The right panel shows a random scan path, sampling various portions of the portrait in absolute freedom and complete neutrality. Which scan path would best describe your eye movements?

fact, when reading an English text, we apply exactly this algorithm, though we may find ourselves spending extra time on unexpected or unfamiliar words, and we would efficiently aim our foveal vision on lines with characters, not on the empty spaces between them. The panel on the right shows the other extreme, with the complete absence of logic, reason, and algorithms. Truly random viewing would also imply an equal distribution of processing resources; if random eye movements keep randomly moving to infinity, the eyes will spend the same amount of time for every pixel in the portrait. In contrast, the middle panel shows a biased mode of viewing. Here, there is no formal algorithm, but a certain level of meaningfulness in the scan path.

Biased viewing—it will be no surprise—is our default mode. It practically defines the human condition; everything we do is replete with biases (Lauwereyns, 2010). We spend more time on some aspects of an image than on others. Some details convey more information—are more useful, more interesting—than what surrounds them. Our gaze finds such details, compulsively returns to them, and processes them more deeply than the rest. In case of the Mona Lisa, as in the case of other faces, we almost inevitably focus on the eyes, the mouth, and the tip of the nose. Specifically in the case of the Mona Lisa, it is possible that we spend a relatively large amount of time fixating the mouth, because the smile of *La Gioconda* remains so enigmatic (even after the compelling account by Livingstone, 2002|2008). More generally, the point is that our gaze shows a massively skewed distribution, spending a vast amount of time on a small selection of pixels.

The scan paths that Yarbus (1965|1967) observed in his experiments consistently showed such biased viewing. There were notable influences of the type of task and the type of image, but the more general conclusion was invariably that the eye movement patterns display preferences within the image. The patterns belong to the type of dynamic that Tsuda (2001) characterized as a "chaotic itinerancy"—the gaze fixations occur near attractors and show sudden transitions (when we make saccades) to other attractors. It is not a random process, and yet it is not determinate either. The unpredictability exhibits boundaries. We can interpret the hotspots and formulate expectations with certain confidence intervals. If I show you the Mona Lisa, I can be more than ninety-nine percent sure that you will spend more time fixating on her eyes than on her forehead (unless I actually give you my prediction, in which case all bets are off—my words undo themselves, and you might deliberately change your strategy simply to prove me wrong).

Informativeness

Which details in an image manage to exert attraction, or create some kind of gravitational pull for the gaze on its chaotic itinerancy? I have just said, perhaps a little too easily, that there can be "a certain level of meaningfulness" in the scan path. What kind of meaningfulness? The first (safe and scientific) answer should be "statistical." We will be able to obtain statistically significant differences among the amounts of time spent gazing at different portions of the image. However, this answer merely confirms that we are in fact dealing with nonrandom, biased scan paths. I also said, equally easily, that "[s]ome details convey more information—are more useful, more interesting—than what surrounds them." This is a big and intolerably vague assumption that would make hardcore cognitive psychologists cringe.

What do I mean by "information"; what counts as useful or interesting? The mere fact that we look longer at one thing rather than another does not immediately, not in and of itself, prove anything about the content. It does not establish that the thing looked at the longest is therefore necessarily the most interesting, useful, stimulating, aesthetically pleasing, or potentially threatening. We are dangerously close to circular reasoning if we take gaze duration directly to reflect the level of "informativeness" of a particular object or detail—it would be saying both "A is informative because our subject looks at it" and "Our subject looks at A because it is informative." We break the spell if we can provide convergent evidence, or an *informed* prediction, about which objects or details may have a special status and would somehow be worth our while, as we allocate our limited resources of information processing. Mackworth and Morandi (1967) and Antes (1974) simply asked one group of subjects which details were interesting in a given set of pictures and then checked looking times of other subjects. The ratings turned out to be consistent with the looking times—obviously, but hardcore cognitive psychologists distrust the obvious and its implicit biases and are happy to point out that scientific progress *is* indeed made by breaking the spell, by escaping the circularity of reasoning.

Loftus and Mackworth (1978) took another tack. They made predictions about informativeness on the basis of the relation between objects and their context. Some combinations were as normal as a phone on a desk in an office—the phone was not informative, did not really add anything critical to the idea of the office, generated by the picture. Other combinations looked as if they were derived from a painting by Salvador

Dalí. The oddities were considered to be informative; they had a critical impact on the semantic implications of the image. They predicted that subjects would more readily fixate oddities in strange scenes (which were only strange *because of* the oddities) than normal objects in normal scenes. The subjects duly, but presumably cluelessly, obliged. Later research confirmed that oddities in a scene influence gaze control, particularly fixation duration, though not necessarily fixation density (Friedman, 1979; the issues were further scrutinized by De Graef, Christiaens, & d'Ydewalle, 1990, and Henderson, Weeks, & Hollingworth, 1999).

Many questions are still unresolved, relating to the relation between informativeness and the gaze. Often the duration and number of fixations go well beyond what would seem necessary for encoding the perceptual structure of the objects. The mind almost literally holds on to the objects that it is processing in more abstract or semantic ways—perhaps it reflects a negative strategy, of not seeing other things, of preventing irrelevant sensory input. But the gesture of pointing with the eyes could have implications beyond the sensory processing via rods and cones. In any case, things remain more easily in consciousness thanks to their continued visual presence, as established by the gaze. I will fully explore this thought in chapters 6 and 7, but for now I would like to note, conservatively, that the gaze does indeed tend to pick informative elements in the field of view. We know this indirectly, by correlating gaze patterns with other data about the informativeness of different elements in pictures. The biased viewing, we can generally state, is oriented to information.

So-called "looking time paradigms" abound in the literature nowadays, well suited as they are as an implicit measure of interest. We might prefer not to ask directly, for instance, when we suspect that verbal responses might deviate from actual looking behavior (see Dixson et al., 2011, for a telling example with human males judging the attractiveness of naked human females—a study that was famous in all of Wellington, New Zealand, not only at Victoria University). The implicit measure is also, naturally, very useful with animals and babies who cannot tell us in words what they are interested in (see Schell et al., 2011, for a recent example with Barbary macaques looking at pictures of group members, and Addyman & Mareschal, 2010, for one with human infants apparently acquiring an understanding of abstract relationships among geometric figures). The looking time paradigms are sound, and safe from circular reasoning, as long as they work on the basis of independent predictions and considerations about what should be, or could be, informative in a given situation.

Apart from working with theoretical predictions and analyses, we may also wish to keep exploring different empirical means of measuring informativeness, alongside the data about gaze dynamics. Alinda Friedman (1979) incorporated memory tests in her paradigm. Differences in gaze control appeared to be associated with the performance on memory tests: Strange objects in a scene produced an increase not only in gaze duration but also in the likelihood of correct recognition. Somewhat in line with this approach, figure 1.4 offers yet another strategy. We can present our gazing subjects with incomplete images, systematically varying the kinds of information deleted. The loss of critical features should hamper recognition as when we block out the eyes, nose, and mouth of the Mona Lisa (left panel). Noncritical features would hardly be missed at all; *La Gioconda* smiles as enigmatically as ever when the three masks are shifted to the hair (right panel). Tests such as these, then, allow us to establish which information is more or less relevant for our cognitive interaction with the visual world before us. Performance measures with deletions can then be correlated with gaze dynamics. The more informative the detail, the more damaging its absence. Details that are shown to be informative in this way will likely be the ones that attract our gaze in normal conditions when no information is masked.

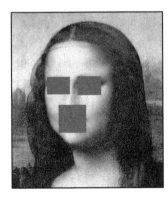 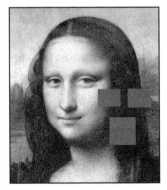

Figure 1.4
An approach to testing the informativeness of particular details. The same stimulus is shown with different areas masked. In the left panel, a roughly human face appears from behind the occlusions, which cover the eyes, nose, and mouth. In the panel on the right, there can be no doubt that the portrait is that of Leonardo da Vinci's *Mona Lisa*, despite the fact that the number of masked pixels is exactly the same as in the left panel (the same three masks were simply shifted to the hair).

The Intrinsic Attraction of News

Skirting tautology again, we may think that, if information does indeed attract our gaze, it must be *attractive*. What is it about informativeness that endows certain objects or details with the power to call our gaze? Some information can be useful in a classic, Darwinian (and also utilitarian) sense, promoting inclusive fitness. Some information gives us the ability to steer away from harm, toward safety, health, well-being—for ourselves and for certain others (loved ones, family, friends, pets, but also strangers, and sometimes even enemies, and old trees, treasured buildings, etc.). Equally obviously, and needless to say, Darwinian processes revolve not only around survival but also reproduction, in the most expansive sense, with the desire and ability to create things and ideas, and little organisms too. "Knowledge is power," sort of said Sir Francis Bacon (see Lauwereyns, 2010, pp. 4–5, for a longer and more exact quote, plus brief discussion). If Bacon's dictum represents indeed a general truth, then knowledge—information—may intrinsically be rewarding. Could it be that humans (and perhaps even other species) come equipped with hardwired mechanisms that naturally connect information with reward—treating information as a goal in and of itself? Do we have a hardwired *desire* for information?

Any new discovery will excite us. I think of Archimedes jumping out of a bath, naked and ecstatic, with a giant smile on his face, knowing exactly how to check the purity of the king's gold crown without melting it down. Do you know how? Do you want me to tell you? If your answer to the first question is "no," I dare you to skip the following explanation and shift your gaze to the next paragraph. Imagine you put an object in a container of water (say the body of a grown-up man in a bath). The water will rise (may even splash out, if it was close to the rim to begin with). This is what Archimedes of Syracuse allegedly observed when he took a bath more than twenty-two centuries ago. He understood right away, jumped out, and shouted "*Eureka!*" ("I got it!") The bigger the bulk of the object, the more the water will rise (or even splash out), regardless of the object's shape. Silver gives more bulk than gold for the same weight. If silver was in the mix, the king's crown would displace more water than a clump of pure gold of the same weight.

Archimedes was happy with his discovery, I would like to believe. Yet not all discoveries are of the enjoyable kind; some will be positively gruesome and depressing (there are most certainly too many of the latter variety in northeastern Japan as I am writing these paragraphs). Still, even the negative discoveries affect us and produce a measure of arousal or excitement, however unpleasant. Moreover, the negative discoveries are equally important for our strategic control of action, our voluntary behavior. To cope with adversity, we need to know. There are positive incentives here as well, in the sense of working toward defense, escape, remediation, closure, or safety (Dinsmoor, 2001)—data or prognoses about catastrophes, personal or macroscopic, may give us a bit of power, or room for thought and action. Bad news would generally be preferable over no news and reinforces our approach behavior, as behaviorist psychologists say. That is, we continue spending effort to obtain the information, today and tomorrow, even if the news is sometimes bad. This is not to say it is always good to know. There are limits, which relate to the relevance and utility of defense mechanisms. Calamitous news can trigger a violent emotional shock with damaging consequences for the self or others—it may be wise in particular circumstances to withhold giving some information or some (graphic or disturbing) portions of the information. I write "withhold," not "refuse"—deliberately shifting perspective from the recipient to the supplier of information. As recipients, we may not be able to refuse information (unless we already had received the general message and then manage in a second step to refuse the gory details), precisely because it exerts such strong attraction.

A very relevant discussion in this regard is busily developing among neuroscientists on the relation between novel stimuli, reward-related processing, and neural activity, particularly in dopamine neurons. A very summary introduction: Dopamine neurons have their cell bodies in the midbrain, more specifically in either the ventral tegmental area or the substantia nigra pars compacta. These neurons project to frontal regions of the brain. There are, roughly speaking, two important routes (Lynd-Balta & Haber, 1994). The ventral route originates in the ventral tegmental area and projects to ventral striatum and orbitofrontal cortex. The dorsal route originates in substantia nigra pars compacta and projects to dorsal striatum and dorsolateral prefrontal cortex. When firing action potentials—"spikes" or nerve impulses—dopamine neurons release the neuromodulator dopamine, a molecule or chemical that interacts with other neurochemical mechanisms to influence the membrane potential of the postsynaptic neuron.

It has been suggested that the short-latency activity of dopamine neurons correlates with novelty detection (Redgrave & Gurney, 2006). Perhaps the dopamine activity is related to the excitement generated by an unexpected or unpredicted event. However, dopamine neurons are also thought to carry signals relating to reward, and particularly reward prediction (Schultz, 1998; Schultz, Dayan, & Montague, 1997). For a while, it appeared as if there were two diametrically opposed schools of thought about whether phasic dopamine activity was tuned to novelty or reward. Data provided by Matsumoto and Hikosaka (2009) suggest that the two families of explanations both deserve territory, literally, in anatomical terms of different neural subpopulations. Matsumoto and Hikosaka recorded dopamine activity in monkeys as they looked at visual cues associated with future pleasant or unpleasant outcomes (i.e., a classical or Pavlovian conditioning paradigm with appetitive and aversive stimuli).

The visual cues implied new information (novelty) about the impending arrival (one and a half seconds later) of either a drop of apple juice (reward) or an air puff (shot through a tube aimed at the monkey's cheek—not painful, but startling and annoying). Two types of dopamine neurons were observed (see figure 1.5). One type was activated by cues associated with a drop of apple juice but inhibited by cues associated with an air puff (left panel). This type of dopamine neuron belonged to

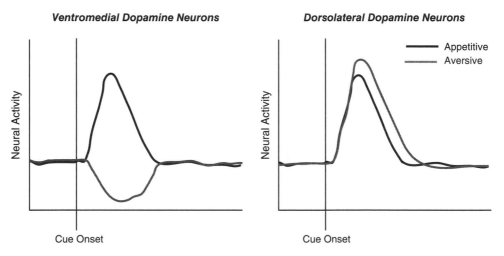

Figure 1.5
Two types of dopamine neuron (modeled after Matsumoto & Hikosaka, 2009). The left panel shows the typical response of dopamine neurons in ventromedial substantia nigra pars compacta (and ventral tegmental area) to cues associated with an appetitive outcome (black line) or an aversive outcome (gray line). The vertical axis represents neural activity (averaged number of spikes); the horizontal axis represents time. The second vertical line indicates the moment of cue onset. The dopamine activity increases for predictions of an appetitive outcome but decreases for predictions of an aversive outcome. The panel on the right shows the typical response of dopamine neurons in dorsolateral substantia nigra pars compacta. Again, the activity increases for predictions of an appetitive outcome. In contrast to the other type of dopamine neuron, however, the activity increases also for predictions of an aversive outcome.

the ventral route. The other type was activated by both good news and bad news (right panel) and belonged to the dorsal route. Interestingly, both types of dopamine neuron appeared to respond in similar ways to information about reward: The likelier the reward, the stronger the dopamine pulse. This was in agreement with Schultz's (1998) proposal that the dopamine neurons function as a homogeneous population with respect to reward prediction. It was the response to bad news that differentiated between the two types of neuron.

Matsumoto and Hikosaka (2009) suggested that the dopamine neurons in the ventral route carry information about reward value, distinguishing between positive and negative. This route would contribute to emotional processing, preference formation, and more complex forms of decision making, especially in situations that require abstract or relative reward processing. In contrast, dopamine neurons in the dorsal route would signal more generally the "motivational salience" or importance of the new information—perhaps a measure of arousal or excitement. The dorsal route projects to the dorsal striatum, an important gateway for mechanisms of orienting and gaze control (I will address this circuitry in full in chapter 2). Phenomenological interpretations here remain speculative at the moment, but speculation is the first step toward formulating empirical questions. Thus, if we are to follow Horace's (and Kant's) *"sapere aude"* ("dare to know," here quoted by heart), we should first dare to guess.

I guess activity in the dorsal route might reflect a sudden rush, a cue-elicited "craving" for information—an acute desire to fully understand what just appeared on the horizon, generating a natural orienting response. The orienting response would be aimed at gathering more information about, or focusing further (conscious) processing on, the novel stimulus. Activity in the ventral route, on the other hand, already implies evaluation and categorization, providing initial readings ("first hypotheses") before additional perceptual data come in. These initial readings would imply decision biases and could be used to control behavior immediately, say, if the circumstances require urgent action. Thus, while the dorsal route is still shifting the gaze, the ventral route is already interpreting what has been seen so far. Both processes are "smart" and likely producers of benefit (making them, in turn, likely winners of Darwinian evolution).

In any case, the paper by Matsumoto and Hikosaka (2009) deserves to be read very closely. In the same year, the same Laboratory of Sensorimotor Research delivered another, perhaps even more compelling, study on dopamine activity and the desire to know. Bromberg-Martin and Hikosaka (2009) again recorded from dopamine neurons while monkeys looked at visual cues associated with different levels of reward magnitude (but no air puffs). This time, critically (and ingeniously), there was a cue before the cue—a second-order cue, which provided information about the trustworthiness of the later cue. The first cue told the monkey whether the next prediction would be true or random. The second cue predicted the magnitude of the reward, which followed more than two seconds later. The reward was a large or small amount of water (throughout the experiments, the researchers carefully monitored the liquid intake to ensure that the monkeys were not dehydrated but were thirsty enough for water to be rewarding).

Figure 1.6 illustrates the main pattern of data. Important is what happens in response to the first cue, the moment when the monkey learns about the trustworthiness of the next prediction. Here the dopamine activity is larger for promises of true information (black lines) than for promises of meaninglessness (gray lines). The dopamine activity after the second cue follows the usual pattern of reward prediction: increased

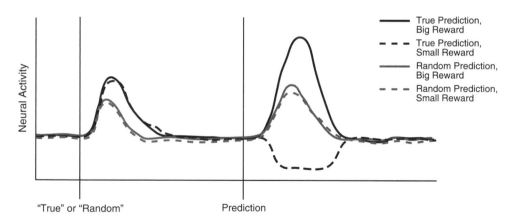

Figure 1.6
The dopamine response to information about the truth or randomness of predictions (modeled after Bromberg-Martin & Hikosaka, 2009). The vertical axis shows the level of neural activity (averaged spike counts); the horizontal axis represents time. Two important events are marked on the arrow of time. The first event is the presentation of a cue that indicates the reliability of the next prediction: "True" or "Random." The second event is the prediction about the coming reward magnitude. Black lines show the activity for true predictions; gray lines represent random predictions. Full lines indicate predictions of a large reward; broken lines stand for predictions of a small reward. News that a true prediction will follow produces a stronger increase in activity than news that the next prediction will be random (cf. the dynamics in response to the first event). The dynamics following the second event show the typical dopamine activity in relation to reward prediction.

activity for a cue associated with hundred percent likelihood of reward (black full line), intermediate activity for cues associated with uncertainty (gray lines), and suppressed activity for cues associated with zero chance of reward (black broken line).

Why is the dopamine activity stronger for promises of true rather than random information? Following Schultz's (1998) understanding of dopamine activity, the data imply that the prospect of true information operated as a prediction of reward—more precisely (technically) speaking, the prospect of true information generated a positive reward prediction error ("the current prediction is better than the previous prediction"), which was larger than the positive reward prediction error generated by random information. In Plain English, the monkey was pleased to know that he would get true information. The experiments by Bromberg-Martin and Hikosaka (2009) also included conditions in which the monkey could actually choose between true or random information. To be sure, both monkey V and monkey Z, the two subjects in the study, opted to know. The behavioral data confirmed that the advance information was something the monkeys were actively willing and trying to obtain. It was not simply aimed at the actual reward. The monkeys received equal amounts of reward, regardless of whether the predictions were true or random. It was the advance information itself which the monkeys were happy to receive and work for. Information was intrinsically rewarding.

Perception for Perception

With information as an intrinsic reward, the function of perception makes a leap. From serving toward homeostasis or other clearly definable utilitarian goals, perception turns to itself, as a function that refuses to be an obvious function. The neural activity in response to reward predictors shifts to indirect predictors—predictors of predictors (see also Bromberg-Martin & Hikosaka, 2011, a follow-up paper that directly compares the different types of prediction in the lateral habenula, a structure in the epithalamus that can suppress dopamine activity). Learning for reward becomes learning for learning. The processing of information requires no additional or ulterior motive; it is indeed the brain's standard response to stimulation, often beyond our control—however active we would like our perception to be, there are passive aspects we cannot deny. Our senses provide us with continuous streams of data, which can be very hard to stop and may require the use of tools like eye shades and earplugs (not trivial on long-haul flights). And even with eye shades on and earplugs in we may find ourselves unable to fall asleep, thinking useless thoughts, helplessly consciously processing the faintest external or internal traces (the ringing in our ears, the virtual blobs against the walls of our eyelids).

Our sensory systems are organized in hierarchical neural circuits that relentlessly supply us with units of information, news about objects and events, and summaries of things as they are. The brain is "a hermeneutic device," as Érdi (1996) put it; much of its activity revolves around information, one way or another, received, shaped, or transmitted. We seek information, constantly, almost compulsively—not just as a reward but as something we need. In an inspiring opinion piece annex review article on curiosity and exploration in *Science*, Berlyne (1966) emphasized that we require, and actively try to maintain, optimal levels of stimulation. Too much induces stress, too little leads to boredom. Referring to a study by Jones, Wilkinson, and Braden (1961), Berlyne (1966, p. 32) notes, "Human beings confined in a dark room with a minimum of stimulation will press buttons to make patterns of colored spots of light appear, preferring those sequences of pattern that offer the most variety and unpredictability." This experiment was conducted long before the arrival of remote control and the Internet, but I can see myself producing similar data in a hotel room, suffering from jetlag and exhaustion, still unable to sleep after a miserable long-haul flight, despite eye shades and earplugs, mulling over the question why I keep coming to the Annual Meeting of the Society for Neuroscience.

Berlyne (1966) distinguished between two kinds of exploration. The button pressing in the dark room would be an instance of *diversive* exploration—Berlyne's bold, but self-explanatory neologism. This type of search is open-ended, is aimless, and occurs when just about any stimulation will do. The alternate type would be *specific* exploration, directed at particular objects, domains, or problems. This more focused exploration, Berlyne suggested, equals "curiosity." It is also, I will remember in my hotel room, slightly invigorated by the positive thought, one of the reasons why I do keep coming to the Annual Meeting of the Society for Neuroscience. I wish to meet my friends, and I wish to explore specifically what they are up to, which new papers are in the making at the Laboratory of Sensorimotor Research and many other labs.

Curiosity will usually be triggered—by the arrival of a novel stimulus, a surprise, or an incongruity, something strange that makes us wonder. Such cues and triggers are likely to appear within our field of view during diversive exploration, so perhaps the two modes of exploration operate less independently than Berlyne (1966) seemed to think. Diversive exploration will naturally turn into specific exploration when the open-ended search for stimulation produces a candidate for further investigation. The different modes of exploration may even be entangled at a microscopic (subsecond) level in ongoing gaze dynamics as we scan the horizon and then shift and lock our gaze to particular objects. Nevertheless, the two modes can and should be distinguished as they imply different computational demands and degrees of freedom for gaze control—a very relevant consideration also for research on the underlying neural mechanisms.

Exploration, whether diversive or specific, aimed merely at obtaining information may also be connected with the more typically human forms of learning for learning. Berlyne (1966) mentions science (especially "basic" or "fundamental" science). Albert Einstein, our cherished icon of scientific genius, claimed simply, "There exists a passion for comprehension" (1954, p. 342). We can further think of the more general human tendency to play and experiment. In its most radical and anti-utilitarian form it is called "art for the sake of art"—an idea that was first shaped in French as *l'art pour l'art*. It was popularized as a slogan in the 1850s and 1860s by the poet and essayist Théophile Gautier (whose name I must have encountered numerous times but only recently really noticed at the beginning of Charles Baudelaire's *Les Fleurs du Mal*, 1857|2010, p. 41, receiving the most honorable mention as an impeccable poet and perfect magician). Gautier did not coin the expression, however.

For *The Dictionary of the History of Ideas* Iredell Jenkins traced the origin of the slogan to Benjamin Constant, who wrote an entry on February 11, 1804, in his *Journal Intime*, in which *l'art pour l'art* was "introduced quite casually to refer to the aesthetic doctrines of Kant and Schelling" (Jenkins, 1973, p. 109). Immanuel Kant had separated cognition, conscience, and aesthetic taste or sensibility. Though Kant was mainly concerned with the first two mental faculties, Friedrich Schiller and many others jumped on the idea of seeing the aesthetic as a separate domain. It was almost, or perhaps indeed, a deliberate misreading in Harold Bloom's sense of the word (1975|2003). The artist became an autonomous agent. Poets began experimenting and promoting self-conscious and vanguard poetics, claiming the right to be concerned with nothing but poetry itself. In the near-ecstatic words of Edgar Allen Poe (1850|2009, p. 1) in *The Poetic Principle* the simple fact is, that, would we but permit ourselves to look into our own souls we should immediately there discover that under the sun there neither exists nor *can* exist any work more thoroughly dignified—more supremely noble than this very poem—this poem *per se*—this poem which is a poem and nothing more—this poem written solely for the poem's sake.

The fact may be simple for Edgar Allen Poe, but even if the poem was written solely for the poem's sake, the life of the poem (if it is a good one) does not end there. The reader reads it, and thereby renews the creation, every reading in a way a variant of the writing. We can distinguish between intention (motivation) and effect (outcome). Darwinian processes operate on the effects. A good poem survives, and keeps being reprinted, because readers are stirred by it, not because the poet wrote it solely for the poem's sake. Perception for perception survives, and keeps being implemented in the neural circuits of new generations, not because the function is inherently pleasing but because it produces valuable outcomes—not primarily intended, but secondarily gained.

Free viewing provides us with information, which more often than not allows us to see (sometimes to foresee) something potentially meaningful, positive or negative, pleasant, beautiful, juicy, noxious, or dangerous. It allows us to adapt our behavior, consistent with the terms of natural and sexual selection. This applies to information for pure and applied reason as well as to sensory patterns that stimulate our aesthetic judgment, to follow Kant's distinctions. Sometimes a new understanding of relations among variables allows us to simplify and organize our data. Information produces mental models and algorithms, opportunities to reapply the knowledge we acquired. It makes perfect sense, in terms of inclusive fitness, for information to be rewarding *because* knowledge really is power. The outcomes of our intrinsically motivated explorations validate Sir Francis Bacon's dictum. Even the ability to appreciate beauty implies functional benefits, particularly in the domain of sexual selection, beauty tending to be associated with, for instance, features that indicate health and various forms of ability, from the athletic to the intelligent. There is nothing neutral about aiming for beauty (see Dixson, 2009, and Miller, 2000, for persuasive functional accounts of our aesthetic judgments, contemplating buttocks and bellies, but also Shakespeare's sonnets).

The functional implications of comprehension and appreciation are that information, however intrinsically pleasing, does move on to a practical beyond. The freedom of viewing is paradoxical. Free viewing is "free" and perceives for the sake of perceiving, in a way that is deeply functional, aimed at information, and therefore implicitly at (natural or sexual) power, which, in turn, is largely antithetical to freedom. Carpenter (1999) addressed a similar conundrum when discussing the variability of reaction time in eye movement studies and, particularly, the notion of procrastination in reaction time. Reaction times, he observed, are often surprisingly slow—much slower than we should expect based on neural conduction times, given the number of steps (synapses) from visual input (at the retina) to oculomotor output (control of the eye muscles). Carpenter concluded that randomness was built in as an essential property of the decision-making mechanism. But why would that be? Randomness might have meaning (p. 20):

If we always responded in the same way to the most probable stimulus, not only would life be extremely boring, but we would never discover anything new. Though by doing something very unusual we may sometimes make mistakes, just occasionally it results in that conceptual, mould-breaking leap that leads to new discoveries and better responses than previously formed part of our repertoire. At a more exalted level it is what we call creativity.

There were other possible advantages. Consistent with game theory, we increase our likelihood of success when we fool our opponents (by being unpredictable). And more generally, variation is an essential component in Darwinian processes: Natural selection works on competing candidates—the more variation, the more select the selection. Extra rounds of random thought *could* produce a benefit. Extra exploration might be wise in hard economic terms.

Indeed, Daw and colleagues (2006) pitched the question of exploration exactly as an economic issue: It is our choice to either exploit what we know or gather information about what we do not know. They designed an fMRI study with the so-called "Four-armed bandit task"—a gambling task with four slot machines that have hidden and varying payoff structures. When the subjects chose to explore, cerebral blood flow increased in the frontopolar cortex and intraparietal sulcus. When the subjects made value-based exploitative decisions, the blood oxygenation level-dependent (BOLD) signal went up in ventral and dorsal striatum and ventromedial prefrontal cortex. To a remarkable extent, these findings match with the divergent dopamine functions proposed by Matsumoto and Hikosaka (2009) in their monkey single-unit study, using a vastly different paradigm. The exploratory activity involved neural structures that had previously been implicated with gaze control and may partially be influenced by the dorsal dopamine route.

The value-based exploitative decisions could be modulated primarily by activity in the ventral dopamine route.

Another monkey single-unit study suggested that the inhibitory output of the basal ganglia (from the internal segment of the globus pallidus) is also differentially active in exploration versus exploitation—being permissive, hardly inhibiting anything, during exploration but suppressing alternate actions when the subject exploits a profitable response (Sheth et al., 2011). Some sort of scheme is ready to emerge, with two routes for exploration versus exploitation, supplied by different dopamine streams and regulated by selective closing or opening of pathways to various responses. No doubt this scheme will be drawn more precisely in the next few years as empirical findings accumulate.

Sting, Speck, Cut, Little Hole

The study by Daw and colleagues (2006) highlights the usefulness of an economic analysis of perception. Information here is the cherished good, the thing of value, the dimension that offers a metric, a currency. At any one moment, we may find ourselves faced with very many sources of information, with different types of sensory patterns, relevant or irrelevant to our various needs and wants. The different types of sensory patterns can be thought of as candidates in a competition for our gaze and our selective information processing. The selection pulls some information to the foreground. This information becomes the object of thought, a thing in our minds. The application of the brain's art of mindfulness is often called "attention" in natural language and counts as one of the forms of conscious processing—one of the faces of consciousness. The word "attention" appears in largely the same, ill-defined sense in *The Principles of Psychology* by William James (1890|1950a) and in contemporary treatises of selective and extensive visual processing (e.g., LaBerge, 1995; Rolls, 2008; Van der Heijden, 2004).

So here is probably an appropriate place to add a note on the trouble with attention. Often this concept is connected with increased sensitivity and improved information processing ("seeing *better*")—an assumption that is not always (or even: usually not) carefully checked in empirical investigations. This sloppiness in the translation of theoretical concepts to experimental variables has produced (almost by routine) a great and terrible number of situations in which phenomena were recognized to be instances of attention even though they did not come with increased sensitivity or improved information processing. Instead, the effects of attention were often due to biases, with heightened anticipation and, indeed, *less* extensive information processing (as in "seeing faster" but sometimes also "seeing things that are not there"; see Lauwereyns, 2010, for a detailed conceptual critique, and Green & Swets, 1966|1988, for the mathematical underpinnings). In other cases, researchers have carefully designed their studies to measure the effects of sensitivity in isolation, free from any contamination by the dreaded biases, but then talked about their findings as if they were true for the operation of attention in general. Yet, the natural language meaning of "attention," I believe, is covered most adequately by including the dynamic and interdependent operations of bias *and* sensitivity mechanisms. So I tend to avoid using the word "attention" altogether, to prevent confusion with the impoverished (sensitivity-centered) construct as it appears in scientific papers. Instead, I prefer zooming in on the dynamics and interdependency of bias and sensitivity, always checking, as carefully as possible, which information is selected, how, and to what extent it is actually processed.

In any case, whether attention or selective information processing, the economic analysis of perception basically revolves around choices: exploration versus exploitation, this rather than that, here instead of there. The informativeness of new information (and its intrinsic attraction) may be pitched against other stimulation, with more obvious (more direct) functional implications in relation to homeostasis and inclusive fitness. Berlyne (1966) mentions the example of a hungry rat taking time to explore before settling down to eat what was already available. We can also think of Orpheus again, his destructive curiosity, looking back into the dark, fascinated perhaps by the unknown, the mysterious—at the expense of losing, and knowing he will lose, his Eurydice. The eternal return of this myth must be fueled by some basic truth about the human experience, its inherent conflicts between relevant and irrelevant information processing, between choosing for something now versus perhaps a bit more if we wait until later.

However intensely we may be engaged in one activity shaped by Darwinian processes—paying (here I will say it) *attention* to what earns us our bowls of rice—we remain susceptible to distraction. We succumb to the sometimes irresistible attraction of novelty and find ourselves helplessly exhibiting the dynamics of curiosity—a behavior also ultimately shaped by Darwinian processes. Not even Darwin would be able to tell who wins the contest between one Darwin and another—the theory of natural (and sexual) selection does not offer, nor did it ever promise to offer, any precise predictions on the microscopic scale of our choices in perception. The best we can try to do is map the probabilities of choice by tracking the biases and sensitivities of particular observers in particular situations, given particular types of stimulation.

An important point here is that the currency of information value is indeed to a large extent observer dependent. My interests are not the same as your interests; my biases are strictly mine. There may be overlap, in some areas, but I do not care for rugby, baseball, basketball, American football, golf, and many other sports, though I am somewhat sensitive to soccer (the real football) and certainly intrigued by sumo (for its rituals as much as for the actual wrestling). Likes and dislikes can be very idiosyncratic, and have a huge impact on the values we (implicitly) place on different kinds of information. Our likes and dislikes determine the informativeness of things and so influence our biased viewing. This biased viewing gives us a very limited understanding of things as they are in front of us. In the same window of the same bookstore I will pick out completely other items than my nine-year-old daughter does. I will never notice there is yet another Rainbow Magic book, focused as I am on the new Damasio.

The limits of our interests inspired (the hugely talented and sorely missed) David Foster Wallace (2003), in his delightful introduction to infinity, to reject even the entire idea that we are intrinsically attracted to information. "One thing is certain, though. It is a total myth that man is by nature curious and truth-hungry and wants, above all things, *to know*" (p. 12). To which he added in a quirky footnote on the same page: "The source of this pernicious myth is Aristotle, who is in certain respects the villain of our whole Story." However, one paragraph later Wallace suggests the disinterest for one thing is offset by the need for another (p. 13): "Theory: The dreads and dangers of abstract thinking are a big reason why we now all like to stay so busy and bombarded with stimuli all the time." This thought rhymes nicely with what Berlyne (1966) offered: "How much excitement or challenge is optimal will fluctuate quite widely with personality, culture, psychophysiological state, and recent or remote experience" (p. 26).

Similarly, Albert Einstein (1954) immediately qualified the passion for comprehension in two ways, one explicit, one implicit. Explicitly: "That passion is rather common in children, but gets lost in most people later on" (p. 342). Implicitly: He refused to investigate it. The meaning of the passion itself mystified Einstein, the way meaning often did: "What is the meaning of human life, or, for that matter, of the life of any creature? To know an answer to this question means to be religious" (p. 11). Such questions were important, he thought, but he felt obliged to relegate them outside science. His passion for comprehension did not apply to them; perhaps they were not compatible with his mode of thought in physics. Thus, the explicit and implicit proposals of Einstein, Berlyne, and Wallace converge on the notion that we all want information, but that these wants focus, specifically for each of us, on particular domains and objects. Informativeness, and with it perception, is indeed, whichever way we look at it, basically a matter of bias.

Yet, one of the most curious aspects of perception is the fact that its biases almost never fail to escape us. Though thoroughly biased, our perceptions continue persuasively to take hold of our minds, convincing us that what we see is really out there—that what we see *is* things as they are. As we look around and take in the visual world, there rests practically something like a taboo on the fact that this visual world is our construction. Seeing is choosing—we select and aim our gaze—but we deny our agency in perception; we keep compulsively believing, trusting, that our self-made perceptions are veridical. I suspect our free viewing, biased as it is, only works efficiently if we turn off our critical thought (our self-criticism about potential biases) and simply "go with the flow," believing the flow is real. Biases do not work if they are caught. Our free viewing, which is inevitably biased viewing, would not work when the biases are brought to the surface. So we delude ourselves and think we are neutral, "just looking." Our gaze finds things, and we see them "popping up," "suddenly there"—as if the object chooses us, a form of exogenous control.

Roland Barthes (1980|1999) introduced a useful pair of concepts to discuss such processes in his strange and fascinating (and nicely short, yet luxuriously written) essay on photography, *Camera Lucida*. Whenever we look at a scene, we will first take in the general gist, the *studium*, meaning "application to a thing, taste for someone, a kind of general, enthusiastic commitment" (p. 26). It is filled with deliberate purpose. But sometimes, especially in photographs that Barthes likes, there is a second element to "break (or punctuate) the *studium*," which "rises from the scene, shoots out like an arrow, and pierces me" (p. 26). This is the *punctum*. It means "sting, speck, cut, little hole—and also a cast of the dice" (p. 27). Barthes describes the *punctum* as an agent of exogenous control, something in the picture that grabs him. But the attraction of the *punctum* can be based on very private or idiosyncratic associations, as in the following description, characteristic of Barthes's inimitable style (p. 45):

However lightning-like it may be, the *punctum* has, more or less potentially, a power of expansion. This power is often metonymic. There is a photograph by Kertész (1921) which shows a blind gypsy violinist being led by a boy; now what I see, by means of this "thinking eye" which makes me add something to the photograph, is the dirt road; its texture gives me the certainty of being in Central Europe; I perceive the referent (here, the photograph really transcends itself: is this not the sole proof of its art? To annihilate itself as *medium*, to be no longer a sign but the thing itself?), I recognize, with my whole body, the straggling villages I passed through on my long-ago travels in Hungary and Rumania.

This particular *punctum* must be uniquely Barthes's. His biased viewing generates virtual images that blend vision with memory. His consciousness intensifies the meaning of what he sees by moving away from the visual details, by continuing the exploration (metonymically, indeed) inside his mind. We may be tempted to claim, somewhat dismissively, that Barthes thereby moves from perception to some other kind of cognitive activity. However, if we wish to understand how seeing works, and how seeing relates to consciousness, we have to account for such processes of intensification and *Sinngebung* (the giving of meaning, with a German word that the thoroughly French Merleau-Ponty also liked to give in German).

Not all *punctum* dynamics begin with private associations. Figure 1.7 gives an example that, my hunch says, will soon exogenously control your gaze as it did mine even though you do not know a single of the pictured ballerinas, nor where or when the picture was taken, nor at which occasion. The *studium* is clear enough. This is a group picture. There must have been a ballet performance. But why did the ballerinas pose in front of toilets? The physical layout of the objects in the scene and the operation of Gestalt laws (such as those of proximity and similarity) cause the abstract icon for men's toilets to stand out from its surroundings. The whole idea of men's toilets seems thoroughly inappropriate here. Can you suppress it, or does it take shape in your mind—the urinals, the tiny traces of mud on the floor, the obnoxious smell of chemicals? How does it influence your reading of the picture? Even if the same *punctum* pricks each of us, as a straightforward consequence of physical features salient in the image, it will expand differently in your mind than in my mind, or the mind of anyone else.

Perception and the giving of meaning must ultimately be understood as a personal experience, intensely subjective in nature. I can never hope to follow or reconstruct the full movie (or poem) of *punctum* dynamics inside your head. Nor even inside my head. However, we can hope to uncover some of the principles and degrees of freedom. Not the poem,

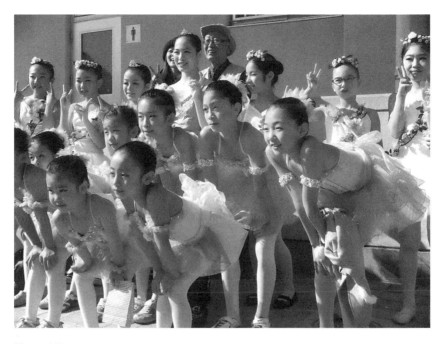

Figure 1.7
Punctum in action. This group photo was taken in Fukuoka, Japan, on November 20, 2010, a few days after a bout of specific exploration at the Annual Meeting of the Society for Neuroscience. Then ready for diverse exploration at a staging of the classic ballet version of *Don Quixote*, the clumsy photographer left room for a conspicuous, *studium*-piercing symbol to emerge near the upper left corner, to the right of the door.

but the poetics. The challenge for the neuroscience of perception will be to address the laws of this subjective nature — not by objectifying (essentially removing or, in effect, denying) the subject but by abstracting it, by properly situating the subject, with a body, a place in the world, certain interests, and certain abilities to move. That is, we need to incorporate the subject's biases as integral components of the process of perception. It is not impossible to do — not even difficult, really. It is already being done, fragmentarily, implicitly, in much present-day research. In making explicit room for the subject's biases operative in experience, neuroscientists will take heed of the valid criticisms by Merleau-Ponty (1945|2008), Gibson (1979|1986), and contemporary proponents of the philosophy of "the embodied mind." It is our project here in this book. For it, we should now take a look at the actual makeup of the body that gives us our active boundaries of vision.

2　A Sensorimotor System

Following the river upstream.
Many willows, many stones; the rush
of rapids. And reeds, which
in the language of this place
sound as they are: reeds
in a gentle breeze.

The walking here almost floats. These words, by the Dutch poet Hans Faverey (1994|2004, p. 104), evoke a *traveling avant* inside my head, to borrow the curious (partly English) term from French motion picture jargon for a tracking shot that moves forward (*into* the scene). I think I like the headstrong combination of different languages in this concept of journeying forward, where it is a very simple mechanical operation (steadying the camera) that produces a fluid sense of movement—a well-oiled sensorimotor system.

In this *traveling avant*, I imagine walking alongside a river in Kyushu—upstream, leisurely, noticing willows (I think I must be in Yanagawa, Kyushu), noticing stones on the riverbank, bluish gray ones, square, with sharp edges. They are on the riverbed as well. My thoughts walk along; the walking and breathing and thinking evolve in convergent rhythms. The thoughts intensify the sensations and add new ones—the syllables and sounds of the words that pop up in my head (Faverey mentions the sound of reeds "in the language of this place," which he finds agreeing with the actual thing, the reeds in a gentle breeze). The poem just keeps moving further forward, the *traveling avant* very smooth indeed—the tracking shot as fluid as can be on silken rails (*Silken Chains* was the title of Faverey's 1983 volume, in which the poem first appeared). I, or we, encounter "An old woman, singing out loud: // to herself, amid / her surroundings." And

A brief greeting, a cough. Then
the singing is resumed, louder
now, it seems. I only catch sight of them
a little further: both her cows,
beside the water.

The moving forward into the scene comes with new visual stimulation, new things appearing within the field of view. These not only enrich the scene but lead to a reinterpretation of what has been seen. Tentative perceptions are revised. Now that we can see "both her cows, / beside the water," we know that the old woman was not merely singing to herself. She was creating a vocal field, an auditory territory, for her cows, keeping them close to her, guiding them, with her song. And the *traveling avant* not only triggers reinterpretation but also produces interaction between the observer and the observed. The walker becomes the object of the old woman's greeting, who then resumes the singing, "louder / now, it seems." Perhaps, having exchanged greetings, she feels less awkward about singing in front of us, the "I," a stranger, and raises her voice. Or it could be that the sound is as loud as before, but the observer listens more intently—Faverey deliberately makes room for this possibility by emphasizing the seeming.

Acquiring (or even eliciting) new visual stimulation by moving into the scene, reinterpreting what has been seen, interacting with the scene—these actions for, and in, perception are vividly present in Faverey's poem, easily tractable and distinguishable. This level of lucidity in tracing the active boundaries of vision is no doubt more common for Faverey's poetry than for our common experience, but the same themes of self-elicited stimulation, reinterpretation, and interaction recur in every act of visual perception. They are integral to the working of the sensorimotor system that allows us to see the things before us. To get an understanding of how this works, we stand to gain by examining the anatomical con-straints—or, positively, the degrees of freedom—of the system.

If we are to give the body its due place in the science of vision, we must be willing to actually consider it. Perhaps the most mystifying aspect of contemporary thinking and writing about embodied cognition, for me, is the conspicuous lack of interest in the actual biology of the body that is supposed to do the embodying. Should we blame Merleau-Ponty (1945|2008) for this? Informed though he was by very detailed analyses of neurological disorders and the effects of brain damage, Merleau-Ponty tended eagerly to proceed with abstract discussions, which then left no room for a return to the body, producing in fact a rather disembodied philosophy. He occasionally made a point of removing the biological—here is an example on page 78: "Even if I knew nothing of rods and cones, I should realize..." But Merleau-Ponty *knew* about rods and cones (very well, actually; the man was an avid and extremely insightful reader). What he would have realized without this knowledge is unnecessary conjecture. Merleau-Ponty had no reason to bypass the anatomical data.

Similarly, in Noë's *Action in Perception* (2004), the body is often treated as a vague set of spatiotemporal coordinates, essentially compatible with the idea that it constitutes a moving point with no extension, as according to the mathematical definition of a point in space (so infinitely small that it does not actually take up any space—a notoriously slippery conception, the stuff of many Zeno-type paradoxes). It is as if Noë dodges Descartes's dualist dilemma by taking the finite for a species of infinity. The move is not neutral. By avoiding a detailed study, or even definition, of the body, Noë creates room for his externalist philosophy, which, in its most defiant moments, appears to even transcend embodied cognition, happening "out of our heads," supersizeable in an (in principle) unlimited way, potentially bordering the esoteric (where the self becomes one with...).

This move is worse than not neutral; it is simply wrong. The body is more than a set (even a specific one) of spatiotemporal coordinates; it has not only extension but also mechanisms and characteristics, biases and sensitivities, needs and preferences—a complex of very clearly limiting factors that influence, shape, and define the active boundaries of vision in various ways that we can study only if we take the body to be what it is: a biological entity. I would therefore urge contemporary philosophers of embodied cognition to follow the lead of their ancestors—seventeenth-century philosophers such as, indeed, Descartes, who actually investigated the finite characteristics of the body, keen to learn from anatomy. Figure 2.1 shows a plate from a book by one such philosopher, Franciscus Aguilonius (or François d'Aguilon, 1613).

The illustration was made by Peter Paul Rubens and appeared in *Opticorum Libri Sex*, Aguilonius's magnum opus, a philosophical and mathematical treatise on optics and vision—partly an adaptation of the work by Alhazen, the great Arab thinker, mathematician, and scientist of exactly a millennium ago. Aguilonius (1613) did more than translate Alhazen, however. Focusing on the idea that visual perception works with the body, Aguilonius made several notable discoveries of his own. He noted, for example, that with two eyes we are better at estimating distances than with one eye (technically: he was the first to describe the

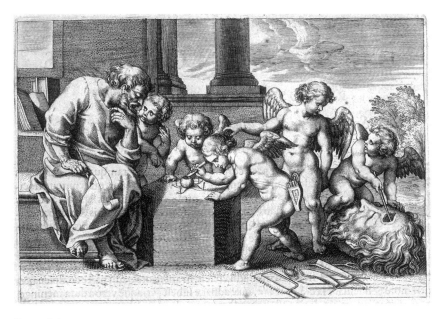

Figure 2.1
Dissection of the cyclopean eye. An illustration by Peter Paul Rubens for book I of Franciscus Aguilonius's *Opticorum Libri Sex* (1613), on the organ, the object, and the nature of vision. The dissection is performed by a group of not-very-fainthearted putti (winged babies, practicing art and science, unlike their counterparts, the cherubs, who busy themselves religiously). Note the ominous-looking instruments next to the giant's severed head and the casual way in which the cyclopean eye is nailed to the hexagonal operating table.

role of binocular disparity in depth perception). For example two, he introduced something akin to the notion of efference copy, proposing that motor commands in the brain should not only activate muscles but also elicit internal monitoring of the upcoming movement—an important topic, obviously, for active vision. Aguilonius, like no one before him, explored the actual implications of the fact that perception is a function of the body. In his work, we find a practical attempt at synthesis of optics (physics, the world) and limited, biological information processing (computation in the brain)—the beginnings of a project that is as at least as valid today as it was (very nearly exactly) four hundred years ago.

Aguilonius did what he did before Descartes and without taking an a priori stance on the domain of the spiritual versus material (or how the mathematical truths relate to, emerge from, or enter into, the human experience). He seemed to have no qualms about frequently moving back and forth between the abstract and the concrete, between equations and movements of the body, in a slightly idiosyncratic way (or, phrased more positively, in a way that displays poetic genius). I see it visualized in an equally idiosyncratic (genius) way by Rubens in figure 2.1, with the concrete images of experimentation and dissection (the cutting and drilling in biological tissue) turning allegorical, the tools in the hands of strange little research assistants, applied to the third eye (the mind's eye?) of a mythical creature. I would like to think the putti and their tools represent the deductive and inductive reasoning of the vision scientist (in a posture that looks remarkably similar to that of Auguste Rodin's thinker, who was initially supposed to be a poet—*Le Penseur*, bronze cast completed in 1902). Body and mind, then, come together in a metaphorical eye, which is really a process, a happening over time and in space, computed (brought into biological being) inside the head.

Aguilonius managed to move back and forth between the abstract and the concrete in other ways as well—in addition to his work as a Jesuit priest, a teacher, a mathematician, a physicist, and a vision scientist, he left his mark on the cityscape of Antwerp (my hometown) as a magnificent architect, designer of the Carolus Borromeus Church (originally dedicated to Ignatius of Loyola). I first encountered the name of Aguilonius in a comment article by Grüsser (1994) in response to a theory by Bridgeman, Van der Heijden, and Velichkovsky (1994) on visual stability (a paper someone picked for a graduate course, I forgot who and which, but I remember the time and place; it was East Lansing, Michigan, the autumn of 1996). At one point I thought I would have to write a novel about or around the figure of Aguilonius, with prominent roles for Rubens and the Plantin Press, set in the city of Antwerp in the seventeenth century. But perhaps the better homage would be what I am working on now, following the lead of Aguilonius, moving back and forth between the abstract and the concrete, between equations and movements of the body, studying the active boundaries of vision. Then we had better talk about things like neural circuits for the control of eye movements.

Oculomotor Control

I take full responsibility for figure 2.2. The four panels on the same (not very concrete and not very abstract) monkey brain are my best approximation of what are, for our purposes, the most important and relevant aspects of the neural circuitry for oculomotor control. It is quite possible to fill entire volumes on the neural circuits that control the movements of the eyes. Wurtz and Goldberg edited one in 1989 (424

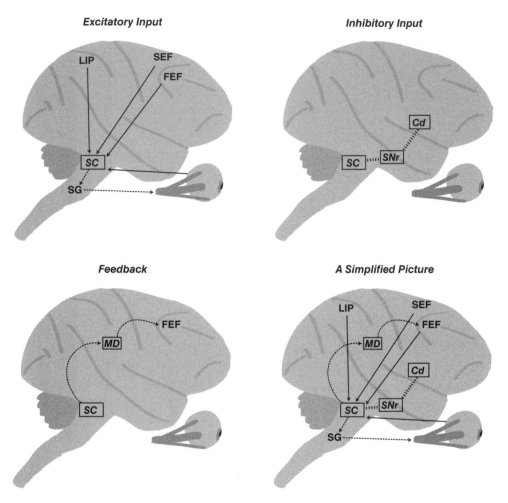

Figure 2.2
Neural circuits for oculomotor control. The circuits are shown on an abstracted shape of a
monkey brain (e.g., *Macaca mulatta*; lateral view of the right hemisphere), taking the superior colliculus (SC) as the crossroads for the planning and execution of eye movements
(inner brain structures such as SC, hidden in the lateral view, are shown italicized and
framed). The upper left panel shows excitatory pathways to SC, from three cortical areas
(LIP, the lateral intraparietal area; FEF, the frontal eye field; SEF, the supplementary eye
field) as well as a pathway of direct activation from the retina. SC, in turn, activates the
saccade generator (SG) in the brainstem to initiate eye movements (i.e., making the extraocular muscles contract). The upper right panel represents inhibitory input to SC from the
basal ganglia (via Cd, caudate nucleus, and SNr, substantia nigra pars reticulata). The lower
left panel indicates a feedback circuit from SC to FEF via the medial dorsal nucleus of the
thalamus (MD). The lower right panel puts the three sets of anatomical projections together
only to note that the result is still very much a simplified picture.

pages), Büttner-Ennever in 2006 (574 pages). My sketches are vastly simplified versions of the myriad circuitry as it has been charted in those and other textbooks. My aim is to give no more and no less than the level of detail relevant to understanding the active nature of visual perception. This is also the reason why I show a monkey brain. The mechanisms for oculomotor control are structurally very similar in monkeys and humans (all the names of neural structures and the types and directions of the projections that I mention here are the same for all primates). The circuitry in monkeys is a bit simpler and easier to draw, and more extensively investigated, than that in humans—hence the inevitable (and, indeed, in this context completely justifiable) choice of monkeys.

Central notions, for our purposes, are the different pathways of excitatory control that initiate eye movements, a set of mechanisms that prevents eye movements, and a type of projection that reports back about eye movements. To show these aspects of the circuitry, I concentrate on the superior colliculus as the proverbial headquarters for the control of (not only, but most importantly) *saccadic* eye movements (the ones that produce an actual gaze shift, jumping from one focus point to another). The superior colliculus (as we call it in mammals) is part of the midbrain; in other vertebrates it is called the tectum, or sometimes the optic tectum. In mammals the superior colliculus is usually said to have seven layers: three superficial layers devoted to sensation, two intermediate layers where things get mixed in various ways, and two deeper layers involved in motor activity.

The superior colliculus (SC in figure 2.2) has all the right connections to be the center of gravity for eye movement control. Direct evidence that movements are actually initiated in the superior colliculus has come from electrical stimulation experiments: By passing a small electrical current to the neural tissue, we can artificially evoke eye movements (see Robinson, 1972, for the modern classic that reestablished this finding). Superior colliculus is not the only brain region in which electrical stimulation can produce eye movements—in fact, there are quite a few, though the level of stimulation required (or the threshold for eliciting saccades) varies across areas. An area with a particularly low threshold, like the superior colliculus, is the frontal eye field (FEF in figure 2.2; I can again refer to a classic paper by David A. Robinson, this time a coauthored one, Robinson & Fuchs, 1969).

Such evidence, by the way, has been around for nearly a hundred fifty years. Robinson (1972) referred to a then exactly one-hundred-year-old paper by Adamük in *Albrecht von Graefes Archiv für Ophtalmologie*, which, unfortunately, I was unable to obtain digitally from where I was sitting (in my supersized mind). However, I did find an even older paper by the same researcher *"aus Kasan"* (I assume from Kazan, the Tatar capital), who was a postdoc in Franciscus Donders's lab in Utrecht, the Netherlands. Dr. E. Adamük (1870) reported that the eyes always move together in the same direction when "irritating" (electrically activating) various points of the frontal hills of the corpora quadrigemina (the superior colliculi; not clear in which species, but probably not human).

The work by Donders and Adamük gets a brief mention in William James's *Principles of Psychology* (1890|1950b, p. 511) in the context of "what Helmholtz calls a *Cyclopenauge*," the notion that both eyes function as one organ—which takes us straight back to Rubens's illustration (figure 2.1). Should we recognize the superior colliculus as the material counterpart of that metaphorical eye on the hexagonal operating table? Doug Munoz, one of the world's leading experts on the neurobiology of the superior colliculus (and, of course, a disciple of Bob Wurtz), once jokingly told me that someone had once jokingly told him that the rest of the brain merely serves to keep the superior colliculus warm. Everything happened inside the superior colliculus; it sat tucked away deep inside the brain for protection.

Of course, oculomotor control is most emphatically *not* localized in the superior colliculus. The first (screamingly obvious) thing to note from figure 2.2 is the distribution of place names and pathways. Localization in contemporary neuroscience is never about attributing a particular function to a particular brain structure but about identifying key components for a particular function. Oculomotor control involves a host of structures in various parts of the brain, so if asked "Where in the brain do we find oculomotor control?" the correct answer is "In the brain." Some philosophy of mind (including, but not only, that of embodied cognition) will find even the question misleading (too restrictive). Yet the control function for eye movement does take place in the brain: Without the brain, no eye movement; without light (and so without visual input from the world) and with an otherwise immobile body, there can still be eye movement. (Of course, the brain would not live without that body, whether mobile or not; there will be movement *inside* an immobile body, the heart beating, blood flowing—the most critical, at present unimaginably difficult, issue for a brain in a vat would be the supply of a lifeline, with all that is needed to let neurons exchange molecules.)

Oculomotor control takes place inside the brain, and we can (and should) be more specific, investigating the circuitry, taking a systems perspective. We can consider the different brain areas involved and how they interact. Around the time when Adamük (1870) stimulated the superior colliculus, and inspired also by the work of Fritsch and Hitzig (1870|2009) on the motor cortex of dogs, David Ferrier (later Sir David Ferrier, a Scotsman in London) embarked on a more systematic investigation, lesioning and stimulating the cortices of monkeys and dogs; he summarized this work in his 1876 book *The Functions of the Brain*. When stimulating near the arcuate area of frontal cortex (what we now call the frontal eye field), Ferrier (p. 143) observed (in italics): "*The eyes open widely, the pupils dilate, and head and eyes turn towards the opposite side.*" Not everyone was happy with these experiments, Ferrier becoming one of the first targets of anti-vivisectionist campaigning, led by "the formidable" Frances Power Cobbe, who forged "a coalition of feminists, abolitionists, vegetarians and anti-immunizers" (Gross, 2009, p. 466; see Elston, 1987|1990, for an essay on anti-vivisectionist action in Victorian England, where women and sentiment were pitched against science and men).

Cobbe chose a conspicuous target. Ferrier was the one person to be singled out by Charles Sherrington for "his many services to the experimental physiology of the central nervous system" (thus the dedication on an unnumbered page at the beginning of Sherrington's classic *The Integrative Action of the Nervous System*, 1906). The Royal Society offers every three years the Ferrier Lecture. The first, in 1929, was (somewhat of a symmetrical gesture) for Sherrington. A few of these lectures went on to become quite famous (like Hubel and Wiesel's of 1971). The list of 28 includes half a dozen Nobel Prize winners and reads (at least until 1974) as a one-page summary of the whole of systems neuroscience (I would agree with the ghost of Cobbe, however, that Wilhelm Feldberg deserved no honors; the list still seems to be hurting from that 1974 error, with an indefensible number of suboptimal choices in the last three decades).

We will be on our guard against complacency, taking the bioethical issues extremely seriously throughout. However, the likes of Ferrier (1876) and Sherrington (1906) deserve full credit. Thanks to their work we can now draw sketches such as those I drew for figure 2.2. To Ferrier's findings that functions are distributed across brain regions, Sherrington added specific ideas about circuitry and excitatory versus inhibitory connections between neurons. The upper left panel of figure 2.2 shows several excitatory projections to the superior colliculus; these can "drive" saccades. There are three important cortical excitatory projections: one from the parietal lobe (the lateral intraparietal area, LIP), and two from the frontal lobe (the frontal eye field, FEF, and the supplementary eye field, SEF). These three areas are all active in the case of voluntary eye movement control (e.g., when we make saccades following a verbal cue). SEF shows more complex types of processing than FEF and LIP, and FEF's workings are more immediately movement related than are SEF's and LIP's. FEF and LIP additionally contribute to stimulus-driven eye movement control (e.g., when we shift our gaze spontaneously to salient visual information). There is also a subcortical excitatory projection directly from the retina to the superior colliculus. This pathway elicits stimulus-driven eye movements on the basis of coarser visual information than what makes LIP and FEF send urgent spikes to the superior colliculus.

Not everything is excitation, however. The upper right panel of figure 2.2 shows an important inhibitory pathway, from the basal ganglia to the superior colliculus. The substantia nigra pars reticulata (SNr, an output station of the basal ganglia) is normally continuously active, with a high baseline, the neurons spiking fifty, sixty, or more spikes per second. These spikes release the neurotransmitter γ-aminobutyric acid (GABA), which hyperpolarizes the membrane of superior colliculus neurons, making these more difficult to activate by excitatory input (e.g., from FEF) — SNr inhibits the superior colliculus. We can imagine a push–pull contest taking place in the superior colliculus, the excitatory inputs trying to outweigh the inhibition from SNr. The two sets of inputs can also work in a complementary fashion, say, if SNr sends diffuse inhibition (inhibiting *any* saccade), and FEF or another excitatory input calls for one particular movement vector (one saccade in a given direction, jumping a given length). Note that SNr itself receives inhibitory input from another basal ganglia structure, the caudate nucleus (Cd). The projection from Cd to SNr forms a direct pathway in the basal ganglia (for simplicity, I skip another direct pathway as well as the indirect pathways in the basal ganglia). The point here is that we can see a double negation in action, with inhibition of inhibition, when Cd tells SNr to shut up so that other voices can be heard (metaphorically speaking), or (in proper Neuroscience English) when Cd removes the inhibition by SNr so that the superior colliculus can more easily respond to excitatory input from the cortical eye fields and/or the retina.

Thus we see the superior colliculus being pushed and pulled by various players. From the superior colliculus there is a downstream projection to the saccade generator structures in the brainstem, which actually lead to the contraction of the extraocular muscles. But the superior colliculus also projects upstream, via the thalamus (see the lower left panel of figure 2.2). There are several of these feedback projections; I show only the one via the medial dorsal nucleus to FEF. This upstream pathway is arguably the clearest anatomical example of the sensorimotor nature of the sensorimotor system that gives us our visual perception. Aguilonius (1613) thought it had to exist; Bob Wurtz and his coworkers charted it (Sommer & Wurtz, 2002; Wurtz et al., 2011). This pathway, if any, makes it possible for us, for the brain, to take the body's own movement into account during perception—surely a mechanism we should like to study, if we are to understand how the self enters into the equation of the active boundaries of vision. I have reserved space for it in chapter 4.

In the meantime, with the lower right panel of figure 2.2 we may begin to appreciate the busy, lively, complex happenings and interactions among the various mechanisms that contribute to oculomotor control. Taking this (abstract and simplified) circuitry as a starting point, we aim to characterize how gaze dynamics are brought about in the brain. We can zoom in on any particular mechanism, analyze the activity of individual neurons, hypothesize about, and test, their contribution. We can trace what kind of signal is projected where and zoom out again, toward reconstructing a system that, as we know from phenomenology, effectively integrates the sensory and motor aspects of our being.

Architecture of Exchange

Even before making an eye movement, during the most stable moment of fixation, motor aspects are indirectly at play in our efforts at perceiving objects. I designed the (slightly trivial, but hopefully effective) tests with figures 2.3 and 2.4 to make the point more easily available as a shared experience for you, the reader, and me, the writer, in our discourse on perception. Focusing your gaze on the black square to the left of figure 2.3, you will have a hard time acquiring specific knowledge of the creature to the right. You may not be able to tell whether it is a dog or a kangaroo, how many limbs it has, and when, if ever, you might have seen something like it before. You may not be able to tell these things even if you ignore my instructions and look straight at the creature. But as you try to play ball, and do indeed keep your gaze locked on the black square, you will *feel* how difficult it is, how unnatural—though not impossible—to prevent your eyes from moving to your area of interest. The difficulty, in neural terms, corresponds to the competition for control over the

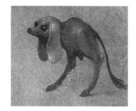

■

Figure 2.3
A test of covert visual processing. Please do not look at the figure until you have read through the instructions. Do you feel the urge to look at the figure? Please do not look at it just yet. Your task will be to keep your gaze focused on the black square and process the creature in as much detail as you can. Would you be able to recognize it in the next figure?

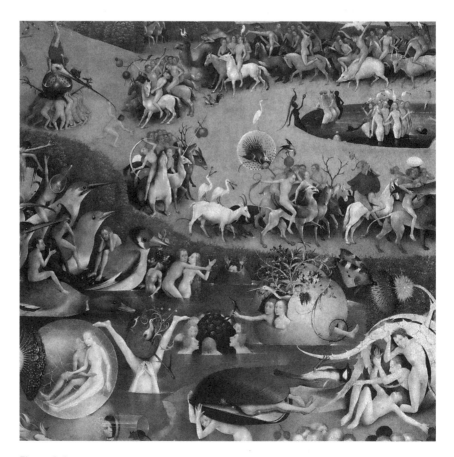

Figure 2.4
A test of overt visual processing. Do you remember the creature from the previous figure? Can you find it here, among the many curious beings and events? The image represents a large segment of the middle panel of *The Garden of Earthly Delights* by Hieronymus Bosch, a triptych from the late fifteenth or early sixteenth century, now at the Museo del Prado in Madrid. Cue: I have adjusted the scale. Second cue: check the top right corner.

superior colliculus, fought between the basal ganglia (following my instructions) and the FEF (urging you to scrutinize the blob). The urge to move your eyes betrays your implicit understanding of sensorimotor logic: If you move your eyes to the blob on the right, you gain access to visual detail.

In normal circumstances, we would apply the sensorimotor logic as a matter of course, exercising our perceptual skills, working from the practical knowledge that center and surround are interchangeable, that what is at this very moment in the periphery can be in the fovea a fraction of a second later; all it takes is one saccade. Even before making a saccade, the objects in the visual field outside the fovea exist as potential detail, as things we can submit to sensory processing via a motor act. Searching for the hybrid dog–kangaroo in figure 2.4, you will experience the need for motor acts as you try to match your memory of the dog–kangaroo with the objects in view. (You may wish you had a more specific template in mind; I will at this point allow you to take a peek at figure 2.3 again, to upgrade your template of the dog–kangaroo.) In a chaotic scene such as that of *The Garden of Earthly Delights*, our eyes seem unable to rest or find one vantage point that provides an overview. Even if you ignore my instructions and simply peruse the scene for pleasure, you will end up making a series of erratic saccades. The scene looks messy (busy, ambiguous, something between paradise and hell, perfectly congruent with Hieronymus Bosch's topic) because it has too many potential targets, laid out in a complex way, difficult to navigate.

If you do me a favor and actually try to locate the dog–kangaroo, you will find yourself persistently, more and more strategically, making saccades, moving from a chaotic to a more systematic search, following my second cue perhaps, focusing on the upper right, and consciously discounting the alternate visual objects one by one. Until you realize (if you have not yet: hereby the third cue) that no one should be trusted, least of all a writer performing an experiment on a reader (the dog–kangaroo actually appeared on a different panel from the same triptych; it is not visible in figure 2.4). I should probably apologize for this deception, and so I do, right now, though adding in my defense that I merely used the deception as a classical psychological tool, to catch you off guard and get good data—with the best of intentions and no harm done? The point is that visual search represents the clearest case of a sensorimotor process, relying heavily on the constant exchange of figure and ground, center and periphery, target and distractor. Every eye movement asks a question about one item in the visual field, "Is this the dog–kangaroo?" If the answer is "No," the next eye movement asks, "This one, then?" We can practically read the dialogue in the pattern of eye movements.

Even when we are, to the best of our abilities, keeping our eyes fixed, fully engaged in the sensory processing of an object in center vision, the motor components of perception remain active in parallel, exerting an influence, virtually, as a potentiality. Even when we are still asking ourselves about the current candidate, "Is this the dog–kangaroo?" we are already picking the next possibility. We do not wait until we have rejected the current candidate. Other objects are likely to be in the neighborhood, somewhere on the horizon. One of these can become the target of our next eye movement. Figure and ground are swapped, actively. Alternate information exists, somewhere, always, waiting in the surround, even if there is nothing but the blankness of white snow or an empty screen. We cannot see a thing without at the same time distinguishing that very same thing from something else. Every definition of a visual object implies the drawing of contours, borders, boundaries, with two sides and therefore, at least partially, a definition of what is outside the object (for every "in" there must be an "out"). Here is how Merleau-Ponty formulated a similar idea (1945|2008, p. 78, completing the quote I rejected earlier for its snubbing of anatomy):

> Even if I knew nothing of rods and cones, I should realize that it is necessary to put the surroundings in abeyance the better to see the object, and to lose in background what one gains in focal figure, because to look at the object is to plunge oneself into it, and because objects form a system in which one cannot show itself without concealing others.

The plunging is a curious image, suggesting something of a metonymic move, from sensation to (associative?) cognition, similar to Barthes's (1980|1999) discussion of *punctum* dynamics—fixing the gaze so that consciousness can perform its meaning-giving operations. However, we will never plunge to the extent that we lose ourselves completely; the plunging does not involve a disappearance, no becoming one with the object. The surround provides anchoring and essential contrast. (Perhaps Merleau-Ponty would in the present day have talked of bungee jumping.) No figure without the contrasting ground. (No bungee jumping without the elastic cord.) The object needs other objects, so they can be concealed. The fixing of the gaze carries meaning by the fact that it can, but does not (or does not yet) shift.

The limits of foveal vision, and the obvious fact that we can have only one focus for foveal vision, ultimately determine the selective nature of

perception. Allport (1987) suggested that selective information processing in vision should first and foremost be thought of as a selection for
action. At least in principle, there are no reasons why the capacity for
information processing should be limited in human cognition, but there
are very undeniable constraints to what we can do, with only two arms,
two legs, one head, and one pair of eyes. Thus we need to make choices.
We aim our actions, our eye and hand movements, at certain objects at
the expense of others. The entire sensorimotor system is structured
around this logic of exchange. "Eye movements bring objects to foveal
vision," would be a standard remark. However, eye movements also take
objects away from foveal vision. Every eye movement brings arrival and
departure, and rearranges the map of possibilities for future action as
well as for information processing. The architecture of exchange implies
that during any fixation, any moment dedicated to sensory processing,
things are not neutral with respect to motor programming. At any one
point in time, there exists a limited set of potential targets for eye move-
ments. Merleau-Ponty (1945|2008 again, now on p. 117) wrote as follows:

> The horizon or background would not extend beyond the figure or round about
> it, unless they partook of the same kind of being as the figure, and unless they
> could be converted into points by a transference of the gaze. But the point-
> horizon structure can teach me what a point is only in virtue of the maintenance
> of a hither zone of corporeality from which to be seen, and round about it inde-
> terminate horizons which are the counterpart of this seeing.

This hither zone of corporeality relates, I think, to Allport's (1987)
notion of selection for action. Points, figures, centers exist as potential
targets for action and so are situated spatially with respect to the body
and its degrees of freedom in movement. The potentiality cuts through
the dichotomy of in versus out. We should speak at least in threes to
specify where things are with respect to the body or, in the case of vision,
with respect to the visual field: in the center, the surround, and beyond.
We have one current focus for foveal vision, several potential targets in
the surround, and an infinite number of points beyond reach. This threesome implies that the architecture of exchange necessarily involves more
than meets the eye. There must be parallel processing for center and
surround. If the object in the center only shows itself by concealing
others in the surround, then this suppression of information can only be
partial. Concurrent (in competition or in concert) with the processing of
foveal information, there will be an unequal distribution of neural activity, dedicated to processing various aspects of the surround, both in terms

of acquiring sensory information and programming future saccades. There is not only sequential but also parallel action in perception.

What versus Where (or How)

Knowledge of rods and cones should be cherished as it sets us on our way to drawing the entire architecture of exchange, with parallel streams of visual information processing. From the different types of photoreceptor cells, and how they are distributed for central versus peripheral vision, we naturally move into separable modes of visual processing, serving functions that may be many things, but not redundant. Figure 2.5 shows the divergent projections from visual cortex, with a dorsal pathway, involving parietal cortex, and projecting to dorsolateral prefrontal cortex (DLPFC), and a ventral pathway, moving into the temporal cortex and from there to ventrolateral prefrontal cortex (VLPFC). The figure uses

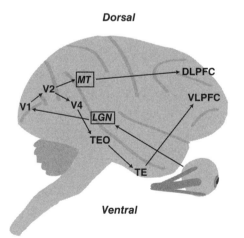

Figure 2.5
The dorsal and ventral pathways for visual processing. The anatomical projections are shown on the same abstracted shape of a monkey brain as in figure 2.2. Visual information from the retina reaches the primary visual cortex (V1, in the occipital lobe, in the back of the brain) via the lateral geniculate nucleus (LGN), a substructure of the thalamus. Area V1 projects to V2, where the projections diverge and create two streams of visual processing: a dorsal stream involved in spatial computations and a ventral stream toward object recognition. The dorsal pathway includes area MT (middle temporal), moves into the posterior parietal cortex, and ultimately reaches dorsal areas of frontal cortex, such as dorsolateral prefrontal cortex (DLPFC). The ventral pathway proceeds via area V4 and area TEO (posterior inferior temporal) to area TE (inferior temporal), down into the lower depths of the temporal lobe. From there, projections go to ventral areas of frontal cortex, including ventrolateral prefrontal cortex (VLPFC).

the same sketchy notion of a monkey brain as the one in figure 2.2 (for up-to-date, more detailed images, see Kravitz et al., 2011).

From the retina the information reaches visual cortex via a relay in the visual input structure of the thalamus (the lateral geniculate nucleus, LGN). Not shown in the figure but good to know is that, at the level of LGN, information from rods and cones moves in segregated ways, in parvocellular versus magnocellular layers. The parvocellular ("small cell") layers receive information that derives from cones and so carry color and fine visual detail with great sensitivity for changes over time. The magnocellular ("large cell") layers are devoted to information from rods, more global, at the expense of high-definition qualitative and quantitative features. Interestingly, four of the six LGN layers are parvocellular, producing something of a "neural magnification" of foveal information, analogous to the cortical magnification seen in, for instance, the primary sensorimotor cortex (where the amount of neural tissue devoted to different areas of the body is famously unequal, our fingertips getting many more neurons per millimeter of skin than, say, the area between our shoulder blades). Already purely anatomically speaking, our visual system is set to work harder on foveal than on peripheral information.

The parvo- and magnocellular layers bring the information, still at least partially segregated, to the cortex. Not surprisingly, then, the visual cortex also divides into different streams, speaking anatomically as well as functionally. Leslie G. Ungerleider and Mortimer Mishkin (1982) established the (very rapidly very widely accepted) concept of two separable visual pathways in a classic paper, reviewing a large literature of lesion studies, including their own. Monkeys with lesions to dorsal areas were unable to figure out which of two choice options was closer to a landmark object. Monkeys with lesions to ventral areas had a particularly hard time learning to discriminate new visual patterns. From these and many similar observations, Ungerleider and Mishkin (p. 549) suggested there are two cortical visual systems in anatomically segregated pathways: a dorsal pathway specialized for spatial perception, locating *where* an object is, and a ventral pathway specialized for object perception, identifying *what* an object is.

Though the idea of two separable visual pathways took firm hold in the neuroscience community, there was, and still is, much less agreement about how the two pathways relate to one another functionally. Goodale and Milner (1992) proposed a dissociation that became just about as popular as the original one by Ungerleider and Mishkin (1982).

Sometimes it takes data from only one person to convince the rest of the world. Goodale and colleagues (1991), in a paper that Merleau-Ponty would have loved to read, observed a strange paradox in the visual behavior of D. F., a woman in her thirties who had suffered brain damage following carbon monoxide intoxication. She was unable to distinguish object qualities such as form, orientation, and size, but when asked to grasp the very same objects, her hand and finger movements betrayed unmistakable practical knowledge of their form, orientation, and size. Most of her primary visual cortex and dorsal pathway had remained intact, but large portions of the ventral pathway were gone. Goodale and Milner (1992) concluded that the ventral pathway might be about conscious recognition of objects—"vision for perception." The dorsal pathway, on the other hand, was not so much processing *where* things are as *how* we can guide our actions. This would be an unconscious or implicit form of visual processing—"vision for action."

The line-up sounded too good to let pass without a funky bit of speculation. So the many readers of *Nature* noted: [ventral + perception + conscious] versus [dorsal + action + unconscious]. Human intellect dictated that it *had* to mean something. And sure enough, it briefly looked as if it would become a sport to expand on the dissociations of ventral versus dorsal processing, toward a yin–yang model of vision, inspired by our most stereotyped hunter–gatherer past (see Silverman & Eals, 1992, for an exotic reference of this variety, riding on the wave of the newest revelations in neuroscience). Ventral processing would be yin, female, nearsighted, making beads, processing emotions, sitting quietly, thinking, happening in the darkest recesses of the brain. Dorsal processing, enjoying a little more sunlight seeping through the skull, would be yang, male, farsighted, analytic, mathematical, throwing spears, guiding actions, going with the flow. Or did I get it all wrong? I bet I did (cf. Sanders, Sinclair, & Walsh, 2007). I will blame the monkeys, for holding their heads upside down, not throwing enough spears, and generally failing to make beads.

No doubt Goodale and Milner (1992) were right in pointing out that the dorsal pathway did more than locate things. However, the contention that the two pathways divided in terms of consciousness was less convincing. A decade later, data emerged showing that the type of visual analysis rather than the amount of consciousness determined the activity in the dorsal versus ventral stream. Very conscious tasks such as mental rotation (Gauthier et al., 2002) or computing the angular difference of line orientations (Fias et al., 2002) produced dorsal stream activation whereas the very same stimuli called for more intense ventral stream processing under other task conditions, no more or no less conscious.

We will have to sacrifice the easy notions and resist the temptation to dichotomize. Any visual feature or type of computation will likely be more dominant in one stream than another, but such differences will be in degree only, no more than relative. The dorsal stream has access to information about color, and the ventral stream will know about motion direction, even though in both these cases the other stream happens to have more of it. Furthermore, such relative differences between the ventral and dorsal stream concerning various visual features do not group neatly for our conceptual convenience. Each neuron, whether in the ventral or dorsal stream, will have an idiosyncratic activity profile in response to a wide variety of visual types of computation. From its activity profile alone, no neuroscientist will be able to tell with Cartesian certainty which structure a given neuron belongs to.

Any functional labeling we wish to impose on ventral versus dorsal processing had better emphasize its relativity as well as the fundamental interconnectivity of the two streams. If pressed for such labels, I would prefer to take the teleological approach to the extreme and look toward the final projections of the two streams. Then we note that the ventral stream tends to project more intensely to ventral than dorsal frontal areas, and vice versa. From what we know of those ventral frontal areas, computations relating to various forms of valuation seem the most prevalent there (e.g., Grabenhorst & Rolls, 2011; Kang et al., 2011; O'Doherty et al., 2001; Tremblay & Schultz, 1999). So rather than a summary "what" system, serving object recognition, I would see ventral processing leading to valuation of potential and actual outcomes (not simply "What is this thing?" but "What does it mean for me?" or "What should I do about it?"). Conversely, the dorsal frontal areas seem to work at solving problems and finding efficient ways to achieve particular goals (e.g., Gerlach et al., 2011; Mansouri, Tanaka, & Buckley, 2009; Sakai et al., 1998; Wallis et al., 2001)—briefly, managing actions and cognitive strategies ("How do I fix this?" or "Which is the best way to get there?"). These ventral and dorsal sets of functions influence, inform, and support each other. Valuation leads to planning, and constraints in planning naturally will factor into valuation. Both sets of functions involve aspects of perception and action, conscious and unconscious processing, and rather more than fewer types of visual features.

Instead of lining up pairs of antonyms (conscious–unconscious, non-spatial–spatial) in supposedly divisive ventral–dorsal (yin–yang) ways, we should ask how the different types of visual analysis in the two streams together contribute to the inherently interactive and dynamic processes of perception *and* action. The aim should be to integrate figures 2.2 and 2.5. How do the different types of processing in the ventral and dorsal stream enable us to generate an understanding of a visual scene and to pick specific details or objects for further scrutiny? This is a question of gaze dynamics. To understand the functions of ventral and dorsal processing in vision, we need to incorporate the movements of the eyes and the position of information relative to the eyes.

Truly Embodied Mapping

To be sure, the control of eye movements, however spatial, is not uniquely, or even specifically, a dorsal task. Put differently, and more strongly, it would be nonsensical to claim that processing in the ventral stream is not spatial. All visual information is spread out over space, defined by contrasts and boundaries between what we have here and what we can see over there. This is obviously true for features such as contour (and more generally, shape), but also for so-called "nonspatial" features such as color (we can easily acknowledge that our experience of one and the same patch changes markedly depending on what surrounds it). We have indeed, as Merleau-Ponty remarked, "reason for holding *a priori* that all senses are spatial" (1945|2008, p. 253).

In Neuroscience English: A crucial concept for sensory neural activity is that of *receptive field*. In (an effort of moving toward) Plain English: We need to realize that any sensory neuron fires in response to only a portion of the information available to the senses. That portion can be defined in various ways, but always also spatially. The question "Which information can trigger a change of activity in the neuron?" can be directed to spatial coordinates: "Where does the information have to come from in order for it to influence the neuron?" In the activity of visual neurons, the spatiality corresponds to a specific region in relation to the retina—computationally the fovea serves as the origin of the spatial dimension. Information from the visual world is mapped in retinal coordinates—most truly embodied, retinotopic mapping. Studying neural activity with respect to visual processing, then, we do well to consider the role of gaze position, in any which situation.

Say, if a stimulus appears in a particular retinotopically defined region, it affects the neuron. We could stimulate the neuron by shining a beam of light straight onto that limited region of the retina (similar to what

Hubel & Wiesel, 1959, did with anesthetized cats), or we could allow light from a complex scene to wander naturally into the eye, so that a portion of it might reach the same region of the retina (in which case we must carefully track the subject's eye position and translate the map of the visual world to retinotopic coordinates). If the stimulus appears outside the critical region, however, the neuron remains oblivious to it. For a given retinal ganglion neuron, a visual stimulus may have to appear within a small zone to the lower left of the fovea for it to elicit an increase in the neuron's firing rate. (All retinal ganglion neurons have different critical zones, together making up the entire visual field.) We can characterize any neuron in LGN or V1 or elsewhere in the visual system in terms of the retinotopically defined region the neuron responds to. We call this region the "receptive field" of the neuron. It is the field from which the neuron receives information.

Even neurons in the ventral stream have spatially defined receptive fields. When we claim that the control of our gaze happens in concert with visual processing, then this must be true for ventral as well as dorsal visual processing, in defiance of any notion that action should go dorsal. Nardo, Santangelo, and Macaluso (2011) found ventral as well as dorsal visual cortical activity relating to (literally) eye-catching events (e.g., human characters appearing) in brief animation sequences of complex and dynamic scenes (e.g., a hotel lobby). The ventral activity responded in a particularly transient way, sensitive to the exact moment a new event occurred in the scene, whereas the dorsal activity seemed to set a continuous baseline against which new events were more or less likely to have an impact. The authors could not (and did well in not trying to) offer any easy interpretation to please proponents of divisive ventral–dorsal schemes. Both ventral and dorsal activity implied spatial processing and contributed to the subject's responsiveness to salient perceptual events. Both pathways played a role in eliciting eye movements. Instead of divergence, the data suggested complementary roles for both pathways, the dorsal pathway providing a continuous ground, and the ventral pathway picking transient focal points.

Further evidence supporting the latter claim comes from a single-unit study by Mazer and Gallant (2003), who recorded activity of (ventral stream) V4 neurons while the subjects (monkeys) performed a visual search task. The monkeys were allowed to make unconstrained eye movements as they searched for a target (a circular patch cropped from a photograph, in black and white, of a real-world scene) among a set of distractors superimposed on a visually "noisy" (complex and meaningless) background. The activity of one in two V4 neurons tended to precede an eye movement to the stimulus in its receptive field. The suggestion is that V4 operates as a retinotopic salience map, indicating where in the visual field we might find information relevant to the task at hand.

Such retinotopic salience maps also provide a straightforward computational solution to the issue of combining visual features into a single object for conscious processing—the infamous "binding problem," which occupied the minds of cognitive scientists in the 1980s and early 1990s. The retinotopic coordinates should in principle allow us to look up all the visual features at the same location. This computational opportunity was exploited most lucidly by Treisman and Gelade (1980) in their influential feature-integration theory that accounts for various phenomena of visual search. Given that the visual system offers separate retinotopic salience maps for each visual feature, we can easily imagine a mechanical operation that integrates (or glues together) all of the features at a selected location in the visual field. Treisman and Gelade dubbed the mechanical operation "attention"—which, I think, is one of the better approximations of this slippery word anywhere in science (precisely because it is formulated so mechanically, which makes it easily refutable —a crucial quality for good Popperians).

The idea that retinotopic mapping could hold the clue with respect to linking up disparate information should please neuroscientists and philosophers of embodied cognition alike. It gives neuroscientists a useful conceptual framework that leads to concrete questions, calling for empirical investigation. How do the receptive fields of neurons line up? How much do they overlap? What is the minimal distance for two points to be distinguishable? How does the spatial sensitivity of the neurons in different brain areas relate to the spatial sensitivity in the subject's behavioral responses? Does activation spread to all neurons that respond to visual features at a given location (no matter which feature, from color to texture to orientation to motion direction to motion speed to curvature to...) or only to those neurons that respond to features that are relevant for the current task (e.g., only color and texture)?

Philosophers of embodied cognition will be happy to note that retinotopic mapping is very much a function of the body, situating all information from out there in the world relative to the body. The body defines space, or once more with Merleau-Ponty (1945|2008, p. 117), "far from my body's being for me no more than a fragment of space, there would be no space at all for me if I had no body." Can this function of the body explain how we integrate information without having to duplicate it to infinity? Perhaps look-up algorithms relying on retinotopic mapping offer an in-brain equivalent to leaving different bits of information distributed (in different brain areas), without having to construct miniversions (tiny mimetic representations) and ending up tumbling forever in infinite regress

The questions about retinotopic mapping and integration of information will naturally keep coursing through this monograph. For now, I would like to add just a few more remarks about this type of mapping before moving on to an exploration of another critical dimension of the sensorimotor system (having thought a little bit about space, we should not forget about time—in fact, two different aspects of time, limited and unlimited, the repetition of events and the continuity of the arrow). Here are just two or three extra thoughts about space, then, to whet the appetite for later chapters.

Retinotopic mapping should be considered first-order mapping only (and not finally). This is how information is initially (at early stages of visual information processing) situated in space. Other, second-order forms of spatial mapping can be derived from the retinotopic through comparison with alternative bodily coordinates and through visual interpretation of objects. Instead of computing from the fovea, we can reference the position of visual items with respect to the head ("craniotopic mapping") or even, though less common, the trunk. Eye-, head-, and trunk-centered mapping are all egocentric (relating to the body). We can also compute allocentric maps, centered on coordinates out there in the world—individual (perhaps even moving) objects or landmarks or relations between objects and landmarks. None of these other maps would exist without the first stage of retinotopic mapping.

The retinotopic mapping itself may show plasticity. The receptive field of any individual neuron does not necessarily have to remain fixed for the visual system to be able to construct a retinotopic map. An important topic of investigation will be the flexibility of receptive fields as a function of context and learning. Rosenbluth and Allman (2002) pointed out that the information about eye position, as implied by receptive fields, can itself become a teaching signal, or support stimulus–stimulus associations (e.g., in accordance with classical conditioning). We should also consider the nature and purpose of complex relations among neurons with different receptive fields across different brain areas. Information may not necessarily be fed forward or back to neurons with overlapping receptive fields. It seems quite possible, for instance, that neurons with peripheral receptive fields feed task-relevant information about specific objects back to neurons with receptive fields centered on the fovea (as argued on the basis of compelling fMRI data by Williams et al., 2008).

With flexibility and complexity, and alternative forms of mapping, we come to the issues that really matter for gaze dynamics and information processing. If the ways of the world were simple and very slow, we probably would not need vision, no faculty to work with active boundaries toward finding out truths about things as they are (the chemical senses might suffice, the way they do for bacteria swimming toward food, even if their chemotaxis does not actually involve anything sentient). Luckily, happily, or merely as it happens, the ways of our world are manifold and change all the time, but not randomly or entirely unpredictably. This means we can put the predictable or systematic variation over time to good use as we proceed with flexible, complex, and various forms of mapping information.

The Context as a Cue

Some things have a habit of returning. In the grandest scheme, they become myths or the focus of entire philosophies. Gilles Deleuze, inspired by Friedrich Nietzsche's concept of the Eternal Return, placed the issue of repetition at the very heart of being and becoming: "Returning is the becoming-identical of becoming itself. Returning is thus the only identity" (Deleuze, 1968|1994, p. 41)—a sameness based on difference, for what is now can never literally (entirely) be the same as what was before. To paraphrase Deleuze's Nietzsche: At the very least the what-is-now is a thing happening after the what-was-before. It would be our task, as thinking beings, to discover equivalences (or notice the return of things) across time and space. It almost sounds like a task of inferential statistics, where we can try to approach truths (various forms of being and becoming) through establishing significant differences and discrediting null hypotheses. The trick is to zoom in on relevant relationships and patterns of data that are meaningful to us. Grouping and categorization are then activities that emerge through the interplay of questions and answers, formulating hypotheses and collecting evidence to reject alternatives— ideally following the logic spelled out by Popper (1935|2002).

Yet in our routine efforts at perceptual grouping and finding the meaningful in daily life—navigating away from harm, toward all that is good for us—we seldom operate as careful Popperians. We do not have the time for it. Instead, we tend to put the null hypothesis second, presuming things to be guilty of projected meaning until proven innocent (see Lauwereyns, 2010, for a detailed account). The projected meaning—the actual hypothesis we have in mind—will depend on only a handful of basic biases in our thinking, shaped by motivation (our desires and fears), familiarity (what we believe or what we know about things), and proximity (what is close to us in time and space). There are at least two advantages that follow from the implementation of such biases: speed and guidance.

First, in terms of speed, the biases enable us to act urgently at any time. The biases provide shortcuts, supplying the best answer in the absence of any evidence. If we assume wishes to have come true and fears to have materialized, we are able to react swiftly, secure the reward, or make a narrow escape. The speed of our reactions is likely to be critical in a world where competition exists in multiple guises at every corner. Second, with respect to guidance, the biases function as cues for search. If given the opportunity for further investigation, the biases will help us narrow down the search area, and reduce the efforts required for collecting evidence. With a detailed target in mind, we are able to look strategically for data that confirm or deny.

In the latter case, we see biases operate in conjunction with sensory mechanisms, improving our sensitivity for critical information, or allowing us more efficiently to extract signal from noise, to borrow the language of signal detection theory (Green & Swets, 1966|1988). This conjunction also influences gaze dynamics. "The focusing of the gaze is a 'prospective activity,'" suggested Merleau-Ponty (1945|2008, p. 269), citing a certain R. Déjean, who went one further, in a 1926 publication on "a psychological study of distance in vision": According to Déjean, the prospective activity would be *of the mind*. For Merleau-Ponty that was too much, though he did not explain why. I would agree with Déjean, I believe. What other thinking or perceiving unit than the mind would there be to engage in prospective activity? I would like to think of the looking ahead as a bias, in the mind, activated in a given context and influencing future processing.

Let me describe an example in more detail. Background information, processed in peripheral vision, might generate the idea (a perceptual bias) that an unclear blob in our visual field corresponds to a particular class of dangerous object—say, a car, about five seconds of biking distance ahead, wrongfully parked by an irrational organism, right on our bicycle path. We might then aim our foveal vision, through the back window, at the back of the driver's seat, to establish whether the irrational organism is presently sitting in the car, in which case we should watch out for sudden movement (the car starting or the door opening). On full alert, bias activated, we will monitor the situation selectively, extracting potentially useful information (e.g., the shape of a human head where, based on the way in which the car is parked, we should fear a lack of reason).

Biases are activated by context. From being latent in our mind, the biases become "occurrent" in a particular situation. Given one thing, we can expect another. This association cuts across time, not only in the sense that the one thing must necessarily come first for it to generate the expectation of another. The association itself relies on prior knowledge, reflects a cognitive mechanism that must have been in place in the mind of the perceiver before the act of perception. When a given context activates a certain bias and guides the gaze, the entire process can tell us something about the perceiver, about the characteristics of the sensorimotor system—the conditions under which particular biases are activated and the ways in which they influence perception. The biases, I believe, are crucial to understanding what happens inside the head of the perceiver during perception. It is only through studying biases that we can hope to understand exactly what it means for processes to be subjective, rather than loosely talking about the subjective nature of perception.

To be sure, many of these subjective processes, linking contexts with biases and acts of perception, are shared across the majority of any random sample of subjects and can be considered "normal" (including "normal" in the prescriptive sense). Most subjective processes are completely mundane—"subjective" is not synonymous with "idiosyncratic," though of course *some* biases will indeed be unique to a particular individual. But to study the mechanisms involved in context-dependent biases, we do well to start with the most common, and investigate perceptual biases that we all share.

One such bias is the expectation that a (living) human body comes with a head on its shoulders. Cox, Meyers, and Sinha (2004) conducted an elegant fMRI study to investigate some of the implications and neural mechanisms involved. They found that severely degraded information of a head (such that none of the facial features were distinguishable), when presented as a natural extension of a human body, produced significant activation in the fusiform face area (a neural structure in the ventral temporal lobe, usually busy in the visual processing of faces; Kanwisher, McDermott, & Chun, 1997; Sergent, Ohta, & MacDonald, 1992).

When the same degraded information was presented alone or below a torso instead of on the shoulders, there was hardly any response in the fusiform face area. Even a highly detailed image of a face, presented in isolation, produced less activity than the degraded face in context, on the shoulders. Apparently, the activity in the fusiform face area was more about interpreting visual information in context (trying to read something as a face) than about processing intrinsic face-related information. Biases played a role above and beyond true face information. The conclusions neatly converged with those of Egner, Monti, and Summerfield (2010), who found that, computationally speaking, neural activity in the fusiform face area was explained better in terms of hypothesis testing than in terms of stimulus feature variation. Put differently, the activity was driven by face expectation versus surprise, not by any physical metric relating to face characteristics.

Moving on from bodies and faces to more accidental contexts, we can study the ways in which complex natural environments lend themselves to strategic search as a function of task (e.g., Peelen, Fei-Fei, & Kastner, 2009; Torralba et al., 2006). Object-specific biases may operate across the entire visual field during briefly flashed images but produce spatially constrained eye movements when we get the time to explore. Given the same photo of a kitchen, our scan paths are different depending on whether we are looking for a mug or for a painting. In landscapes and cityscapes, there are plausible and less plausible places for cars and people. Our search is guided by these kinds of plausibility.

Contextual cueing can work quite subtly, outside our awareness according to Chun and Jiang (1998). Repeatedly searching through complex arrays of elements, subjects are able to pick up certain embedded regularities. They can learn to expect where a target might appear, given a particular background. If I would make you search for our little dog–kangaroo through the same Hieronymus Bosch painting several times, you would learn to navigate it efficiently (see figure 2.6). Or let me describe it in the way Chun and Jiang studied the process. Say I would use two categories of paintings as potential search displays: one set of five familiar paintings (each of which I show in ten percent of the trials) and a large set of novel paintings (each of which I show only one time). On half the trials, the dog–kangaroo is in the picture. For the familiar paintings, if the dog–kangaroo is in the picture, it will always be in the same place (say, for painting 1, always in the top left corner; for painting 2, always in the bottom right corner; and so on).

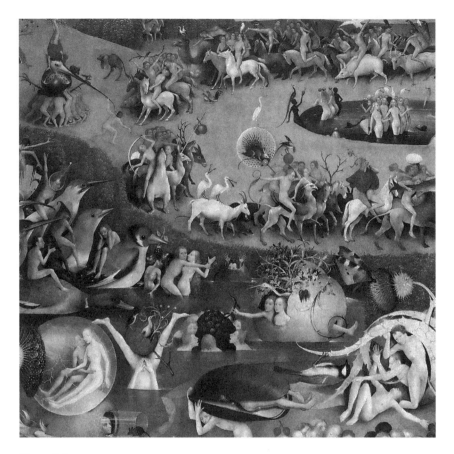

Figure 2.6
A demonstration of contextual cueing. Do you remember the image from figure 2.4? It is
the very same large segment of the middle panel of *The Garden of Earthly Delights* by
Hieronymus Bosch. This time the dog–kangaroo is really in the picture, in the top left
corner. You might see the outline of a square superimposed on the original image—evidence of my clumsy pasting. Now, once you have found the dog–kangaroo, it will be easy
for you to find it again, any time you return to this figure. Try it. Close the book, open it,
and look again for the dog–kangaroo. The background lets you navigate to the target in a
fraction of a second. This is what contextual cueing does.

Now, if you keep searching for the dog–kangaroo under these conditions, the context may help you on your way with the familiar paintings.
For the novel paintings, there can be no hope of shortening your chaotic
itinerancy, no way to predict where the target might show up. However,
for the familiar paintings, you might learn that, given painting X, the
target, if present, will be in location Y. So as soon as you detect the
context, you can make an eye movement to the relevant location. Chun
and Jiang (1998) found that subjects can acquire such search skills, even

though they are unable to tell the experimenters how they do it—Chun and Jiang argued that it represents a type of implicit learning. Chun and Phelps (1999) further suggested that the hippocampus and the adjacent medial temporal lobe play a critical role in this implicit usage of contextual information. Amnesic patients with damage to these brain areas showed normal implicit skill and perceptual learning but no evidence of contextual cueing.

Another line of work appears to corroborate the findings on implicit contextual cueing and hippocampal involvement. When subjects are asked to study images of complex scenes and then tested with exact repetitions versus slight modifications, they tend to gaze disproportionately at the manipulated regions. This happens even when the subjects are unable to explicitly recognize the changes (e.g., Hayhoe et al., 1998; Henderson & Hollingworth, 2003; Ryan et al., 2000). Our gaze appears to precede our full awareness of the changes, as if the visual system is already processing something funny before the rest of the brain catches on.

Inspired by such findings, Hannula and colleagues (2007) developed a paired association paradigm, relating complex scenes to specific faces. They found that the scene cue elicited eye movements to the matching face in a subsequent choice display, despite the fact that the scene cue provided no spatial information about where that matching face might occur—a rapid influence from memory on eye movements that preceded, and exceeded, the influence on the explicit (manual) responses. Intriguingly, Hannula and Ranganath (2009) provided fMRI evidence with exactly this paradigm to suggest that hippocampal activity predicts the contextually guided eye movements to the matching faces. The relevant target would be signaled by hippocampus first, putting out a call for the visual system to confirm. Explicit realization would kick in only after the gaze provides convincing evidence.

The contextual guidance of the gaze is a pervasive theme in the operations of the visual system. Time, and therefore memory, comes into it. Without memory, we cannot exploit the context to guide our gaze. Perceptual processes that are extended over time, with a series of actions aimed at tracking or finding objects, do not only tell us that vision integrates sensory and motor mechanisms. This integration must have something to do with memory, with content-bearing information in the mind.

Integration across Views

"As soon as I raise my eyes / the invisible has slipped away / and I begin to see what I see: / memories of what I have seen // and whatever I will see." This is a quote from Hans Faverey's 1988 collection *Against the Forgetting* (1994|2004, p. 136). The poet never doubted that time comes into it. Seeing relates future to past, at the microlevel of hundreds of milliseconds, before and after an eye movement, as well as at the macrolevel of days, months, years, or an entire lifetime. Every vision works toward recognition—a bringing back to mind—and may (with emphasis on the potentiality) lay down a memorial trace for future recognition, in which case we will happen to see again at a later time what we are seeing right now.

The business of recognition, the very act of re-cognizing, happens inside the mind. This is not so much a theory from neuroscience or psychology as a matter of linguistic praxis. Re-cognition is a return to the mind, by definition. That is simply what the word "recognition" means. At its most basic (micro) level, every perception involves the cognizing of a thing over time, across movement, even if we disregard all semantics: "[I]n order to perceive a surface ... it is not enough to explore it, we must keep in mind the moments of our exploratory journey and relate the points on the surface to each other" (Merleau-Ponty, 1945|2008, p. 281). The disputes among scientists and philosophers start only when we ask *how* perception works, what is actually cognized in the various cognitions, and which kinds of physical and computational processes it involves.

Neuroscientists would simply charge ahead and say that this is an empirical question. How do we manage to recognize objects from among the huge amount of variation in their retinal images? Some philosophers might start grumbling, saying the word "images" sounds too representational, but most neuroscientists would continue without batting an eyelid and ask to see the data from neurons in the inferotemporal cortex. Neurons there show a remarkable selectivity in their firing rate for particular objects and yet a fair amount of "tolerance" for different views of these objects—the neurons respond most strongly for their preferred objects despite considerable changes in position, size, and orientation (e.g., Hung et al., 2005; Ito et al., 1995; Logothetis & Sheinberg, 1996; Vogels & Orban, 1996).

One intriguing idea, championed most persuasively by Li and DiCarlo (2008, 2010), is that the tolerance relies on the temporal contiguity of objects in vision. Given that real-world objects are likely to be *somewhere* in the visual field for seconds or longer, it should make good sense for the visual system to work from the assumption that changes in retinal images are due to some kind of motion, either of the object or of the viewer—that is, it pays to implement a bias in favor of ascribing a blob at time t to the same object as a blob at time $t + 1$. The main computational issue for the visual system would be to learn just how tolerant it should be for changes in retinal images (or what should constitute a significant difference between two views of blobs). Li and DiCarlo showed that this tolerance in inferotemporal cortical neurons adjusts dynamically as a function of natural visual experience. When objects start swapping more easily, the activity patterns of the neurons gradually show a reduced tolerance to changes in retinal images.

Though the underlying algorithms remain unclear, the notion of dynamic tolerance to changes is a promising one, which deserves further exploration. I particularly like the idea that the visual system uses time as an implicit teacher. Objects only deserve to be called objects insofar as they represent stable structures of some kind. The stability refers to temporal contiguity. With this property of objects in mind, we can start computing. Anything that looks like an object right now should have a certain degree of stability (and so temporal contiguity) and still be an object one moment from now. What level of dissimilarity can there be between two views of the same object? Our task, toward the perception of objects, is to zoom in on efficient assessments of the temporal contiguity.

With time as the implicit teacher, our perceptual system would adopt a minimalist approach, relying heavily on bias, assuming that multiple views belong to the same object unless there is compelling evidence to the contrary. Minimalist approaches will be likely winners in many arenas—evolutionary, philosophical, and computational. The gesture toward minimalism will be appreciated by just about any thinker and experimentalist interested in perception, but much is left to clarify. What is the nature of the representations used in the comparison between old and new views? What kind of algorithm is employed in the actual comparison? Is there perhaps even a problem with the very notion of "representation"?

Virtual Content

Some philosophers would say "Yes, there is a problem" and might add "A big one." How does what we see in the inferotemporal cortex prove that information is actually represented there? Neuroscientists, of course, would point to the wealth of empirical data showing that, of all brain areas, particularly inferotemporal cortical regions produce the best neural correlations with visual object stimulation. However, "brute correlation" (Noë's phrase, 2004, p. 210) does not convince philosophers. Some thinkers about the mind find it problematic that we plunge straight into empirical investigation, say, in the inferotemporal cortex, without acknowledging, or even realizing, the contentious nature of our assumptions about the visual system—particularly with respect to the role of representations, duplicates, or "pictures in the head."

The problem runs deeper than most neuroscientists would admit (to others or even to themselves). Sometimes we think we have eluded the problem when we really have not. A good example can be found at the very beginning of Richard L. Gregory's *Eye and Brain* (Gregory, 1966, p. 7; still the same wonderfully rich page I already quoted from in chapter 1). "There is a temptation," Gregory writes, "which must be avoided, to say that the eyes produce pictures in the brain. A picture in the brain suggests the need of some kind of internal eye to see it—but this would need a further eye to see *its* picture," the classic challenge of infinite regress. Gregory seems to be a hundred percent aware of the issue but then writes, at the end of the same paragraph: "When we look at something, the pattern of neural activity represents the object and to the brain *is* the object. No internal picture is involved."

Gregory warns us against internal pictures, but in the same breath assures us that representations of objects do in fact exist in the brain. Philosophers shall be forgiven for finding this just a tiny bit fishy. How are those representations different from the notion of internal pictures? Do they not call for an internal mind to contemplate the representations? Does this really save us from infinite regress? We need to think about it more carefully, with Alva Noë (2004, p. 2), for instance:

[W]e ought to reject the idea—widespread in both philosophy and science—that perception is a process *in the brain* whereby the perceptual system constructs an *internal representation* of the world. No doubt perception depends on what takes place in the brain, and very likely there are internal representations in the brain (e.g., content-bearing internal states). What perception is, however, is not a process in the brain, but a kind of skillful activity on the part of the animal as a whole.

Daniel C. Dennett was the first philosopher to fully articulate an alternative, in *Consciousness Explained* (Dennett, 1991). Instead of constructing an internal representation of the world, we might just leave the world where it is, out there—let the world be its own representation. Noë (2004) took the idea one step further, making it the core of his enactive view of perception. We do in fact experience a visual world in extreme detail, Noë acknowledges, but "[t]he detail is experienced by us as *out there*, not as *in our minds*" (p. 33).

Noë has a point there. Take figure 2.7, with the frontispiece of Aguilonius's (1613) *Opticorum Libri Sex*. If we glance quickly at the left panel,
we will have the impression of high visual detail, a complex compilation
of objects and words, available for us to process. Yet, we know from
experience, and from chapter 1, that we cannot absorb the meaning of
the whole scene at once. We need to make eye movements, perhaps following a pattern such as that indicated in the right panel. As we do so,
we will be able to take note of specific items, label them, and think about
them. In tutorials on eye movements and perception, teachers often blur
the background (as I have done in the right panel of figure 2.7) to give
an impression of the degree to which information is actually processed
in peripheral vision. Yet, even if I keep my eyes fixed on any single point
in the right panel, I can immediately see that the image is distorted. The
blur bothers me. It feels palpably like a lie.

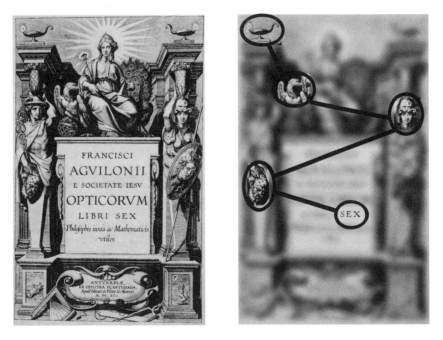

Figure 2.7
The frontispiece of Franciscus Aguilonius's *Opticorum Libri Sex* (1613), designed by Peter
Paul Rubens. The left panel gives a photographic (external) representation of the image.
The right panel illustrates a possible pattern of eye movements, focusing in turn (and not
entirely randomly) on an oil lamp, an eagle, a living person's face, a decapitated head (of
a man who might have suffered from the bubonic plague), and the Latin word for the
digit that comes after five and before seven. I have blurred the background for expository
purposes as is done routinely in tutorials that discuss the role of eye movements in
perception.

The pedagogical trick may work efficiently to show the extent of visual detail that we can process consciously at any one point in time (in the fovea), but it fails miserably in conveying our preconscious sense of the rest of the scene. In natural viewing, we experience richness of visual detail in peripheral vision—our visual system tells us *that* the richness is there without giving us much in the way of concrete information about it. Noë knows about this, and argues as follows (Noë, 2004, pp. 66–67):

The enactive, sensorimotor approach offers an explanation of how it can be that we enjoy an experience of worldly detail that is not represented in our brains. The detail is present—the perceptual world is present—in the sense that we have a special kind of access to the detail, an access controlled by patterns of sensorimotor dependence with which we are familiar.

We can epitomize this phenomenological insight as follows: The content of perceptual experience is *virtual*.

This passage is my absolute favorite in *Action in Perception*. I completely agree with it. "Access" is a crucial word, here, for me. In vision, we know we have access to rich visual detail in the world before us. Unfortunately, Noë goes on to nearly extinguish my enthusiasm for the quote by writing the following elsewhere in his book: "If the content of experience is virtual, in this way, then there is *a sense* in which the content is not in the head" (p. 214). Apparently, Noë understands "virtual" and/ or "represented" to mean something different from what I would naturally read into it. My liking of the passage must have been promoted by lexical ambiguity, leaving room for the wonderful magic of projective verse (following Charles Olson's [1967, pp. 15–30] concept). The present monograph being an explicit effort in the service of science, however, I must try to throw more light on the issue, so we can see the differences in theoretical positions more clearly.

I think the virtual content of visual experience should be located *in* the head. The sense of access to rich visual detail is a sense we have inside the brain, working with (among other things) sensorimotor coordinates of potential targets for the gaze. Let me explain. To begin with the obvious, just to be sure, I will focus on experience first, before moving on to the trickier issue of virtual content. Experience, in the sense of conscious processing, is a function of the mind that, for very good reason, we believe to be in the head. I have no doubt that Noë will agree with this, but it may be safe to spell it out (for my own train of thought, if for no one else's). Take away the head, no experience of any kind. Proposition from the Far Side: We have a massive amount of causal evidence to suggest that decapitation leads to the removal of a subject's experience (sure, a decapitated body can still show reflexive action for a few seconds, but it is not likely the locus of any experience; instead, the severed head might still register its predicament for an awkward moment before all experience extinguishes). Thus, I hypothesize (along with probably every sane neuroscientist and possibly the majority of sane philosophers) that having a head is a necessary condition for experience. Mike the Headless Chicken might at first look like an interesting challenge to this notion, but he still had what he needed most from his brain, and even an ear, so I would be willing to accept he enjoyed, or rather suffered, a minimal amount of experience (see Lloyd & Mitchinson, 2006). Even Andy Clark (2008), developing the most radical notion of mind leaking out into the world, places experience *in* the head, reserving the supersizable part of the supersized mind to unconscious information processing (I will come back to this in chapter 3).

Now, what about the "virtual content" of experience? "Virtual" would be (paraphrasing the Oxford Dictionaries Online) the content that does not actually or physically exist but shares with such actual content the appearance (cf. the etymology of "virtual" in late Middle English, "possessing certain virtues"). My best guess is that Noë thinks of the world as possessing the physical energy that could generate actual experience in the mind and, for this reason, claims that the potential, virtual content of our experience exists out there, in the world, out of our heads. I naturally agree with the idea that the world's energies possess the power to generate experience in our minds. However, I prefer to see those energies as actualities outside our heads—not virtual content but actual presence.

The content of our experience, actual or virtual, I would see as a function of the mind/brain. All content of experience, I suggest, would be in the head, depending on "internal representations in the brain (e.g., content-bearing internal states)," which Noë (2004, p. 2, already quoted above) concedes are "very likely." The virtual content, in my view, corresponds to the brain's active and passive "anticipations of perception," to appropriate a Kantian concept (Kant, 1781|2007). The virtual content reflects the brain's active and passive biases in perception and decision making. Imagination and expectation can activate such biases; learning and previous experience produce passive biases. The biases in perception and decision making are content-bearing internal representations that can be ON or OFF or anything in between (ON meaning that the underlying neural circuit is maximally active; OFF meaning that the underlying neural circuit is at baseline). Virtual content can become actual content by interaction with the world—the world's physical energies have the power to convert virtual into actual or to generate actual content without any prior virtual content in the case of truly novel experience. But I think it is wrong to say that the world's physical energies *are* the virtual content of our visual experience.

I will have to expand on these ideas, of course. This entire monograph works toward that expansion. I am only at the beginning of my construction, but it will revolve around internal virtual content. It will take representations not as actual re-presentations or duplicates of objects in the world but as incomplete, abstract code that makes predictions about the world and revises its predictions on the basis of interaction with the world (see Berkes et al., 2011, for successful empirical work that takes a similar approach). At present, I would like to note simply that we *can* accommodate the notion of virtual content in the head. It can be done without representation of the world but with access to the presentation of the world—all from within a worldview *à la* Spinoza (1667|2001, p. 100), as per the scholium under proposition 2 in the third part of his *Ethics*, "Origin and Nature of the Affects," where he states that "the mind and the body are one and the same thing, conceived at one time under the attribute of thought, and at another under that of extension."

In the same movement, I believe an approach of virtual content from within a worldview *à la* Spinoza offers a valid strategy against the ever-dreaded charges of dualism that philosophers and neuroscientists like to throw at each other. Offense may be the best defense against dualism, grabbing it by the neck, thoroughly absorbing it, inhabiting it—learning completely to incorporate dualism in the application of perspective. If one and the same thing looks like *this* from one angle and like *that* from another, it is up to us to understand the angles (a quick flash forward: with John Keats we need to exert our negative capability, and with Slavoj Žižek we need to dance with the parallax). We should not try to negate the dualism of perspectives, but negotiate it, supplement it, with second-order perspectives, of the third kind. It must be possible to relate the two first-order perspectives to one another, translating from one to the other, moving between them, back and forth.

Moving back and forth, with virtual content in the head, I would like to think in the beautiful words of Wallace Stevens that "Description is / Composed of a sight indifferent to the eye. // It is an expectation, a desire, / A palm that rises up beyond the sea, // A little different from reality" (Stevens, 1954|1984, pp. 343–344, in part II of *Description without Place*). The description (or representation) changes the physical energies into something a little different from reality, an expectation of what comes next, a bias in favor of one thing rather than another. Making such descriptions in the head *is* what perception does. Of course, for this to happen we need objects out there in the world to supply us with the physical energies that can generate and influence the internal representations, expectations, biases. However, if we are to understand the sensorimotor system, we had better look for the content of vision *inside* the brain, with degrees of freedom controlled by the gaze. The moving retina is a good place to start.

3 The Moving Retina

As he paces in cramped circles, over and over,
the movement of his powerful soft strides
is like a ritual dance around a center
in which a mighty will stands paralyzed.

Only at times, the curtain of the pupils
lifts, quietly—. An image enters in,
rushes down through the tensed, arrested muscles,
plunges into the heart and is gone.

How much can we make of these words? To what extent do our autonomous mechanisms of interpretation allow us to "read" the scene? Do they (i.e., we?) even engage in an effort of trying to understand the words? Context, as we have seen in the previous chapter, can cue our expectations, give cognition a head start. For those compulsively needing some context here, I will add that the scene was composed by Rainer Maria Rilke (1995, p. 31) in Paris, 1903, or possibly late 1902, around the time he worked as a secretary for Auguste Rodin. The creature hopelessly pacing is a panther, locked up in the zoo of the Jardin des Plantes in an age well before humans started caring about enriched environments for caged animals. However, rather than expanding on the topic of contextual influences, I would like to take a closer look at the dynamics of visual processing "from the bottom up," as psychologists like to say, focusing on perceptual mechanisms that appear to work in a machine-like fashion, deriving complex information from naked sensory data. What happens when "the curtain of the pupils / lifts" while the "mighty will stands paralyzed," the body moving back and forth without any deliberate or consciously engineered plan?

"An image enters in, / rushes down through the tensed, arrested muscles," writes the poet, a nice metaphor, which has made implicit, if not intuitive, sense to several generations of psychologists and neuroscientists but must be recognized quite simply as utterly wrong. The image "plunges into the heart and is gone," adds the poet, and this idea I like very much. The reference to the heart goes with poetic license—Rilke does not play hide-and-seek; his poetry is never less than generously lyrical. But the plunging and being gone is what binds me to the poem, the fleeting nature of the image-induced rushing that is swallowed up by the heart—effectively a vanishing. Could this be an idea to explore further? Idea: that the visual world in all its richness lives extremely briefly between stimulating the eye and vanishing in the heart. Our minds would not look at pictures but swallow them.

The panther's vision, writes Rilke in the lines following the quote, "from the constantly passing bars, / has grown so weary that it cannot hold / anything else." The caged animal sees only that it ("he") is caged, or not even that. What would it see if it were roaming somewhere in the wild? Do ecological psychologists predict an entirely different perceptual experience? Or do we have some reason to think that vision is never about *holding* anything? And how many lovely questions should one little poem be allowed to offer us? With science, let us wander along, and wonder.

Absurd in the Highest Degree

Even with our mighty will paralyzed, we cannot help but be washed over by the richness of the visual world. As soon as we open our eyes, the various colors of countless surfaces come to us without any effort. To fully block out the autonomous processes of the visual system, we have to take radical measures, turn out the light or close our eyes. Vision gives us a forceful experience of things out there. It is a strange and magnificent gift, food for wonder all right and heated debate at times—to the point of sparking a religious war of sorts, between creationists and scientists (or perhaps I should say "most scientists," acknowledging the existence of curious hybrids). Creationists have been known to inoculate themselves against Darwin with Darwin, quoting the following passage from the beginning of chapter VI on "Organs of Extreme Perfection and Complication" in *On the Origin of Species* (1859|1866, p. 215):

To suppose that the eye, with all its inimitable contrivances for adjusting the focus to different distances, for admitting different amounts of light, and for the correction of spherical and chromatic aberration, could have been formed by natural selection, seems, I freely confess, absurd in the highest degree.

It is possibly the most frequently quoted sentence of *On the Origin of Species*. Many of these frequent quotes prove poor or malicious readership, suggesting Darwin gave up on the eye as a product of natural selection, thinking "I have an eye—therefore God exists." Perhaps Darwin really did believe in something he wished to call "God," but he did not for that reason take the miracle of the eye to be incompatible with the theory of natural selection. In fact the passage about the eye is now also gaining a second (or is it third?) life as a textbook example to illustrate the fallacy of quoting out of context—or, when done intentionally, the praxis of "quote mining." Here is how the text continues (still on p. 215):

When it was first said that the sun stood still and the world turned round, the common sense of mankind declared the doctrine false; but the old saying of *Vox Populi, vox Dei*, as every philosopher knows, cannot be trusted in science. Reason tells me, that if numerous gradations from a perfect and complex eye to one imperfect and simple, each grade being useful to its possessor, can be shown to exist; if further, the eye does vary ever so slightly and the variations be inherited, which is certainly the case; and if any variation or modification in the organ be ever useful to an animal under changing conditions of life, then the difficulty of believing that a perfect and complex eye could have been formed by natural selection, though insuperable by our imagination, can hardly be considered real.

We note Darwin's clever appeal to the Copernican revolution, the great paradigm of scientific victory over the Catholic Church. He urged us to go beyond intuition and immediate experience—toward a deeper phenomenology, reflecting on the hidden connections between things as they appear. The challenge was to search for evidence of variations and gradations in the complexity of the eye. Wonder should be the start, not the end of exploration.

No one rose better to the challenge than Richard Dawkins. What seems insuperable to our imagination will be suddenly within easy reach for anyone who reads *Climbing Mount Improbable* (1996|1997). In the chapter on "The Forty-Fold Path to Enlightenment," Dawkins sketches a plausible and very sensible account of slight variations and gradations in the structure of many different types of eye. The story takes special care in making sure that every eye, every gradation, however crude or far from perfection, gave its owner, however tiny or simple the organism, some kind of practical benefit.

Dawkins is one of that rare breed of teachers who can properly open our eyes to never-seen vistas; his texts are a treat, unafraid of a bit of verse. I do not think I would have ever strayed into a creationist camp, but I will readily admit pre-Dawkins fogginess in thinking about eyes evolving. He sees just about anything that might be relevant (of course, he also discussed the fallacious quoting of Darwin; or more to the point, I first learned about the case in *Climbing Mount Improbable*). He even comes achingly close to something like an enactive view of perception, early on in that beautiful chapter (1996|1997, p. 144):

Photons arrive at random times, like raindrops. When it is really raining properly we are in no doubt of the fact and wish our umbrella hadn't been stolen. But when rain starts gradually, how do we decide the exact moment when it begins? We feel a single drop and look up apprehensively, unconvinced until a second or a third drop arrives.

Here, the analogy with raindrops suggests that perception is a decision-making process that involves hypothesis and testing via skillful sensorimotor control with actions that strategically produce relevant sensations. However, rather than pursuing the very promising theme of sensorimotor processing and decision making in vision, Dawkins leaves the "we" behind and zooms in on the issue of capturing every possible photon. The more photocells, the more photons captured, Dawkins reasons. The idea of decision making is not really his idea at all (1996|1997, p. 146):

The essence of seeing a patterned image is that photocells in different parts of the retina must report different intensities of light and this means distinguishing different rates of pattering in different parts of the photon rainstorm.

Dawkins treats the eye as a tool for reporting and does not venture beyond lenses and photoreceptor cells. Of course, there is already plenty to be said about lenses and photoreceptor cells (and Dawkins does it brilliantly), but that does not give us the sum total of the eye, let alone the essence of seeing a patterned image. Dare I conclude that Dawkins's readership, however impressive, is still not perfect? His focus on lenses and photoreceptor cells in the mid 1990s was not abnormal. Noë had not yet written *Action in Perception*. Dennett's *Consciousness Explained* had not yet sunk in. Dawkins spoke with the neuroscience and biology of a previous generation. In that context, it was understandable that he glossed over the "inimitable contrivances" of the eye, which, according to Darwin, included higher functions, such as "adjusting the focus to different distances," "admitting different amounts of light," and even "the correction of spherical and chromatic aberration."

This last contrivance sounds like an oblique reference to what we now know as the topic of object constancy. Correcting spherical and chromatic aberration—it takes us back to chapter 2 and our ability to attribute various appearances in color and shape to different views of the same object. No doubt this is not done by the eye alone. Could it be that Darwin used the word "eye" to mean more generally the system with which we make visual contact with the world? Our awe and wonder, shared even with creationists, was first and foremost directed at the magnificent gift of vision, not specifically only the curious balls in the front of our skulls.

Nevertheless, I promise it will be worth our while to keep the focus on the eye (the actual organ that we call "eye") a little while longer and ask which kinds of higher functions it might perform. If Darwin attributed too much and Dawkins too little, then where is the appropriate middle, what is the correct attribution? Which higher functions are performed by, let us narrow it down, the retina? To begin with, Dawkins must know the retina is very much more than an array of photoreceptor cells. The relevant information has been vivid and explicit for well over a hundred years, thanks to the fabulous drawings of Santiago Ramón y Cajal (see figure 3.1 for an example). Masland (2001), in a modern reexamination of the structure of the retina, identified more than fifty different cell types, in five categories (still the same as those identified by Cajal, 1893): photoreceptor cells, horizontal cells, bipolar cells, amacrine cells, and ganglion cells. Why do we have so many different types of cells in the retina? What warrants their existence?

Perhaps the truth will listen to a little phenomenology. Merleau-Ponty (1945|2008, p. 184) boldly stated that "no layer of sensory data can be identified as immediately dependent on senseorgans: the smallest sensory datum is never presented in any other way than integrated into a con-figuration and already 'patterned.'" The activity of retinal ganglion cells, or the output from the eye to the brain, will imply configuring and pat-terning already—visual interpretation before the brain gets a chance to play with the data. Does this imply a form of cognition in the eye? The eye as an apparatus for visual thought?

What Is an Apparatus?

We loosely and easily use the term "visual system" in neuroscience, psy-chology, and philosophy of mind. Chapter 2 carried "system" in the title, and I have argued for a systems perspective in considering the function of vision as well as the underlying anatomy. But should we think a bit more carefully about the implications and assumptions, the hidden mean-ings and pitfalls, when we use a word like that? What exactly qualifies as a "system," and more specifically *the visual system*? Just now I was about

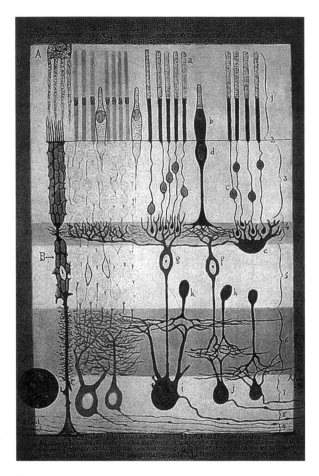

Figure 3.1
Different cell types in the retina. This is one of the most famous of the many wonderful drawings by Santiago Ramón y Cajal, made in the course of research reported in Cajal (1893) and dozens of other papers and monographs. Identified (in lowercase letters) are the following components and cell types: (a) outer segment of a rod, (b) outer segment of a cone, (c) nucleus of a rod, (d) nucleus of a cone, (e) horizontal cell, (f) and (g) different types of bipolar cell, (h) amacrine cell, and (i) and (j) different types of ganglion cell.

to write, "more specifically a visual system," but the indefinite article sounded wrong in my ears. An indefinite article comes with the implication that there might be other visual systems—multiple visual systems in the mind. I cannot subscribe to that. The visual system, I would like to think, is one thing, responsible for all of our vision, one unit of sorts, composed of multiple mechanisms and subsystems. The eye is part of it, one of the subsystems. How does it relate to the mind?

Let me backtrack for a second, and explore the notion of a system a little bit before moving on to situating the visual system, the eye, and the mind with respect to one another. A quick visit to the Oxford Dictionaries Online tells me that a system is (1) "a set of things working together as parts of a mechanism or an interconnecting network; a complex whole," and (2) "a set of principles or procedures according to which something is done; an organized scheme or method." There is a (3), and a (4) as well, but they are less relevant here. The first two definitions, however, look perfect to me. But how does this work for the visual system, or the system that gives us vision—the system with which, tradition tells us, we see. Who actually does the seeing? Does the system do the visual processing and we get to do the seeing? How does the visual system relate to *us*? The definitions of "systems" are rather noncommittal about who does the work and why. The first definition ("a set of things working together as parts of a mechanism or an interconnecting network; a complex whole") says the system does the work, but not why or on whose command. The second definition ("a set of principles or procedures according to which something is done; an organized scheme or method") is even more noncommittal, suggesting a system is a way of doing this, regardless of who does the doing.

Can philosophy help us out? Here speaks Giorgio Agamben (2009, p. 14), grand master of contemporary Continental philosophy, about the cognate term "apparatus," or actually, as per the original text, the French term "*dispositif,*" which can also be translated as *device* or *mechanism*: "I shall call an apparatus literally anything that has in some way the capacity to capture, orient, determine, intercept, model, control, or secure the gestures, behaviors, opinions, or discourses of living beings." Agamben's examples include tools such as pens and computers but also cultural systems such as prisons and factories and also language and (oddly or quirkily) cigarettes. The visual system certainly fits in the list. More interestingly, Agamben (still on p. 14) then tells us that he distinguishes between "two great classes: living beings (or substances) and apparatuses. And between these two, as a third class, subjects." In the next sentence, he calls "a subject that which results from the relation and, so to speak, from the relentless fight between living beings and apparatuses."

I am not sure whether I agree, but the thought tickles me. Agamben basically suggests that systems and living beings together define subjects—it is only through the interaction that subjects become what they are. For Agamben (p. 14), this also implies that "the same individual, the

same substance, can be the place of multiple processes of subjectifica-
tion," or the subject is only a subject in relation to a particular apparatus—the subject does not equal the living being; it is only one of its
functions. Applied to vision, this means that the subject, the observer (the
one who sees), emerges from the interaction between the visual system
and the living being. It is a thought I will wish to return to in the following chapters. I certainly like the idea of studying subjective processes (the
observations of an observer) as the result of the interaction between a
living being (a human body) and the visual system (a set of algorithms
and mechanisms for visual processing) if I can take this interaction to
mean that the visual system becomes active in the living being. I think
Agamben's concept is also compatible with Dennett's (1991) multiple
drafts theory of consciousness: We would all be various (parallel and
competing) subjects in one body, where subjects are functions that
emerge from specific interactions with systems.

Such systems would be quite crucial in making what we are: "[A]ppa-
ratuses are not a mere accident in which humans are caught by chance,
but rather are rooted in the very process of 'humanization' that made
'humans' out of the animals we classify under the rubric Homo sapiens"
(Agamben, 2009, p. 16). Of course, tool use and language are among the
usual suspects when it comes to hypothesizing about what it is that makes
us "special." However, I do think that Agamben's idea of subjects' being
shaped by their systems is an original one and worth contemplating.
Some impatient neuroscientists might at this point sigh, "But why should
we bother with that Continental fog?"

Why should we bother? Thoughts of a different order, outside our
comfort zone, can challenge us, give us a chance to rise to the challenge,
and thus to *rise*—to change or sharpen our own ideas. Do we have the
power to cut through the fog? In the study of vision, we can translate
Agamben's ideas to the possibility that the visual system helps shape
the subject who sees. I like this proposal (no longer Agamben's, but one
I obtain via Agamben) better than the classic notion that we use the
visual system to see, which sounds a bit as if the visual system would
somehow be an object outside "we." The visual system is part of us, is
part of what makes us who we are. If I say that I am a person who can
see, then the visual system must be part of the "I." When used loosely or
carelessly, the term "visual system" can seem to imply that it is something
that produces representations, or even images, which should then be
analyzed, looked over, or interpreted by the mind. Such implications
are fundamentally wrong; they put us on the slippery slope to infinite

regress and inexplicable homunculi who must do all the magic work of consciousness.

Instead, we should try to see the visual system as an integral part of the mind. I promised I would situate the visual system, the eye, and the mind with respect to one another. It is quite simple. The excursion via Agamben helps me see it more clearly. The eye is a subsystem of the visual system, and the visual system, in turn, is a subsystem of the mind. The mind itself is a system, which can be a subsystem for other systems (family, sports team, city…). Some systems overlap partially with others; the relations among systems are not always clear. In vision, I think the threesome of eye, visual system, and mind is unambiguously organized vertically, with layers of different levels of complexity, the higher encompassing the lower. So we move from relatively simple (the eye; yes, my Darwin, the *relatively simple* eye) to the most mind-bogglingly strange and difficult (the mind!). This means the eye *is part of* the mind. The thinking about the actual features of visual objects starts already in the eye, not in the visual cortex or any other brain structure.

Note in the previous sentence that I slipped in the "actual features" of visual objects. This is to avoid the fallacy of the input–output structure (Hurley, 1998) in vision. The thinking about visual objects does not necessarily start in the retina. Indeed, in many cases it does not, with some kind of bias active in the brain before the arrival of photons in the retina. The visual system, I have argued in an entire chapter, is a sensorimotor system (here the indefinite article is appropriate; we have other sensorimotor systems); its actions do not run solely from retina to cortex. However, the processing of the actual information carried by photons does really start with those photons' affecting photoreceptor cells. In figure 3.2 the photons have bounced off an image of a snake. If we zoom in to the level of pixels in the image, we can imagine photons coming from four neighboring pixels, and reaching four different photoreceptor cells. What happens next?

The typical, extremely sketchy textbook explanation of vision suggests that the retina acts as some kind of spatiotemporal prefilter, with essentially a 1:1 mapping from pixels to photoreceptor cells to the retinal ganglion cells that send their signals into the optic tract (toward the LGN and the superior colliculus, and from there to the rest of the brain). The drawings by Cajal already told us that this idea must be wrong, but that did not keep it from surviving, at least implicitly, in the heads of most neuroscientists. Worse than merely wrong, it is the kind of redundant processing that simply shifts the task of interpretation forward. It gives

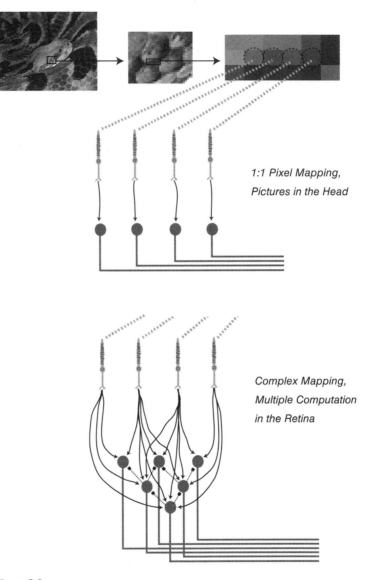

1:1 Pixel Mapping,
Pictures in the Head

Complex Mapping,
Multiple Computation
in the Retina

Figure 3.2
Information processing in the retina. Looking at a digital picture of a snake, we zoom in on a string of four individual pixels. Let us imagine that the photons bouncing off from these pixels are captured by four different photoreceptor cells (the rod-like objects standing for rods). Ultimately the activity of these cells will influence the retinal ganglion cells, whose axons find their way into the brain. Which photoreceptor cells influence which retinal ganglion cells (after mediation and modulation via bipolar, horizontal, and amacrine cells)? The top scheme suggests 1:1 mapping, preserving the detailed structure of the image and implying that all interpretation is left to the brain. The bottom scheme suggests complex mapping, with multiple forms of computation in the retina and a highly processed and diverse set of signals for the brain.

us tiny little viewers inside the heads of viewers that forever pass the information on until (if ever) some infinitely tiny little viewer finally actually looks at the picture (which is now so degraded from all the copying that the last homunculus has nothing to look at and declares, in what almost sounds like philosophy, that there never was anything out there in the first place).

We can do better than that. We must revise our textbooks—with the title of a stimulating review by Gollisch and Meister (2010): *Eye Smarter than Scientists Believed.* I feel tempted to add an exclamation mark. The retina is structured, via complex mapping, to support multiple types of computation in parallel. The mechanisms of active perception are fully at work already at the level of the retina. We may consider it the first, most typically machine-like stage of visual processing, answering best to our conventional ideas of what a system does. The retina receives no feedback signals from downstream brain areas and, for this reason, can be considered to function in a strictly autonomous or "bottom-up" fashion. However, research over the past decade or so has shown time and again how advanced the information processing is in the retina. I will highlight some of these feats in the following paragraphs.

The upshot of taking the eye to be an integral part of the mind is that explaining the computations in the eye amounts to explaining some of the picture viewing that homunculi had to do in old theories of vision. Already at the level of the retina, the mind bypasses the use of detailed pictorial representations. Such detailed pictorial representations would anyway be a waste of time, a waste of effort. I write these words with a slight flavor of melancholy in the mixture, realizing that this indictment applies most forcefully to one of my cherished predecessors, someone I wish I could have met, though of course I was, and he died, too young. From the very beginning of his *Vision*, David Marr (1945–1980) had it completely wrong (1982|2010, p. 3):

What does it mean to see? The plain man's answer (and Aristotle's too) would be, to know what is where by looking. In other words, vision is the *process* of discovering from images what is present in the world, and where it is.

Vision is therefore, first and foremost, an information-processing task, but we cannot think of it just as a process. For if we are capable of knowing what is where in the world, our brains must somehow be capable of *representing* this information—in all its profusion of color and form, beauty, motion, and detail.

Elsewhere in the book, Marr acknowledged the need for useful representations but reckoned that "that requirement is rather nebulous"

(p. 31) and insisted on engineering toward highly detailed pictorial representations with information "in all its profusion." Ironically, his pragmatic attempt to analyze the visual system as a machine—his efforts at demystifying the computations—ultimately relied on homunculi to appreciate the highly detailed pictorial representations.

Today we enjoy Marr's *Vision* for its boldness, its clear concepts, and its hands-on approach to modeling and actual problems of computation. It remains a source of inspiration in its clarity about different levels of understanding, the distinctions between variables and operations, objects and events, representations and processes. The trouble with Marr is not in his approach but in his assumptions—not how he works, but where he starts and what he works toward. He allowed himself a simplification—a crucial error—assuming that the input (at the level of photoreceptors) is an array of image intensity values, a pixel-by-pixel representation to be decoded by the brain.

Marr did not consider fovea versus periphery and so failed to acknowledge that there should be different kinds of "pixels," with different sizes, different resolution. By the same token, he failed to acknowledge the need to make eye movements to reorient the fovea or to obtain the relevant "image intensity values." He had no interest in saccadic eye movements and concentrated only on papers about visual cortex. I find it particularly painful to read (on p. 14 of *Vision*) that in the 1970s "[n]o neurophysiologists had recorded new and clear high-level correlates of perception."

Marr completely ignored the massive series of four papers on "Activity of Superior Colliculus in Behaving Monkey" by Wurtz and Goldberg (Goldberg & Wurtz, 1972a, 1972b; Wurtz & Goldberg, 1972a, 1972b). The papers showed, among other things, that visual responses of superior colliculus neurons depended on what the monkey intended to do, whether the monkey had to make an eye movement to a visual stimulus or ignore it. It was the first time that anyone obtained something like a potential neural correlate of consciousness (if we briefly adopt a fuzzy layperson's notion of "consciousness"). If Marr had read these papers, if he had not limited his view to visual cortex, he would certainly have spent a moment or two thinking about the role of the gaze, and more generally the role of action, in perception—Marr would have realized the retina is really a *moving* retina.

Missing the fovea, and therefore eye movements, was one thing. However, Marr was also fundamentally wrong about the purpose of vision. We do not look to know what is where in all of its profusion. Marr had read, and even appreciated, some of J. J. Gibson's work but refused to properly incorporate the ecological perspective. He explicitly rejected the notion that validity, or value of information, has a decisive impact on our visual processing. To paint detailed pictures is not *the* goal of the visual system. We look to know where to go and what to do. Occasionally we look to appreciate or savor particular aspects of the scene before us, or we let curiosity reign. Very occasionally we look indeed to paint a detailed picture. The one-line truth is that there are multiple goals, with different priorities. The priorities depend on the circumstances. We will need a bit more of J. J. Gibson (coming in chapter 4). In the meantime, let us take a look at some of the interpretations that the retina does perform—some functions of the mind carried out autonomously by the eye.

Change Vision versus Cluelessness

We do not construct detailed internal representations of the visual environment to know what is where. Striking behavioral evidence to this effect emerged a decade after Marr passed away. In the 1990s philosophers and psychologists became entranced by the fact that we are surprisingly poor at detecting changes between two images of the same scene. Try it with figure 3.3. Do the two images at first glance look the same? How long does it take for you to notice the difference? (I promise there is one, no more and no less than exactly one.) You will probably need at least two or three eye movements, perhaps even several seconds. In some cases we take an embarrassingly long time to spot changes that in hindsight seem so obvious (Grimes, 1996; Levin & Simons, 1997; Rensink, O'Regan, & Clark, 1997; see Simons & Rensink, 2005, for a critical review of the phenomenon and its implications).

What surprised me most about this kind of research when it burst on the scene was not so much our own cluelessness about the visual world but the fact that it took till very near the end of the second millennium (and my first years as a graduate student) before researchers caught on about something I already knew as a nine-year-old child from the comics and brainteasers page in the newspaper my family used to subscribe to (carrying plenty of sports and very little else). There would often be a "Spot the Seven Differences" assignment with two line drawings side by side, showing the same ordinary scene (say, a living room or a supermarket). The drawings initially looked completely identical but gradually revealed variations in fairly conspicuous places. I usually spent a few

Can You Spot the Difference?

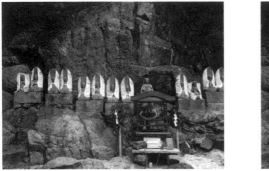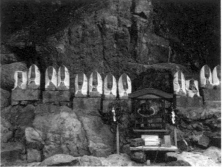

Figure 3.3
A little change detection task. Do you notice anything added or deleted in the right image? It may take a few eye movements before you can give a confident answer. People are surprisingly poor at detecting changes when the dynamics of the change are masked (e.g., by quickly swapping the images while the observer is making an eye movement or by flashing a noise pattern that covers the entire visual field). When the changes occur during normal gaze fixation, they are glaringly obvious. Here, once you have detected the change, you will be able to shift your gaze very easily back and forth between the little Jizo Bosatsu's being-there and being-not.

minutes scrutinizing the drawings before getting bored and giving up. I would find three, four, perhaps five of the differences, but very rarely all seven. Then I checked the answers, printed on a different page. It never ceased to amaze me how obvious the differences actually were, once I had confirmed them. I could not get my head around how I had missed them.

Every time I opened the newspaper I knew I would be amazed; I looked forward to being amazed. The paradox (of course, I did not know the word "paradox") was positively bewildering. I was absolutely sure I could see things clearly, and yet the evidence proved with certainty that I did not. As a nine-year-old, I was, I freely confess, unable to move beyond the superficial beauty of the mystery. As a beginning graduate student, I nodded my head in tune with the sounds of philosophers and psychologists that suggested we simply do not make internal visual representations; we leave the world out there, we let the world be its own presentation. In my mind this brilliant meme belongs first and foremost to Daniel C. Dennett (1991). Later, Alva Noë (2004) seemed even more radical—perhaps too radical, suggested the like-minded Andy Clark (2008, p. 141): "Confessions first. In one area at least, fans of radical embodiment *have* almost certainly overplayed their hand in a way that unjustifiably downgrades the contribution of the biological brain." The area was change blindness.

Clark (2008) was careful to point out that several psychological studies have shown some visual details to be carried over from one gaze fixation to the next, particularly those belonging to objects that are actually foveated (Hollingworth & Henderson, 2002; Hollingworth, Schrock, & Henderson, 2001). Sometimes it appeared that a few bits of information relating to visual changes were still active in the subject's mind even if she or he was not able to explicitly identify the changes as such in a change detection task (Mitroff, Simons, & Levin, 2004; Silverman & Mack, 2006). These are important observations that go some ways toward indicating the multiplicity of information active (encoded and accessible) in the brain during viewing, across saccades. I note with special interest that the gaze plays a critical role in determining what gets encoded. But for now, I would like to focus on a different way in which fans of radical embodiment have overplayed their hand—by forgetting about the retina.

I started developing a fascination for change *vision*. Philosophers and psychologists have largely ignored our ability to detect changes in normal conditions. Clark (2008, p. 141), for instance, notes that change blindness occurs whenever the changes themselves are masked: "Just about anything that takes out the motion transients that typically draw our attention to a locus of change seems to do the trick." Clark knows what typically happens in response to motion transients but chooses to focus on those contrived cases in which the blindness occurs—the flicker paradigm, with huge flashes that wash over the screen, or the transsaccadic paradigm, with images that are strategically swapped while the subject is making an eye movement. Scientists have been able to engineer a number of ways to conceal the transients. However, from a computational viewpoint, the more intriguing message should be that motion transients *can indeed* typically direct our gaze (or our covert selective information processing) to a locus of change.

Not being able to do something should be relatively easy to model—zero achievement being the default. It is not necessarily all that interesting. But how come we are so good at detecting changes when they suddenly happen in plain view? Which processes using what kinds of representation allow us to orient urgently to the locus of change? Not only are these more interesting computational questions than blindness. They are also ecologically more relevant. How often do we have to deal with mysterious appearances out of nowhere, which somehow occur during the fraction of a second while we are making an eye movement?

In natural vision, with the physics on planet Earth, the overwhelming majority of changes a typical animal might be confronted with do occur in plain view. No animal stands to gain much from neural mechanisms that can deal with the types of changes studied under the rubric of "change blindness." Instead, such neural mechanisms would likely be too costly, in terms of the amount of energy required and the increased potential for interference with other, more important types of information processing. We are probably better off with brains that do not bother about trying to detect changes in the absence of motion transients. Indeed, the motion transients are excellent indicators of changes, which is why they reward computational efforts that focus on them.

Such motion transients are computed already in the retina, on the basis of what must be a fairly extensive internal representation living extremely briefly in retinal circuitry (at most a few tens of milliseconds). This internal representation is not a neat array of image intensity values; it is not anything like an exact copy of a real-world scene at all but is a messy, noisy, rich spatiotemporal pattern of activity that supports extensive parallel computation. This messy pattern is not passed on. The infinite regress is broken at the very first step, as Dennett required (1991, p. 53), but this step must be located *in* the eye, not out of the head. Instead of passing on this extensive but very costly richness, the retina immediately economizes and derives various potentially relevant signals from it. I think of it as a process of diverging reductions: from extensive richness to a multiplicity of potentially useful readings, all of which together are much less expensive (measured in energy needed for neural processing) than the initial richness.

One class of retinal ganglion cells, the "Y-type," responds when a textured image moves across the retina (Demb et al., 1999; Enroth-Cugell & Robson, 1966; Petrusca et al., 2007). The texture motion implies dynamic patterns of light intensity increasing and decreasing; retinal circuitry affords the integration of such local changes. In figure 3.4 we go one step further. My sketch presents the gist of findings by Ölveczky, Baccus, and Meister (2003), which show that signals from retinal ganglion cells already imply the segregation of background motion from object motion. The first hint at the existence of cells that respond selectively to differential motion was given by Jerome Lettvin and his colleagues in famous work, part of which was published under the flippant title "What the Frog's Eye Tells the Frog's Brain" (Lettvin et al., 1959; Maturana et al., 1960)—work that inscribed the concept of "bug detectors" in our collective unconscious. The early findings and the discourse that went

Two Moving Objects against a Moving Background

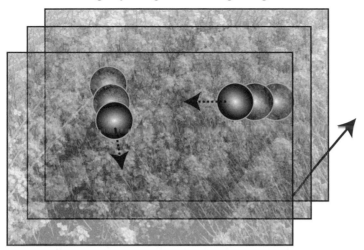

Recording from Four Retinal Ganglion Cells

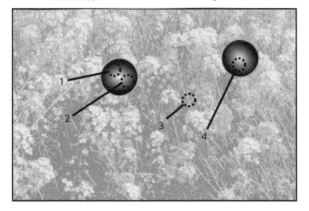

Spike Trains of the Four Retinal Ganglion Cells

Figure 3.4
Segregation of object and background motion in the retina (modeled after Ölveczky, Baccus, & Meister, 2003). Two balls (globes, planets) are flying in different directions against a drifting (or jittery) background (the flower field). We consider the activity of four retinal ganglion cells with different receptive fields, labeled 1 to 4 in the middle panel ("Recording from Four Retinal Ganglion Cells"). The lower panel shows spike trains for these four cells. Cells 1 and 2 have their receptive field in areas covered by the same object; both cells have a high firing rate with spike trains that are strongly correlated. Cell 3 has its receptive field somewhere in the background; it has a low firing rate. In the case of cell 4, the receptive field is covered by the alternative object. It has a high firing rate, but not strongly correlated with cells 1 and 2.

with them were frowned upon by later generations, who demanded better controls, more carefully collected data, and a more restrained language.

Contemporary work has vindicated at least the complexity of the computational processing suggested by Lettvin and colleagues. Some retinal ganglion cells do not fire in response to global motion (of the entire background) but show vigorous activity when their receptive field is stimulated by an object that moves in a different direction relative to the background. Presumably, these cells receive excitatory inputs similar to those of Y cells and inhibitory inputs from amacrine cells, activated by global motion. If the excitatory inputs synchronize with the inhibitory ones, the retinal ganglion cells remain silent. If the inputs are asynchronous, there must be differential motion; the retinal ganglion cells fire (Baccus et al., 2008; Ölveczky, Baccus, & Meister, 2003). This kind of neural signal provides retinal coordinates of a local change and so may well play a crucial role in our ability to spot a sudden appearance (or disappearance) in plain view. It can support change vision; it can direct our gaze. In this way, the retina is able to control its own movement. And so the very least we can conclude already is that the retina manages some mighty computation.

Functional Promiscuity

Circuits in the retina support a multiplicity of computations. Individual amacrine cells contribute to more than a hundred independent microcircuits (Grimes et al., 2010)—we could call it a type of "functional promiscuity." The organization of microcircuits promotes highly specific types of computation. The math is in the architecture. A good example is the asymmetrical inhibition from so-called starburst amacrine cells, which supports selectivity to particular motion directions in retinal ganglion cells (Briggman, Helmstaedter, & Denk, 2011; Euler, Detwiler, & Denk, 2002; Fried, Münch, & Werblin, 2002). This asymmetric inhibition emerges rapidly in early postnatal development, following an initial stage in which random inhibitory connections are established (Yonehara et al., 2011). The development occurs even under conditions in which retinal activity is blocked (Wei et al., 2011), suggesting an autonomous developmental program, unlike the experience-dependent development of direction selectivity in the visual cortex (Li et al., 2008).

Zooming out, I note that this research highlights the autonomy, complexity, and sophistication of the eye as a subsystem of the visual system. It also reinforces the validity of converging operations in biology and engineering to study the eye as a biological mind-machine (thus in the same movement vindicating Darwin's optimism). We live in a particularly exciting time with plenty of new discoveries that gradually demystify the eye as an organ of perfection. The lesser need for divine intervention does not have to imply a descent into secular depression. We can continue wondering about, and being positively excited by, the magnificent intricacy of the eye. Some of the computations performed by the retina look particularly impressive, well beyond mere "sensation" of physical information. Let us zoom in on two of these—two retinal types of computation that I would naturally have thought to be instances of cognition. Figure 3.5 shows the detection of approaching motion; figure 3.6 presents a neural response that implies pattern recognition.

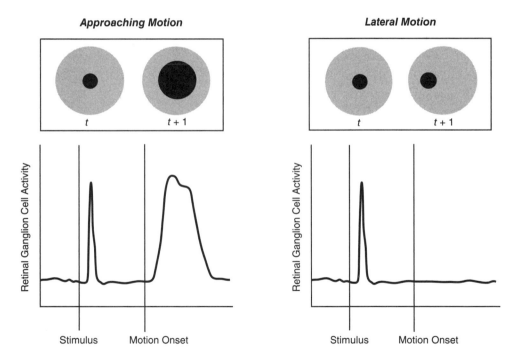

Figure 3.5
Retinal ganglion activity to approaching motion (abstracting the data of Münch et al., 2009). The left panels present data relating to approaching motion, with an object progressively covering larger areas of the visual field. The right panels show data relating to lateral motion, with an object moving from one side to the other without changing in size. The retinal ganglion cell activity is presented with respect to two important events: the first appearance of the object and the moment when the object starts moving (as always, vertical axis: activity level; horizontal axis: time). The first appearance of the object produces strong transient activation. The motion onset leads to a longer-lasting response in the case of approaching motion but no response in the case of lateral motion.

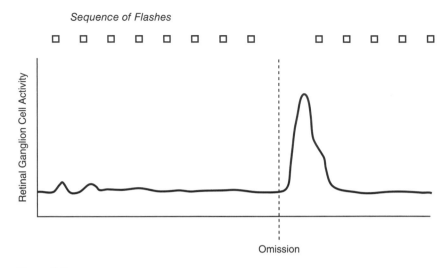

Sequence of Flashes

Omission

Figure 3.6
A retinal mechanism of expectation (zooming in on the conclusions by Schwartz et al., 2007). A sequence of very brief flashes (forty milliseconds each) is presented to the retina (*only* the retina—a bit of tissue is "isolated"; that means cut out and kept working in a dish). The retina can be from either a larval tiger salamander or a mouse; the two species produce similar data. Some ganglion cells show evidence that the retina supports prediction. When a flash is omitted from a regular series, the critical (non)event elicits a vigorous burst of activity.

Approaching motion is arguably one of the most behaviorally relevant stimuli for any creature. Things that come nearer should be assessed with special urgency for the animal to be able to respond efficiently, to make an escape, to engage in confrontation, or otherwise to try and benefit from the impending encounter. An approaching object casts an ever greater shadow (or set of reflections) on the retina of the observer. Münch and colleagues (2009; the paper after which I modeled figure 3.5) showed in mice that retinal ganglion cells with an OFF-type response fire for an expanding dark spot but not for lateral motion. Such retinal ganglion cells essentially offer the rest of the brain already a highly interpreted reading of the visual scene, indicating in retinal coordinates the presence of something on course to make contact with the observer— a very meaningful alert.

This ability to detect approaching motion adds to the family of different types of motion processing already known to exist in the retina. All of these readings concern the same visual scene, analyzed from a specific computational angle. The readings are not redundant and not merely reductionist either. The retina engages in something that again makes me think of the perhaps slightly nerdy notion of "functional promiscuity" (apparently a fairly common expression in molecular biology). Vision does not involve a one-track mind painting a detailed, comprehensive internal representation but a variety of processes and mechanisms that converge, diverge, partially overlap, and generally serve a number of goals. The multiple visual signals are relatively open-ended, shaped to be maximally useful—for the important tasks first, but not only. The signals are sent in parallel to the brain where they afford yet other, more complex forms of information processing, including sensorimotor mechanisms such as reorienting the gaze toward an approaching object.

My favorite retinal computation is anticipation on the basis of pattern recognition (see figure 3.6; after Schwartz et al., 2007). "Anticipation," "pattern recognition"—do my words sound too contentious? What would be the appropriate vocabulary? Retinal ganglion cells respond with a burst of spikes to the omission of a flash in a regular sequence. The response to omission implies that there was some kind of prediction, however rudimentary. Given a periodic stimulus, somehow the retina manages to factor in the oscillation. When the periodicity breaks down, its internal trace continues and creates a mismatch with photoreceptor input. Superficially, such neural mechanisms resemble cortical processes in response to infrequent visual targets embedded in a sequence of distractors; say, the P300 component in brain waves recorded from the scalp (e.g., Courchesne, Hillyard, & Galambos, 1975). Speaking with Marr, we can note at the computational level, or at the surface, that the cortex and the retina perform the same pattern analysis; beneath the surface, at the level of material implementation, we can suspect that the algorithms are different.

Does the retina really anticipate visual information on the basis of pattern recognition? If the eye is part of the visual system and therefore part of the mind, does this mean that our anticipation is based on the retina? It does. My language is certainly not very adventurous as compared to, say, that of Rizzini and colleagues (2011), who talk (almost polemically) about plants' perceiving and responding to ultraviolet-B to optimize their growth and survival (in a paper published on the first of April, but some of the same authors have used similar language on other days). Adventures in language serve their purpose. Yet I do wish to be as precise as I can with words; the adventures should be meaningful, not a matter of cheap tricks. "Our anticipation *is based on* the retina," I claim. This is not the same as saying that, when a predicted flash fails to materialize, our visual experience of a gap in the pattern *exists in* the retina.

The retinal computation is not a sufficient condition for our visual experience. It might not even be a necessary condition for it, given that similar computations appear to be computed in the cortex. However, the retinal computation *can* be part of our visual experience—neither necessary nor sufficient, but useful, a building block, a candidate cogenerator of our visual experience of "something missing."

Retina 2.2

The retina, in and of itself, does not harbor experience. The retinal ganglion cells that worked on the basis of pattern prediction (Schwartz et al., 2007; figure 3.6) did so in patches of "isolated retina," well and truly out of the head and completely unconscious. Still, I think the retina deserves to be regarded as a little mind-machine of its own, part of the bigger mind-machine that gives us—that *constitutes*—our mind. The beginnings of the miracle of mind from matter, of visual thought from biological tissue, happen already in the retina. The mind, however, does not equal experience. Not all of cognition is conscious. If the eye is a subsystem of the visual system, which in turn is a subsystem of the mind, this does not say anything yet about consciousness. Of course, to work toward a complete understanding of vision, we will have to incorporate consciousness, not reluctantly or as an awkward add-on, but as the beginning and end of what makes vision meaningful to us: access to real-world objects and events in a way that feels intense and personal, and enables us to do things as we wish. For those of you who are particularly sensitive about the notion of free will, I add: regardless of whether such wishes actually cause the doing.

Consciousness must get its rightful place. In this section, I will make a few preliminary remarks while we are on the topic of the mighty and autonomous retina. I have dubbed this section "Retina 2.2" in homage of *Galatea 2.2*, the unforgettable novel by Richard Powers (1995) about a neural network come to life (or rather a neural network come to *consciousness*, or to *a mind of its own*). The fictional network invented by Powers started by being smart and encyclopedic, only to become achingly aware of not being embodied as a human. In a roundabout way, the novel raises an issue that all too often remains hidden in works on or from the philosophy of mind, particularly the "embodied mind," sometimes also called "embodied cognition" or "situated cognition." In *Galatea 2.2*, Powers explores the being of a mind without a body (or I should say more precisely, without a biological body). To really be a mind like ours, does the neural network need a limited (individual) perspective? Say that all the intellectual bits can be programmed, all the smarts. Does such a supersized mind need some constraints for experience to be possible — constraints that are, in a sense, debilitating?

Neither the fictional character (Richard Powers) nor the author (another Richard Powers) offers any easy answer. Superior novels never do. But the questions resonate — have been resonating for centuries, ever since Descartes reinvented the philosophy of mind with "Cogito ergo sum." Yet the questions resonate slightly differently in *Galatea 2.2*. We are coming to an age in which artificial intelligence is less fanciful, less exotic. For an interesting case in point, see Markram, 2006, and note the discrepancy between the popularizing rhetoric behind the Blue Brain Project and the prosaic nature of the decent research papers that it produces. Philosophers have started contemplating the implications of the various types of computation that take place out of our heads but seem to form an integral part of our thinking (Clark, 1997, 2003, 2008; Noë, 2004, 2009). What *are* the boundaries of the mind? With Andy Clark in *Supersizing the Mind* (2008, p. 138),

[W]here ongoing human activity is concerned, there are usually *many* boundaries in play, *many different kinds* of capacity and resource in action, and a complex and somewhat anarchic flux of recruitment, retrieval, and processing defined across these shifting, heterogeneous, multifaceted wholes.

The boundaries of our minds are active, Clark argues. Philosophers and scientists disagree vehemently about where the boundaries are. When we use a computer program to analyze a data set and receive a diagnostic, should we think of the program as an epistemic tool or as a part of our extended mind? If it plays a causal role in our train of thought, if it fills a cognitive gap in our thinking, does it mean that the computer program is thinking for us or that it performs a cognitive function? Is there a difference? What *is* the difference?

They are certainly tricky, perhaps even uncomfortable questions. If we do not have any answers, at least the questions challenge us to further thought and experimentation. Let us say we *can* extend our minds artificially, not simply by using epistemic tools but by incorporating them as integral subsystems of the cognitive system that makes the mind. Is this a crazy idea? Crazy ideas may help us stretch our imagination. We do not have to marry bizarre or outlandish theories to benefit from them. "We should not feel locked into some pale zero-sum game. As philosophers and as cognitive scientists, we can and should practice the art of flipping among these different perspectives, treating each as a lens apt to draw attention to certain features, regularities, and contributions" (Clark, 2008, p. 139).

Would you consider a prosthetic limb to be a part of your body? What about a pacemaker? Say you suffer from a sleeping disorder, and some handy bioengineer invents a slow-wave oscillator for you. You get it implanted in your brain. Whenever you need some sleep, you press a button; the slow-wave oscillator orchestrates your brain's sleep cycles. Is the oscillator part of your mind? Or another example, closer to current reality: What about a deep-brain stimulator to help you walk (say you have Parkinson's disease)? Is that stimulator, with its intracranial electrode that stimulates the subthalamic nucleus, part of your motor system? And therefore part of your mind?

At first I would be inclined to answer, "No." These things are tools, and we can simply keep calling them tools even if they are integrated in the body. But then I think about organs being transplanted or, better yet, neural grafting. Say I have Parkinson's disease twenty years from now; I get stem cells (from an unidentified but human source) grafted into my poor striatum; the stem cells become functional dopamine neurons (a feat already realized in rats; Kim et al., 2002). My new neurons lift me out of my depression and help me control my motor actions. Are they part of my brain, my mind?

Of course they are. But then if I accept another person's stem cells to extend my mind, does this not put me on a slippery slope to all kinds of mind extensions? What if the stem cells are from a monkey or a pig? And if I allow nonhuman stem cells to extend my mind, then why not that deep brain stimulator? Why would an artificial retina (Retina 2.2) be any less a part of my mind than a real retina if it somehow managed to send signals about light patterns into my optic tract? The idea of such things extending the mind does not necessarily sound altogether unreasonable to me. However, it could lead to new problems. If the mind can be supersized by incorporating all kinds of devices, programs, and tools, does this not mean that the mind is being extended without obvious boundaries, perhaps all the way to infinity (or certain kinds of infinity)? Is this infinitely extendable mind no longer bound to anything material?

Clark never speaks about supersizing the body in parallel with the mind. I am not sure whether this is a deliberate tactic to avoid difficult questions or an innocent blind spot in the theory. I see two possibilities, both of which are troublesome. Option 1: The body should be supersized along with the mind. In this case the body is in danger of being unlimited, unsituated, and disembodied—no longer properly speaking *a body*. Instead of denying the existence of consciousness, might a new breed of skeptics start denying the existence of the body? Option 2: The mind and the body should be considered disentangled, uncorrelated, disconnected—surely the clearest form of Cartesian dualism?

What is obvious from Clark's writings is that he thoroughly embraces the philosophy of the embodied mind. Is there a paradox in this fascination? Or does the paradox with unbound minds and all-important bodies reflect an inherent weakness in the theories about embodiment? Let me be up-front. I have never liked the term "embodiment." I have always been suspicious of any combination with the adjective "embodied." I disagree with the dynamics that it implies—the direction of evolution, with the putting of something into a body. It sounds as if there was something first (a mind) and that this "initial something" then materialized (was bound to a body). Immaterial and infinite minds find a temporary vehicle in the body—another form of Cartesian dualism?

Sometimes Clark does sound eerily similar to (or compatible with) Descartes. I mean this not as a disparagement. I believe there is still plenty to like about Descartes when we look beyond the obvious errors toward the nobility of thought, the clarity and elegance of writing. I reread *A Discourse on the Method* every so often to replenish my energies (just a couple of weeks ago I read it in a new translation by Ian Maclean; Descartes, 1637|2006). Reading the works of Clark (and those of Noë, for that matter) has the same effect on my energies. We are not finished with "Cogito ergo sum" or with cognition outside of our heads. There is something truly beyond the material about the Cogito (the thinking being), in the memes that continue to speak to us, via books and texts, across time and space. The Cogito might simply be the voice of the author, captured in text (like the sayings of Mr Cogito in the intriguing poems by Zbigniew Herbert, 2007). Somehow the extended mind connects to the Cogito. It will be worth exploring such ideas, the relation between memes and active thoughts in a human mind, or how memes become embodied (activated) in a living mind/body. Yet I do not think anyone really wants to revert to Cartesian dualism. In fact, Cartesian dualism is something like the stock accusation that we throw at each other to discredit theories we do not agree with. Here is a quote from Noë (2004, p. 215) scolding contemporary neuroscientists:

They treat the mind as standing to the body as a pilot does to his ship and they deceive themselves into thinking they've eliminated mystery because they use the word "mind" to refer to the brain. The brain, thought of in this way, is less material mind than spiritualized matter; instead of eliminating the mystery from the mental, they've simply concocted a mysterious account of the physical.

Embodied mind or spiritualized matter? Which is worse? Both concoct a mysterious account, with an abrupt add-on, from merely mind to embodied mind or from merely matter to thinking matter. The concocting of mysteries can equally be lamented, but I do think the contemporary neuroscientists have at least the direction right. From merely matter to thinking matter, that is how our minds evolved. That is what needs to be investigated. The other direction is for fairy tales and science-averse religions. It is not where philosophers want to be.

The biggest problem with the philosophy of embodied mind is that, despite the lip service, it does not give the body its due. It still sounds too much as if the body is merely there to serve the mind, to support it, to give it a home, a bed, a situation. It is no accident that philosophers like Noë and Clark are ready to drop the body at the first turn and think about the mind spreading out in the world. Such spreading involves memes and artifacts, *products* of the mind (and products *for* the mind). I believe we are still better off thinking with Spinoza that the mind and the body are one and the same thing, considered from different perspectives. The crux for neuroscience is to explain how the mind gradually increases in complexity, along with complexity in neural circuitry, all the way to a point where we can look back and note that somewhere between then and now we must have become conscious—even if we cannot draw an exact line between the conscious and the unconscious (for instance, because there is no straight line, but a complex set of active boundaries).

How, then, do I relate to my body? We need to acknowledge the full implications of the Copernican revolution that was set in motion by Darwin. The body does not revolve around the mind, even if that is what our phenomenology tells us. Neuroscience will make more progress by working from the hypothesis that it is really the other way round. The conscious mind (the Cogito, or the being that thinks it is an "I") is no more and no less than a subsystem of the mind. This subsystem may flatter itself into thinking that it owns the body ("I have a body"), but this is at best a very late hijacking in the evolution of human beings. It is also not correct to think that the conscious mind is the same as the body ("I am my body"). Indeed, I repeat, the conscious mind is only a *sub*system of the mind. So at best we can claim "I am a part of my body," or "My body has me."

In this view, the conscious mind evolved (at least in primates and perhaps in other mammals as well) to serve the mind/body in particular ways, performing fairly abstract and adaptive computational tasks such as flexible decision making, complex problem solving, and long-term planning. Language and identity formation probably enhanced these functions exponentially in humans, who began telling themselves stories about who they are and what they went through. The conscious mind, then, started out as a slave to the body, but at some point the power balance shifted, such that the subsystem thought of itself as "the Special One." This belief, in turn, would have easily seen itself reinforced since the subsystem did have some kind of access to the body's mechanisms of motor control: It could decide to go left or right, to eat a banana or save it for later. It actually became the boss, a very fine self-fulfilling prophecy.

Of course, it is not my intention here to compose a detailed theory about the evolution of consciousness. I only wanted to sketch a brief scenario that allows us to think about consciousness as a subsystem of the mind. This subsystem naturally emerged as a useful player for the mind/body as a whole. The conscious mind partially overlaps with other subsystems, one of which is the visual system. Some visual processes will also be conscious processes. We will need to consider the overlap, where and how it occurs. To understand vision, we must study all of the related subsystems and their interactions. These interactions determine the active boundaries of vision—boundaries like those between the conscious and the unconscious. In response to the philosophy of embodied mind, I argue that we have to concentrate on the actual mechanisms in the body to understand how vision works. The body is ultimately the best place to handle the parallax, the double perspective on cognition and neural circuitry, computational function and material implementation. Let us take the perspective of the body as thoroughly as we can.

Above all, this means we have to consider the body's limits. The limits are there; they determine what is possible and what is beneficial or harmful for the body. The body's limits also imply limits for the mind. To the extent that the mind can be supersized, the body will have to be supersized along with it. I will only consider mind extensions to be a sensible concept insofar as they can be connected with parallel body extensions. Otherwise I will prefer to call all kinds of epistemic tools simply "tools." I am very happy to accept that some cognitive functions happen outside our heads, in service of our heads. However, this gives us no urgent reason to consider them to be fully (and literally) incorporated in our minds. I will in most cases, though not always, resist such incorporation, not out of attachment to old ideas about the human body but because I prefer a minimalist stance, thinking it is good for the body to have limits (the limits actually give meaning). We do, however, have urgent reason to study how the various out-of-body mechanisms interact with our brains, or which kinds of neural processes they elicit. Indeed, the crux, as ever, is in the interaction.

The Orienting Response

Talking about the retina, the mind, and things outside the body, the clearest (most easily traceable) instance of interaction is that of gaze orientation to a salient stimulus. When retinal ganglion cells signal the presence of a moving object, the rest of the mind will urgently respond in various ways. The animal may freeze and orient its processing resources so as to acquire more information about the motion stimulus, about the potential threat or treat it implies. Such orienting mechanisms are likely to be hardwired and certainly appear to operate in a machine-like fashion. Theeuwes and colleagues (1999), for instance, showed that human observers often are unable to prevent making an eye movement to an abrupt visual onset even when they are instructed to ignore such onsets and look for a color singleton. This kind of involuntary response, in opposition to the observer's goals, must surely qualify as an "exogenous" mechanism, under stimulus control, determined by physical properties.

The Russian behaviorist Evgeny Nikolaevich Sokolov (1963; Sokolov et al., 2002) concentrated on the idea that orienting plays a crucial role in the development of conditioned reflexes. Sokolov, of course, was trained in the great Pavlovian tradition. Ivan Petrovich Pavlov himself had observed that his dogs tended to make eye movements and adjust their ears in response to cues that predicted the arrival of food. The dogs developed "conditioned reflexes" to these cues; they started salivating to the ring of the bell even before the desired beefsteak dropped in the bowl. But did the eye movements and ear adjustments contribute to the making of connections? Sokolov was convinced that they did, and he conceptualized arguably the first truly sensorimotor theory of perception.

Sokolov (1963) saw the orienting as a reflex that heightened the subject's sensitivity to the stimulus. Curiously, Sokolov's language in this respect was more precise, and more compatible with mathematical modeling, than Posner's (1980) work that borrowed the concept of orienting for application in cognitive psychology. When Posner introduced his immensely influential location-cueing paradigm, he spoke of the "orienting of attention" in a way that allowed him to distinguish overt attention (accompanied by behaviors such as eye movements) from covert attention (hidden mechanisms of information processing, independent of behavior). Unfortunately, and unnecessarily, in the same movement he blurred the distinction between bias and sensitivity (Downing, 1988; Lauwereyns, 2010). We can and should appreciate mechanisms of sensitivity as different from those of bias.

In Sokolov's posthumous work of 2002, through the mediation of coauthors interested in neurophysiology, the orienting *reflex* morphed into the (more agreeable) orienting *response*, a component of exploratory behavior. Here, the interaction is brought into full view. The orienting response begins under exogenous control with autonomous processes in the retina that signal the presence of something that should be investigated. We might say that the signal evokes a bias for oculomotor control, or an increased likelihood of an eye movement targeted at the retinotopic coordinates of the new stimulus. This gaze bias to new information can itself be seen as an instance of the more general bias toward meaning and intentionality (or "aboutness" as Dennett, 1987, 1991, sometimes calls it).

The mind is anatomized to expect that the new information could be meaningful in some ways, that it could add something critical, or at least nonredundant, to knowledge of what is going on at the moment. New information warrants inspection exactly because it *could* be relevant. The economics of the situation are probably such that it is wise to check the new information, just in case it does turn out to carry an important meaning. Indeed, in most cases, the information processing itself is not very costly—nothing very valuable will be lost by the act of checking the new stimulus apart from a bit of time and a bit of energy. Instead, ignoring important information could be extremely risky, in some cases even life threatening, say, when the presence of a predator goes unnoticed.

If the gaze actually fixates the new stimulus, the foveal processing provides the observer with more detailed visual information. Thus the orienting produces a clearer, sharper understanding of the stimulus. The observer's sensitivity to the stimulus increases. The interaction that constitutes the orienting response, then, involves not only an interlocked series of sensory and motor events but also a dialectics of bias and sensitivity. In a way, this interaction implies autonomous control by the eye: The retina feeds the brain with information that actually induces the higher-order control that produces shifts of gaze, which make the retina move. It is an indirect form of feedback that helps shape the action in perception.

The orienting response does not work only for abrupt visual onsets. Figure 3.7 presents data from my own laboratory (Weaver & Lauwereyns, 2011) about gaze control in a change detection task using displays with four different types of visual objects (faces, clothes, appliances, and musical instruments). Subjects tend to shift their gaze faster to faces than

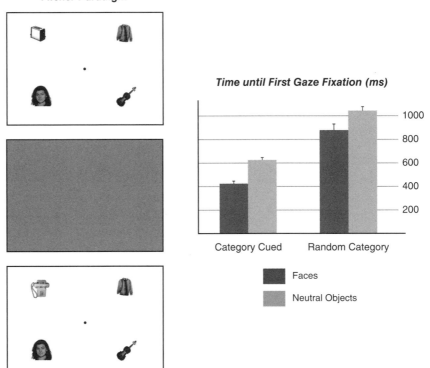

Figure 3.7
The orienting response to faces (reported in a different format in Weaver & Lauwereyns, 2011). The three panels on the left show screenshots of a change detection task (a flicker paradigm, in which images alternate with a blank gray screen). Observers are asked to detect changes to any of the four objects in the display (always from the same four categories: faces, appliances, clothes, and musical instruments). There is a fifty percent chance of a change in the display (in the example here, there is one, swapping the toaster for the phone). Sometimes a label at the start of the trial tells the observer which category to concentrate on (this is the "Category Cued" condition, as opposed to the "Random Category"). The data on the right show the time until the observer's gaze fixates the changing object in trials with a change (the error bars represent standard errors of the means). The eyes always go faster to faces.

to other visual objects. The fact that faces enjoy a privileged status as visual objects of interest was of course no news (e.g., Ro, Russell, & Lavie, 2001). Our study showed that this privileged status effectively influences the processes of oculomotor *capture*, that is, the actual orienting of the gaze toward the face (not merely oculomotor hold, or the fixation duration once an object happens to be visited by the gaze). Even when subjects know beforehand which kind of object to look for, they move their eyes as much as two hundred milliseconds faster to faces than to the other types of visual object. Somehow our eyes are, literally, drawn to faces.

Such gaze bias toward faces is not likely to work on the basis of retinal processing alone. The average initiation time of eye movements to faces in the fastest condition (around four hundred milliseconds) was roughly twice as long as that to abrupt visual onsets in the study by Theeuwes et al. (1999; around two hundred milliseconds). It is safe to say that in the orienting to faces we can expect a role for cortical processing, particularly in the fusiform face area (Kanwisher, McDermott, & Chun, 1997). Quite possibly, this processing occurs autonomously. The mere appearance of a face in our visual field might be sufficient to prompt its own analysis (Lavie, Ro, & Russell, 2003). More generally, it will always be an open, empirical question which kinds of stimuli elicit an orienting response under what circumstances for which observers.

Some stimuli, like faces, will naturally have priority for most humans because they provide important social information (Kanwisher & Yovel, 2009). Primates, including humans, may have evolved a processing module that prepares them for fear of snakes—something like a potential instinct that is activated or suppressed as a function of experience early in life (Öhman & Mineka, 2001). The orienting response, I propose, is biased toward meaning—toward things that tend to matter for the observer. The mind is programmed to be interested in certain kinds of information. Some of the programming code may be installed without any need for experience (as was argued by Wei et al., 2011, for the direction selectivity in motion processing by retinal ganglion cells). Other code (I would venture to say *most* of it) depends on the mutual interaction between genes and context, with the limits of our bodies influencing those of our worlds, and vice versa.

On the Shaping of Reception

Biases such as those for face or snake processing involve dedicated neural circuitry able to detect and monitor the prized types of stimuli with little effort and great speed. Expertise and training have a huge impact on such mechanisms of specialization. Though we have good reasons to think that the priorities of faces and snakes exist from the outset as potentialities in our DNA (with the role of context and learning merely that of activating a preprogrammed module), other biases are more structurally dependent on experience. Nobody is born into the world with a prepared module for recognizing *Pokémon* characters ("Pocket Monsters," Japanese anime) or Japanese rhinoceros beetles (my five-year-old son in both cases being the exception that proves the rule).

We become experts in such intensely personal or idiosyncratic domains of knowledge by internalizing the relevant structural descriptions—a form of learning that might (or might not) include an initial stage of explicit (language-mediated) instruction but eventually surely will turn implicit. Indeed, expertise can often be characterized as a mode of operation that allows us to relegate certain components of task performance outside consciousness, thus freeing up thinking space for other levels of thought (Berry, 1987; Berry & Broadbent, 1984; Hart, 1986; Lauwereyns & d'Ydewalle, 1996). My son does not need laborious conscious analysis to categorize his different rhinoceros beetles; his thoughts go immediately to predicting which beetle is more likely to push the other off the rock in a little sumo contest (there is no end to the creativity of the Japanese entertainment industry).

Interestingly, Gauthier and colleagues (2000) showed that such idiosyncratic expertise in recognizing visual objects (their subjects included bird-watchers and car fanatics) produces neural activity in the fusiform face area. This is not to say that the activity *is the same as* that for faces. Rather, some of the neural circuitry useful for face processing may also come in handy for other types of highly skillful object recognition—it would be another case of functional promiscuity. Does this sound a little contradictory? Can neural specialization and functional promiscuity go hand in hand? They can. The specialization refers to the entire neural circuitry involved in a particular type of recognition. The functional promiscuity happens at the level of single neurons that work for multiple independent circuits. The data of Gauthier et al. suggest that some neural activity in service of face recognition also works for highly skillful bird recognition. My preferred hypothesis would be that different circuits within the fusiform face area support the routine combination of visual elements—something like a fixed visual integration to complete an expected pattern (two eyes above a nose above a mouth in the case of a face, or a head, a chest, wings, and claws in the case of a bird), thereby making the visual experience more holistic.

The ability to detect and monitor the prized types of stimuli with little effort and great speed, however, comes at a cost. The biases allow us to work with minimal information by working from assumptions and expectations. The shortcuts come at the expense of occasional false alarms when we too easily take things to be in fact as we thought they would be all along. The biases prompt us to draw conclusions that can turn out to be premature. In *The Anatomy of Bias* (Lauwereyns, 2010, pp. 105–116) I discuss the mechanisms that underlie learning-induced specialization in some detail. The main point for present purposes is that, at a descriptive level, we can note that neurons in visual cortex become *tuned* to specific information. It is a form of cortical plasticity that creates a structural bias in information processing.

The tuning is akin to the notion of receptive field (see chapter 2) or actually extends this notion toward a variety of properties beyond the retinal coordinates of visual information. The reception can be specific for any combination of spatial position, line orientation, task context, and so on. It is now well established that neurons in the primary visual cortex of adult monkeys adapt in highly specific ways to training and task contexts (Crist et al., 1997; Gilbert, Sigman, & Crist, 2001; Schoups et al., 2001). Often this involves a combination of sharpening and softening, of strengthening and weakening. Neurons that used to respond to specific stimulus features do so even more vigorously and specifically when these features become more valuable or behaviorally relevant, say, predicting a reward or indicating the imminent danger of an unpleasant event. Conversely, other neurons may show a slight shift in their firing pattern, being activated more easily by stimulus features that in the present context are particularly relevant.

In Neuroscience English, the slope of the tuning curve increases for neurons that code task-relevant features. For neurons originally tuned to other features, the tuning curve may become flatter, start showing a second peak, or generally be bent out of shape a little bit, depending on the similarity between the originally preferred feature and the now-relevant feature—the greater the similarity, the larger the shift in the tuning curve; if the features are dissimilar enough, the tuning curve may remain entirely unaffected.

Back to Plain English: The plasticity involves rewiring. New synapses grow such that progressively more neural tissue responds to information that holds special value for the observer. Ecological validity, of course, gets a say in the matter. The relevant features literally get more weight; more neurons are ready and waiting to fire for them. The biases are inscribed in the anatomy. They become, properly speaking, *structural*.

This also means that the biases operate implicitly and autonomously. With built-in biases, the processing is done before consciousness gets a chance to kick in. However, this does not prevent consciousness from being able to play a part in the follow-up. As with the autonomous retinal mechanisms that call an eye movement to an abrupt visual onset or some kind of motion, we are likely to find the highly specialized (learning-dependent) cortical mechanisms elicit orienting responses to gather more information.

The implicit biases for important information serve to alert us quickly to the possibility of something relevant. This allows us to shift our gaze to the item in question. We can then scrutinize it at length and construct as detailed a visual description as we like or as we need. This conscious processing, facilitated by the gaze, will improve the quality of the signal reception. In this way, we get the best of both worlds, both bias and sensitivity: The implicit biases give us speed and minimalism; the conscious follow-up increases our sensitivity and allows us to confirm or disconfirm the first thoughts and initial hunches. This dialectic sets us on our way to seeing and grasping things with maximum efficiency.

Lightfall, then, is couched with reasons, to more or less quote from a poem by Hans Faverey (1994|2004, p. 56; see below). The observer's thoughts and associations (cognitive biases) run wild at a peripheral glance of a knife (perhaps "that hungry kitchen knife" from *Song of Joy*, written by Nick Cave, on the 1996 album *Murder Ballads* by Nick Cave and the Bad Seeds). But then consciousness focuses the gaze on the actual object, the source of the cognitive noise, and sees it for the mere thing it is, "reduced in view of itself."

Lightfall:
couched with reasons,
the standstill opens
of something else than

housed in this blade, glinting

as it is, not yet tempted

and seduced by blood,
as if it were all a vision
already unsure of itself,
reduced in view of itself
to its source.

Move that barn a little to the left
if you would

and that memory of a barn
a little to the right

until they coincide.
That's good.

This tiny poem, entitled "Move," comes from Michael Palmer's collection *Thread* (2011, p. 32). The quiet and effective humor derives in surrealist tradition from the implication of two absurdities, both of which extend our good honest intuitions beyond the boundaries of (human) nature: the idea that vision would be a form of grasping, and the idea that memory has access to detailed representations of the past. Recognition, says the joke, would be like moving two pictures, the old and the new, until they overlap perfectly. We imagine Magritte's little helpers, men in gray suits wearing bowler hats, moving the current landscape and the one in memory. We smile, we understand the absurdity right away, the humor is unmistakable, but where does the joke really begin and where does it end? Can we actually specify the boundaries that the poem obviously crosses?

As is typical of Michael Palmer's poetry, and more generally of all good poetry, there is much more to it than what dominates in the first reading. Here is not the place to talk about the subtle music of the poem (but let me insert a few sneaky pointers parenthetically: the hidden rhyme, *would* and *good*, that wraps around the more salient assonance, *right* and *coincide*; the alternation with two sets of repeated but varying structures, one itself based on alternation, *a little to the left* and *a little to the right*, and one based on recursion, *that barn* and *that memory of a barn*; all set in a plausible, and pleasing, rhythm for thought). I could say a couple of

things about that barn, and about the situation of the poem in the collection, but I should probably come to the point as soon as possible.

The goal here, in chapter 4, is to rethink the bidirectional moving in
perception, the spatial translation from past to present and from present
to past. Presented in a surrealist light, the absurdity of this idea strikes
us. However, thinking about our biases for meaning, and how "lightfall"
(speaking with Faverey) is "couched with reasons," we must come to
terms with the relativity of what we see, the inherent self-relatedness. We
must account for the manipulative nature of vision, a grasping that shapes
the graspable before it is grasped. Bidirectional movement will turn out
to be very real indeed, the stuff of science as well as poetry.

The Poetics of Space

Can we find a common ground in the study of vision? Is there a minimum,
a basis, to which we all agree, regardless of our backgrounds, practical
insights, theoretical leanings, and intuitions, however deep or shallow?
Vision has something to do with light, the processing of light. This processing is about gathering information. Thus, I venture my least controversial statement about vision—*it lets us know about things.* It performs
a function in the service of cognition. Sure, we will quickly get into
trouble with definitions and boundaries. Is vision an aspect of cognition
or rather a faculty independent of, but cooperating with, cognition? In
chapter 3 I have argued for vision as an aspect of cognition. However,
before digging into our (various) areas of disagreement, let us dwell a
little while longer on our universal understanding of vision as a way of
grasping the visual presence of objects and events.

The grasping should naturally be thought of as a figure of speech, a
metaphor. But given that we happen to be dwelling in a precious zone
of agreement, would it be worth our while to explore this peculiar word,
"grasping?"—how it resonates with literal meanings, with all kinds of
manual gestures and manipulation. We can always disagree later, but in
the meantime why not try and stretch our imagination, following Michael
Palmer's lead? What if we see the grasping not merely as a cognitive
process of passively receiving information but more radically as a physical act, a material form of making contact with *res extensa*? This could
be less silly than it sounds at first.

In one sense at least, we find that vision and actual grasping—manual
grasping—are tightly coupled. In a task in which subjects had to grasp a
bar and move it to press a switch, Johansson and colleagues (2001) found

the gaze leading hand movements. The gaze naturally focused on places where critical task events were about to occur. The gaze contributed to manual motor planning by indexing key target positions and by monitoring how well the hands were moving on with their task. In high-acuity tasks such as threading a needle we may even make strategic microsaccades to monitor our task performance (Ko, Poletti, & Rucci, 2010). The gaze sets the goal; it does not focus on the hand but on what the hand has to achieve. The visual input via the gaze is converted to manual action in a way that allows us to state, exactly, that the gaze initiates the grasping. It would be a trivial step for engineers to close the motor loop mechanically with the gaze as a physical control device for action in the world.

In another sense, we also find visual processing in the brain focused on manual grasping with specific coding of visual input within reach (e.g., Brozzoli et al., 2011; Duhamel, Colby, & Goldberg, 1998; Graziano, Yap, & Gross, 1994). We mark out what is in our zone. However, the notion of vision as literal grasping may go still further to the core of what things are. Perhaps vision does not simply access predefined physical objects and events. The most radical and intriguing idea would be that vision in a very proactive sense defines and delineates objects and events. This idea calls into question what *objects* are, or which physical boundaries serve to segregate things as units for vision. It will be a question that runs as an undercurrent throughout this entire chapter. Could it be that *we* pick those physical boundaries? Objects may only become objects because we decide to see them as units. Physically speaking, there may not always be obvious boundaries that are given to us, or impose themselves on us, as the unequivocal borders of objects. Certainly at the microscopic level, any composite of materials that we think of as an object (a car, a mountain, a flower, a comb, a river, a face, a bird) may not sharply or precisely be separable from its surroundings.

When we start looking for exact definitions, we may find the task surprisingly hard. We may in this or that case have few clear-cut rules for deciding what is, and what is not, part of a particular object. Some combinations that we consider to be objects are physically more heterogeneous and discontinuous than others that we do not see as objects. In practice we usually do not care about such boundaries and only call them into question when there is particular need for precision. Instead, we let our gaze roam, we fixate points, and the points we fixate serve as the indices of objects. The indices effectively become our practical handle on the visual definition of objects.

This would be vision's most active, most literal form of grasping: We index objects by gazing at them. We *create* the objects by indexing them with our gaze. That is, objects would come into existence only because we treat them as visible things, as "graspable" units in vision. Of course, by this I do not mean that vision literally bends, plies, or otherwise sculptures wood, iron, or any kind of meat in any fancy form or shape we like. Vision does not physically change the materials. The point is that objects are units of thought. Their definition speaks virtually, as a cognitive collection of features. It is the unit of thought which can then be translated to, or be found to correspond with, a certain physical mass, a given composite of physical materials. Our concept of a mountain helps us define where the foot begins. Our ideas allow us to impose boundaries on the physical.

Does vision really *create* objects? It sounds like a poetic function, to borrow a phrase from Roman Jakobson (1960)—a self-reflective function, one that gives what it takes, focused on the very thing that it makes. This harks back to our notes in chapter 1 on perception for perception as a process not unlike that of art for the sake of art. Etymologically, we derive "poetics" from the Greek *poiein* ("to make"). With this in mind, I read Gaston Bachelard's *The Poetics of Space* (1958|1994) and find myself convinced that there is indeed a certain depth to the idea of multiple connections between vision, our making, and the structure of the world. "At the level of the poetic image, the duality of subject and object is iridescent, shimmering, unceasingly active in its inversions," writes Bachelard (p. xix). The poetics of space involves bidirectional influences; we create the objects, and the objects that we create in turn shape our being as subjects. But how does this actually work?

In figure 4.1, looking back and forth between the two shots of Minoru Tsukada walking toward me in a New Zealand landscape, I cannot help but be struck by how much of my visual understanding relies on "extravisual" information, on things that I remember, infer, imagine, and read into the scene. The two shots, and the obvious spatiotemporal relations between them, make me realize with extra vigor that I do not perceive space or time as such. Space and time, we know well enough, are constructs of infinity. I do not *see* them. I see bodies, substances, and notice differences. Different things occur at the same location at different times (in another set of two shots I see a neutral face and, after the joke, a smiley face). Different things occur at the same time at different locations (in one and the same shot I see here a tree, there a dog about to pee). Ultimately my grasping of the spatial and temporal metrics of these

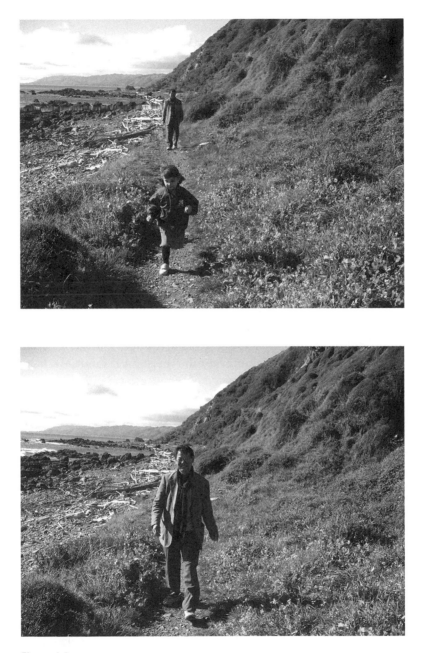

Figure 4.1
The extrapolation of spatiotemporal dynamics. These two photos were taken in the space of a few seconds at Pukerua Bay, New Zealand, on May 6, 2006. Minoru Tsukada is seen leisurely following a pigtailed creature that wishes not to be photographed. The landscape stays more or less constant. We can easily imagine the flow of events between the two static images, Minoru Tsukada steadily approaching while the little white rabbit hops out of sight. Does our imagination poeticize space? Does it contribute to active perception?

differences is anchored on the bodies and substances that I see. Thus, I read time and space. "It makes sense," insists Bachelard (1958|1994, p. 14), "to say that we 'write a room,' 'read a room,' or 'read a house.' " The notion is echoed, in a more aggressive tone, by Gibson (1979|1986, p. 3):

> I am also asking the reader to suppose that the concept of space has nothing to do with perception. (...) The doctrine that we could not perceive the world around us unless we already had the concept of space is nonsense. It is quite the other way around: We could not conceive of empty space unless we could see the ground under our feet and the sky above. Space is a myth, a ghost, a fiction for geometers.

The doctrine that Gibson refers to is, of course, that of the a priori pure forms according to Immanuel Kant (1781|2007)—a doctrine that has received explicit support in neuroscience from O'Keefe and Nadel's classic work on the hippocampal cognitive map (1978), with the bold suggestion that this map reflects an innate system that serves as a scaffold for representing experience about the environment (see Langston et al., 2011, and Wills et al., 2011, for recent evidence from rat pups upon their very first explorations). Does such an innate tendency to map the world indeed imply the kind of synthetic a priori knowledge Kant was after? My hunch is not, but in truth the question is moot. We will never know what Kant would have made of the recent rat pup data, nor do we know enough about hippocampal spatial representation to even make the question intelligible to the greatest Kant scholar alive, whoever that may be.

Researchers of hippocampus and related neural structures easily speak of "place cells," "direction cells," and "grid cells" as if these cells contribute to a so-called allocentric map of the environment, that is, a map anchored on external information (landmarks or sensory cues about where things are). The neurons, however, usually appear to code something about the animal relative to the environment and its sensory cues: either the place the animal visits (as in the case of hippocampal "place cells" and, in a more convoluted way, also in the case of entorhinal "grid cells") or the head direction of the animal relative to the environment (as in the case of subiculum "direction cells"). A true allocentric map would show activation for events somewhere in the world regardless of what kind of event it is or who takes part in it. The vast majority of research on place cells, direction cells, and grid cells works on the basis of the animal's own interaction with the world. Thus we cannot quite exclude the possibility that the neural activity really reflects the kind of experiential construction of space that Bachelard and Gibson had in mind. Even the first spike of a place cell in a particular place may actually be composing the opening line of verse in the poetics of space.

Perhaps the debate of pure forms versus construction, Kant versus poetics, can only lead us astray. Of course experience matters in vision. And naturally the biological hardware that gives us vision is a product of genetics. We can, and we do, think of pure forms. We certainly have the ability to entertain the supreme fiction of geometers, the infinities of time and space. As always, the more interesting questions in vision will focus on the interaction. How do our ideas and experiences emerge from the way we, human animals, live in the world? This question is as valid for Gaston Bachelard as it is for John O'Keefe—as it is for anyone interested in perception.

One important corollary of the interaction, with respect to the poetics of space, is that vision does not have the final say. Vision does not in and of itself establish the existence of what we take to be out there. Even if vision creates objects, even if we read and write space, the creations and our poetics in vision are bound by the world. Reality belongs to the world—only what is actually out there can validate our take on things. The poetics in vision works with, or toward, the world. The reading and writing of space aims to be truthful; the poetic function of vision has evolved to be extremely efficient in providing us with veridical information about things in the world—to the point that most of the time we can happily remain oblivious to the fact that what we see is the product of our making.

In the vast majority of cases, what we see is actually out there, but sometimes it really is not. We make mistakes. Occasionally we judge too fast, we have perceptual illusions, or we get confused. Our errors in vision tell us something about how the visual system works inside our heads—the biases and shortcuts, the weaknesses, the issues in our information processing. Even highly trained visual artists, working diligently, using whatever tools they have at their disposal, have been known to make conspicuously faulty readings of space—figure 4.2 shows a famous example from Caravaggio. Look at the right hand of the disciple with extended arms, and compare it to his left hand. The right hand, though a good deal farther from our vantage point, is actually painted slightly bigger than the left hand. The contemporary artist David Hockney (2001) attributed this curious lapse to clumsy reliance on lenses. Caravaggio would have traced details such as the hands with the help of lenses, but failed to take into account the implications of shifted perspective when moving the lens to focus on a different detail.

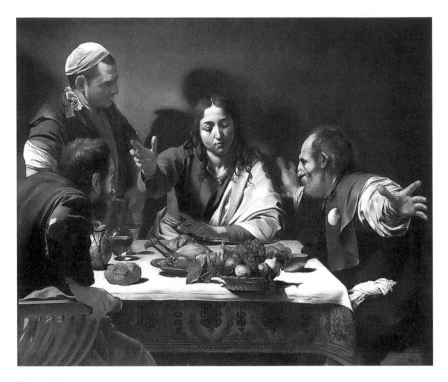

Figure 4.2
Supper in Emmaus, painted in 1601 by Michelangelo Merisi, better known as Caravaggio (collection of the National Gallery, London). The scene is based on a passage in the Gospel of Luke, 24: 30–31, in which the resurrected Jesus Christ is recognized by two of his disciples, one of which is identified as Cleopas: "And it came to pass, as he sat at meat with them, he took bread, and blessed it, and brake, and gave to them. And their eyes were opened, and they knew him; and he vanished out of their sight" (quoted from the King James version of the Bible, Anonymous, 1611|2004). Note the supersized right hand of the disciple on the right, with arms extended.

If Hockney is right, Caravaggio's mistake was that he relied too much on his tools and not enough on his eyes, assuming perhaps that the tools were less likely to make mistakes. Even if Hockney is wrong, and Caravaggio for some obscure reason intentionally enlarged the hand, it is still obviously a violation of perspective. Whichever way we look at this painting, no matter how we read and write its details, the supersized hand stands out as an anomaly, a problem, a scar, a rupture. Yet the painting still counts as a masterpiece (thinking *à la* Roland Barthes about photography, we might see the hand as the very *punctum* that makes the painting larger than life). Let us marvel at it, and appreciate how fiercely the poetics of space in vision is dedicated to the truth.

The Parallax View

Space may be a figment of the geometer's imagination, but the world definitely offers a very real dimension of depth with rather robust physical laws governing how light bounces off surfaces—extremely robust at the Newtonian level, which, to be sure, is the only one relevant for human vision, at least in terms of light stimulating the retina. The optics can be processed correctly or incorrectly; truths exist, the quality of representations can be rated "objectively," in reference to reality (the facts, the absolute ways of the world). Vision aims to harmonize with the optics and the spatial layout of bodies and substances it comprises. The poetic nature of this process—the reading and writing required to achieve the harmonization—dawns most clearly on us when we heed the fact that even slight shifts of perspective can have a noticeable impact on what we observe. Our perspective determines what we see.

Figure 4.3 shows how the point was already understood some four hundred years ago. Aguilonius (1613) described, and Rubens illustrated, the fact that even the two views of our own eyes are markedly different. Binocular disparity produces parallax when objects appear to shift position as seen with the left eye alone compared to the right eye alone. Occasionally an object may disappear from view entirely in one perspective, but not the other. The dramatic influence of perspective, down to the level of a single eye from the same observer, emphasizes once again that vision works with relative data—necessarily and fundamentally related to the position of the observer. This relativity condemns us to poetics, whether we like it or not. We have no choice but to read and write the visual world on the basis of our limited perspective, our intrinsically relative data. Yet vision aims to transcend our limits and make contact with truths about the world.

The easiest way to move beyond the limits of one perspective is to take a look at what can be seen with another. In a very basic way, the visual system achieves such transcendence by taking advantage of the fact that we have two eyes, two slightly different perspectives. Aguilonius (1613) was the first vision researcher to note that with two eyes we are better at reaching for objects—estimating depth—than with only one eye. On this point (as on several others) our man in Antwerp was able to include a few insightful notes of his own in *Opticorum Libri Sex*—a work that otherwise borrowed heavily from the treatise on optics by the genius protoscientist Alhazen, or Ibn al-Haytham, written in Arabic seven hundred years earlier (see Smith, 2001, for a partial translation

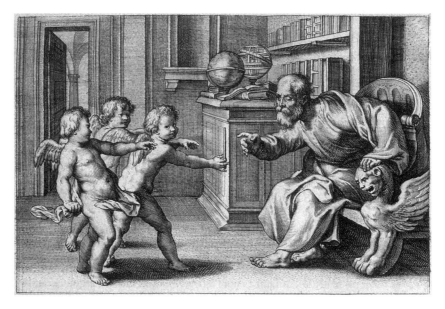

Figure 4.3
A demonstration of parallax with putti. An illustration by Peter Paul Rubens for book III
of Franciscus Aguilonius's *Opticorum Libri Sex* (1613). The bearded thinker peers with one
eye at the three putti before him (or is there really only one putto?). Switching from one
monocular view to another, the pioneering psychophysicist notices the putti apparently
changing position relative to one another. Aguilonius not only understood the phenomenon of parallax but also argued that we exploit the difference between the views with the
left eye versus the right eye (i.e., the binocular disparity) to improve depth perception.

and critical introduction). Aguilonius learned from Alhazen, and we, in
turn, may learn from Aguilonius—science itself being an enterprise that
derives depth from different perspectives.

If binocular disparity does indeed provide us with an opportunity to
improve our perception of depth, it is because we are able to integrate
or synthesize the information obtained from different views. The combination probably takes the form of some kind of averaging or merging,
though the exact computations involved are not yet known (Bridge &
Cumming, 2008, make a specific plea for more data collection). Somehow
we abstract depth from the different perspectives. We construct a single
understanding of the spatial environment, which is no longer tied to
the nature of the sensory input. Different sensory sources are allowed
to speak to the same issue. For instance, at the level of parietal cortex
(to be precise: in the caudal part of the lateral bank of the intraparietal sulcus, CIP), some neurons fire selectively for a particular three-
dimensional surface orientation regardless of whether the visual cues for

depth are obtained by looking with only one eye at the texture gradient (e.g., how lines converge toward a vanishing point) or by relying on binocular disparity (Tsutsui et al., 2002). Here, the completely different computations on the basis of texture gradient and binocular disparity both contribute to the perception of depth by activating the same internal code—the firing of neurons in CIP.

Such convergence toward a shared position is not always possible between different perspectives. True parallax has something paradoxical about it: One perspective says A, another says B, and there can be no meaningful compromise AB. For the contemporary psychoanalyst Slavoj Žižek, who has an insatiable appetite for all kinds of reversals and a sixth sense for the obscene, the notion of incompatible perspectives is quite crucial to virtually all domains of human knowledge. According to the back cover of *The Parallax View*, Žižek (2006|2009) seeks "a rehabilitation of dialectical materialism," and on p. 4 of his book, we read that it involves "the occurrence of an insurmountable *parallax gap*, the confrontation of two closely linked perspectives between which no neutral common ground is possible."

Žižek (2006|2009) finds such gaps everywhere, but the most intriguing one would be that of body and mind (and, of course, I agree): "Does Spinoza not formulate the highest parallax? The substance is One, and the difference between mind and body, its two modes, is purely that of parallax: "body" or "mind" are the same Substance perceived in a different mode" (p. 42). Žižek spends the middle third of *The Parallax View* on this highest parallax, noting that "different versions of the emergence of consciousness, from Dennett to Damasio, all seem to 'get stuck' at the same paradox: that of a certain self-propelling mechanism, of a closed loop of self-relating, which is constitutive of consciousness" (p. 177). Žižek's wager (explicitly stated on the same page): The missing concept is "what German Idealism called self-relating negativity and Freud called 'the death drive.'"

The thinkers in contemporary neuroscience, in Žižek's eyes, seem to have done a reasonable job with respect to the first business, that of emphasizing the self-relating and the feedback loop it implies. Favorable citations are reserved for Metzinger (2004, p. 337) on redefining the self or the subject ("What exists are information-processing systems engaged in the transparent process of phenomenal self-modeling") and for Taylor (2001) on relating our current sensations to the past, effectively *re*-cognizing so that our experience can become what it is. Žižek (2006|2009) repeatedly connects such ideas with Hegel and the notion of positing the presuppositions—deciding that what accidentally happens to be a certain way should in fact necessarily be that way from now on: "[T]he only way to account for the emergence of the distinction between 'inside' and 'outside' constitutive of a living organism is to posit a kind of self-reflexive reversal by means of which—to put it in Hegelese—the One of an organism as a Whole retroactively 'posits' as its result, as that which it dominates and regulates, the set of its own causes" (p. 205).

According to Žižek (2006|2009), the problems for neuroscience arise after this Hegelian step, after the looping and self-relating. Neuroscience would fail to move beyond the body—the organism's biases, the self-interested reactions to disturbances of the homeostasis. In a surprising way, Žižek's criticism rhymes with the gist of proposals such as those by Noë (2004) and Clark (2008), moving from embodied cognition to supersizing the mind (but not the body) and reaching out of our heads. It is as if, after all the Descartes bashing in the last few decades, some thinkers are starting to get ready to wonder about the Cogito as a free agent that escapes the "control of solid earth," as Žižek puts it (2006|2009, p. 213). Here is a relevant sample of sublime Žižekolalia, complete with new affects for the undead Cogito (p. 227):

The chain of equivalences thus imposes itself between the "empty" *cogito* (the Cartesian subject, Kant's transcendental subject), the Hegelian topic of self-relating negativity, and the Freudian topic of the death drive. Is this "pure" subject deprived of emotions? It is not as simple as that: its very detachment from immediate immersion in life-experience gives rise to new (not emotions or feelings, but, rather) affects: anxiety and horror. Anxiety as correlative to confronting the Void that forms the core of the subject; horror as the experience of disgusting life at its purest, "undead" life.

Poor Cogito may wish to find a way back to the body. Žižek's words here sound like incomprehensible poetry (of a variety that, I confess, tickles me in a pleasant way). What can we take away from it that might be relevant even to neuroscientists?

Transmitted to the Internal Sense

Somewhere along the line, Žižek got lost. I think it was relatively early in his argument, leaving the notion of looping and self-relating unspecified. Žižek is right, along with most neuroscientists, to adopt the idea that some kind of return of information structurally underpins consciousness. Information brews, somehow it crystallizes into an explicit thought, and this crystal, the emergent organization, in turn influences information processing. The internal sense works with recurrent information transmission. At the very general level, there must be some truth to such descriptions of the reflexive arc of consciousness. Žižek then disparages neuroscientists for merely describing the arc, not explaining it (a criticism to which the addition of the death drive offers no solution).

Neuroscientists deserve to be disparaged, but not for trying to describe. The problem is that our descriptions are not thorough enough. We have failed to emphasize several key aspects. The looping takes time and energy. The looping is not done for all information. The looping itself changes the information. Many of the underlying mechanisms of selection and computation involve prospective activity—biases and projections. These key aspects of consciousness imply that any casual talk about looping and self-relating, or the Hegelian act of positing the presuppositions, will be entirely off the mark. Perhaps the loop and the reflexive arc are not good metaphors for consciousness after all. Information moves and changes in different directions and at different levels of abstraction in a highly interactive system. Loops and reflexive arcs lead us into endless reverberation. The thing about consciousness is that it does *not* reverberate.

More interesting, I think, is Žižek's basic idea of parallax view, the idea that perspectives, even closely related ones, may not show any correlative order that can be neatly projected to a common ground. Perhaps we tend too easily to look for integration and merging in information processing, when it comes to working with multiple sources of information. Sometimes compromise is not the answer. Sometimes we need to take sides and judge which perspective is more appropriate, what angle gives the best view. The issue for consciousness is to move between perspectives, to grab useful bits and discard others. Rather than getting stuck at thinking about loops, we do well to concentrate on the selective movements of consciousness. Describing those movements in detail, we will discover no simple loops but chaotic itinerancies (Tsuda, 2001). The trick will be to find ways to track the degrees of freedom of such itinerancies, how and when they switch from one attractor to another, from one information source to another.

At present, the relevant focus for neuroscience is on the working with multiple sources of information—how and when do we make use of which kinds of information? We can make use of the parallax view to keep our minds open to shifts and reweighting of information. At the same time we should bear in mind that leaving information as it is (even out there in the world) may often be a better strategy than compulsively trying to represent everything, either as it is or in honestly synthesized averages. Thus I read, with doubled interest, a paper like that by Guo and Raymond (2010) on the reweighting of sensory inputs when monkeys learn to make less variable eye movements without losing accuracy in a task that requires tracking a compound visual–vestibular stimulus. The monkeys learn to rely mostly on vestibular information. Does this still involve integration somewhere in the brain? Should we think of it as a weighted integration? Perhaps the parallax view is simply a special case of weighted integration, in which one source gets a weight of zero? How is the weighting achieved at the neuronal level? These are the questions we must ask.

When juggling perspectives and allocating weights to information, we need to keep track of where we are at in our perceptions, our thoughts, our reasoning and decision making. We need to do this consciously as well as unconsciously. The sensorimotor processes can only produce sensible outcomes if they relate back, in a systematic and organized way, to the perspectives and the information that shape the sensorimotor processes in the first place. I may not be keen to call it "looping," or to go Hegelian on it, but somehow the systematic and organized relating of information will need a point of reference—the idea of a body, the basis of a self. The information and the perspectives will derive their relevance—their weights—from this systematic organization. Without it, there can be no observer, no subject, no soul, and no self. Without it, there can be no meaning to anything. There must be transmission to an internal sense.

Aguilonius (1613) realized as much. It should not surprise us (but it may please us all the same) that the same vision researcher who first talked about the advantages of binocular disparity was also the very one who first considered the need for internal monitoring of our own movement. Both topics, after all, are about accounting for perspective in active vision. The following quote, proposition 20 of book I from *Opticorum Libri Sex*, was translated by Grüsser (1994, p. 263):

Since the force to move the eyes is controlled from the soul and the soul is free in this control, it is not only a necessary natural law that the movement of the eye is excited. It is also necessary that the signals about this movement be transmitted to the internal sense. If the soul did not sense the motion, how could she be able to achieve that the movements sometimes stop by command. What would happen if the soul widely ignored whether that which was commanded was executed as requested.

Aguilonius in this quote relates the internal monitoring to the issue of self-control and, particularly, inhibitory control of movement. There are in fact several uses for internal monitoring beyond the voluntary guidance of movement. Wurtz (2008), in an important review of a vast literature, makes an explicit connection to visual stability—that is, a perceptual function, referring to our general sense of a stable visual world despite the fact that we make frequent eye movements, implying huge variability in the mapping of the world to points on the retina. Monitoring the eye movements we make would allow us to deal with their sensory consequences—online, in the full flow of perception. This would be a perfect example of extreme sensorimotor interaction, with the threesome of movement, signals about the movement, and dynamic visual input converging on the world as we know it—always out there, no matter how frantically we move around in it.

Though otherwise a fan of all kinds of action in perception, Noë (2004) has strong objections to such a view of sensorimotor interaction. The issue for Noë is with the notion of internal monitoring—this sounds too much as if all kinds of things should happen inside the head, such as compensation for retinal shift. The counterargument, first offered by Bridgeman, Van der Heijden, and Velichkovsky (1994), would be that visual stability is actually never in danger from eye movements as long as we do not construct retinotopic internal representations of the world. With the discussion from chapter 3, we might even allow for detailed retinotopic representations that live extremely briefly: during a single fixation. Noë (2004), invigorated by such ideas, bites hard in proposals to explain visual stability that rely on special mechanisms of compensation for changes in position. They are "guilty of committing the homunculus fallacy," he writes (p. 47). They fall for "a problematic conception of the need for pictures in the head" (p. 48). Instead, Noë urges us to seek other kinds of account—we get no clues for direction, but presumably the search should be for anything but the internal.

Ironically, this call for open-mindedness exhibits an unjustified prejudice against the internal life of the brain. As it happens, the internal plot is thickening with very interesting data that do speak for a close relationship between signals of movement intention and visual stability. Figures 4.4 and (in the next section) 4.5 are devoted to such data, which deserve, I believe, a few paragraphs of background and explanation. The idea that we rely on internal signals of our movement was, as mentioned, first raised by Aguilonius and then picked up by Descartes and many others, including most notably Hermann von Helmholtz (1910|2000). Much of the early thought was based on anecdotal observations, including the notion that the visual world seems stable when we make deliberate (active) eye movements but jitters when we push against our eyeballs,

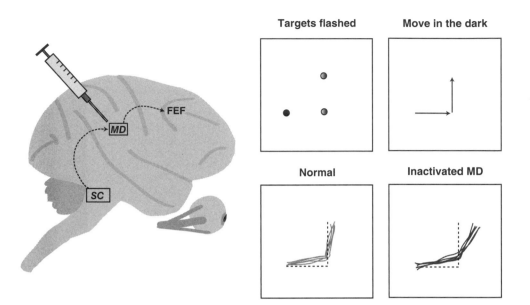

Figure 4.4
A thalamic pathway for internal monitoring (following Sommer & Wurtz, 2002). Muscimol, a drug that increases the inhibitory action of the neurotransmitter γ–aminobutyric acid (GABA), is injected (via the awesome syringe on the left) into the medial dorsal nucleus of the thalamus (MD) to inactivate the feedback circuit from the superior colliculus (SC) to the frontal eye field (FEF). The left upper panel shows the visual stimuli that are presented to the monkey; the right upper panel indicates the required eye movements: a double-step task. The lower panels represent the kinds of eye movements the monkeys actually make, when all things are as normal as they can be in the lab (lower left panel) versus after the injection of muscimol (lower right panel). The inactivation of the thalamic pathway leads to erroneous eye movements, particularly for the second step. The monkeys seem to lose the ability to adjust for their own movement in the computation of the second saccade.

forcing unintended (passive) movement. Interestingly, the opposite is true for visual afterimages: They move along with intended eye movements but seem to remain in place under passive movement. These observations suggest that the intention of movement has a strong impact on perception, rather than retinal position or physical movement alone.

More systematic experimental evidence started emerging in the first half of the twentieth century. The modern vocabulary arrived on the scene: von Holst and Mittelstädt (1950) talked about "efference copy"; Sperry (1950) preferred "corollary discharge." These terms essentially indexed the same concept. The experimental evidence implied the existence of something internal, a signal that represented the movement instruction—when a neural structure sent a motor command downstream (i.e., efference), it would in parallel (as a corollary) send the same information to other structures in the brain so that they could adapt to it, monitor it, or factor it in for decision making, control of action, perception, and so on. Efference copy and corollary discharge both remain current terms. We could debate whether the "copy" in efference copy implies that it should be an exact duplicate; Sommer and Wurtz (2002) preferred the term "corollary discharge" because it remains noncommittal about the degree of precision in duplication. I would agree with that and add that it also remains noncommittal about the input–output structure. This way we can respect Hurley's (1998) point and consider the multiplicity of signals without buying into any preconceived direction in terms of perception and action.

Without a doubt the most dramatic experimental evidence relating to corollary discharge was collected with humans undergoing paralysis—unable to move, but wide awake, some researchers blur (or activate) the boundaries between heroism and insanity. Solely in the interest of science, John K. Stevens, of Stevens et al. (1976), underwent complete paralysis via succinylcholine, "very unpleasant but bearable" (p. 93)—not once, but thrice (in addition to another two sessions under curare, which did not quite suppress all eye movement). He noted a vague sense of displacement in the direction of his intended eye movement but thought this perception was "not necessarily visual in nature, and found it very hard to describe" (p. 95). Stevens tried harder than anyone else. His predecessors, as reported by Siebeck and Frey (1953), had merely observed that the paralysis prevented eye movement without producing perceptual illusions.

More useful and only slightly less crazy were the sessions that weakened the extraocular muscle activity, effectively creating a mismatch between motor commands and actual eye movements—either by injecting a local anesthetic (e.g., Kornmüller, 1931) or by giving low systemic doses of curare (e.g., West, 1932). In these conditions, subjects consistently made errors in localizing visual stimuli and reported striking apparent displacement in the direction of eye movements. John K. Stevens noted that these illusions were far more "jumpy" and conspicuous than the vague sensations under complete paralysis (Stevens et al., 1976). Matin and colleagues (1982; including our insane hero) further investigated what they called the "oculoparalytic illusion" by examining how well subjects (grunting to the best of their abilities) linked the locations of visual and auditory stimuli when under the influence of curare.

The task was performed either in complete darkness or under normal room illumination (giving a "structured visual field," or a relatively rich visual environment). The illusions of displacement in the direction of intended eye movements occurred only in darkness. Apparently, the subjects were able to use information from the world to clear up the confusion inside their heads. Intriguingly, however, the errors in linking the visual and auditory stimuli remained. These are two important pieces of the puzzle, for you and me to keep in mind as we try to move toward a general understanding of what corollary discharge does for perception.

In the meantime, though, it should be noted that the work by Matin and colleagues (1982) did not actually prove that curare interfered with internal monitoring on the basis of corollary discharge. Indeed, the researchers were careful to point out that they examined the use of extraretinal eye position information, "whether derived from motor commands directing gaze or proprioceptive feedback from the orbit" (p. 198). The study did not tease apart whether the brain operates on the basis of a signal in parallel with the motor command (before moving the eye) or on the basis of feedback from the extraocular muscles (after moving the eye).

Guthrie, Porter, and Sparks (1983) provided tantalizing evidence in favor of corollary discharge. They eliminated the feedback from the extraocular muscles by sectioning the relevant fibers (there were no human volunteers for this experiment) and found that monkeys were still able to aim their eye movements correctly despite perturbations from electrical stimulation in the superior colliculus. The data suggested that, somehow, somewhere, corollary discharge allowed the visual system to compensate for the stimulation. Sommer and Wurtz (2002) went one further, actually pinpointing to the corollary discharge in the brain (see figure 4.4). In the medial dorsal nucleus of the thalamus, they recorded from neurons that were activated by electrical stimulation in the FEF (against the direction of the anatomical projection or "antidromically") as well as by electrical stimulation in the superior colliculus (in the direction of the anatomical projection or "orthodromically"). In Plain English, these neurons were part of an upstream pathway from a midbrain structure involved in motor control to a frontal lobe structure in charge of eye movement planning. The neurons were relay units that showed an increased spiking rate right before the monkey made a saccade—evidence in favor of corollary discharge, not proprioception or any feedback after eye movement.

Next, Sommer and Wurtz (2002) sought to obtain causal evidence of a functional role for this corollary discharge. They injected muscimol in the sites where they had recorded relay neurons—enough to partially and temporarily inactivate the region. The monkey was asked to perform a double-step saccade (see figure 4.4, upper panels on the right). The trick in this task is that two stimuli are flashed briefly and simultaneously, but the monkey has to shift his gaze to the remembered positions in two steps. For the first eye movement, the required vector is given by the retinal coordinates of the flashed stimulus. However, for the second eye movement, the vector should be straight up from the new starting position, not diagonally as according to the initial retinal coordinates. To perform the second step correctly, then, the monkey has to take into account his own movement. In the control condition, without muscimol, the monkey can perform the task all right, but when the thalamic pathway is inactivated by muscimol, the second eye movement goes astray—it seems to follow the initial retinal coordinates, suggesting that the critical corollary discharge went missing.

What we have, at this moment, is clear evidence of a signal transmitted to the internal sense—corollary discharge. This signal is needed to carry out a task that requires self-monitoring (see Wolpert, Ghahramani, & Jordan, 1995, for a solid computational argument based on a different paradigm). On the other hand, we know that curare produces perceptual illusions. The mismatch between intended and actual eye movements disrupts visual stability, at least in relatively poor visual environments. How can we close the gap? How do we move from a signal that looks like corollary discharge to implementing the information in a mechanism that promotes visual stability?

Predictive Remapping

An important clue to the connection between corollary discharge and visual stability actually existed already about a decade before Sommer and Wurtz (2002) published their instant classic. The clue came from close to home for Wurtz: from his own Laboratory of Sensorimotor Research. Figure 4.5 represents the basics of the phenomenon of predictive remapping as coined and discovered by Duhamel, Colby, and Goldberg (1992). They recorded from neurons in the LIP as the monkey performed a simple saccade task, following jumps of the fixation point. As it happened, the LIP neurons did something funny that violated the classic concept of a visual receptive field.

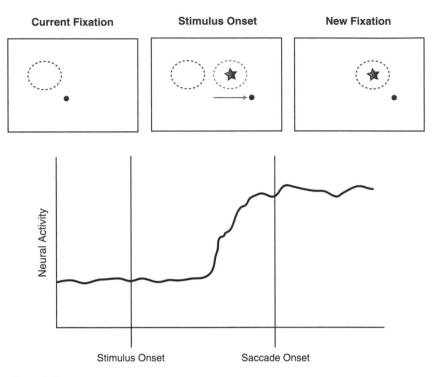

Figure 4.5
Predictive remapping of the receptive field (based on Duhamel, Colby, & Goldberg, 1992). The top left panel represents the receptive field (black dashed ellipse) of a neuron in the lateral intraparietal area (LIP) as the monkey gazes at a fixation point. In the middle panel the fixation point jumps to a new location. At the same time a second stimulus (a star) is presented in the "future" receptive field (the gray dashed ellipse), that is, the receptive field of the LIP neuron after the monkey has completed the required eye movement to the shifted fixation point (result shown in the right panel). The activity of the LIP neuron (bottom graph) increases well before the monkey actually initiates the intended saccade to the shifted fixation point. Such data suggest predictive remapping in the brain, allowing neurons to respond already to information that will soon be in their receptive field.

Things used to be straightforward in visual neuroscience: Visual neurons had receptive fields—regions in the visual field to which they were sensitive. If a stimulus appeared there, they would fire. If the stimuli appeared elsewhere, the neurons would not fire. The LIP neurons behaved in exactly this way during a preliminary fixation task when the monkey just gazed at a static fixation point. But then Duhamel, Colby, and Goldberg (1992), in a brilliant move, made things forever more complex: Together with the fixation point, they presented a second stimulus elsewhere in the otherwise blank visual field (see top panels of figure 4.5). The second stimulus (a star) was visually distinct from the first (a point) and irrelevant to the task. It was positioned in the *future* receptive field of the LIP neuron, that is, the receptive field as according to the situation after the eye movement to the shifted fixation point.

As a result, textbooks had to be rewritten. The LIP neurons started responding after the presentation of the new visual display but before the eye movement—at a moment in time when there was no stimulus in their visual receptive field. The neural firing preceded the saccade, but only if the star was placed in the future receptive field. For all purposes, it looked as if the LIP neurons had access to visual information in their receptive field even before the retinal coordinates had physically changed. The receptive field had been remapped by means of prediction. Duhamel, Colby, and Goldberg (1992) argued that the retinotopic spatial representation was updated in advance as a function of the intended eye movement. The data implied a role for an internal signal about the intention—corollary discharge. With information about the upcoming eye movement, the receptive field could be addressed to the future retinal coordinates.

The phenomenon proved to be very robust and easily replicated. Carol L. Colby dedicated a significant portion of her research to investigating the neural circuitry of predictive remapping (e.g., Berman et al., 2007; Merriam, Genovese, & Colby, 2003; Nakamura & Colby, 2002). Would it be possible to collect more direct evidence of a connection between corollary discharge and predictive remapping? What if we used Sommer and Wurtz's (2002) approach in combination with something along the lines of Duhamel, Colby, and Goldberg (1992)? Sommer and Wurtz (2006) set themselves to exactly this task. They targeted the predictive remapping in FEF (as first observed by Umeno & Goldberg, 1997) and found that the spatiotemporal dynamics of the thalamic corollary discharge neatly predicted the receptive field shifts. Moreover, inactivating the thalamic relay neurons disrupted the receptive field shifts in the FEF. The corollary discharge was necessary for predictive remapping. Computationally, it now seems very plausible that the corollary discharge can indeed be factored into a neural model that simulates the receptive field shifts.

However, what exactly is the role of predictive remapping in visual stability? I remember being truly amazed, and also slightly suspicious that the argument was not entirely correct, when in the mid 1990s (in a very dreary winter in Michigan) I first encountered the wonderful work by Duhamel, Colby, and Goldberg (1992). Especially the drawings in their conceptual figure 1 smelled of a sleight of hand. The actual experiments used very simple displays (a point and a star in an otherwise empty visual field), but the conceptual figure explained everything with drawings of a complex scene: a tree, the sun, a cloud, and a mountain—a rich image of the world. The implication was that, to contribute to our sense of visual stability, the remapping should occur for the entire visual scene, however complex. This did not seem quite right. I had just been reading a number of articles on "exogenous capture" by abrupt visual onsets (e.g., Jonides, 1981; Theeuwes, 1991; Yantis & Jonides, 1990) for a review I was working on (Lauwereyns, 1998). Human observers cannot help but notice sudden flashes, especially if these appear in a relatively poor visual environment.

The star in the experiments by Duhamel, Colby, and Goldberg (1992) was not an innocent bit of information somewhere on an extensive visual map. It was one of only two sudden onsets—arguably even the only onset, considering the fact that the other one (the fixation point) could be interpreted as a shifted stimulus. The star was a highly salient visual element that stood out and demanded "attention" (or *selective* information processing) even if it was irrelevant to the task. In fact, a few years later Michael E. Goldberg himself, with two new associates, provided evidence that LIP neurons respond selectively to such abrupt visual onsets (Gottlieb, Kusunoki, & Goldberg, 1998). The LIP neurons represent salience, was the lesson—and it applied to the star in the 1992 study.

Where does that leave the argument about the role of corollary discharge and predictive remapping in visual stability? The remapping probably does not occur for the entire visual scene at once. Bays and Husain (2007) even argued that the remapping contributes very little to perception though their alternatives sound like close neighbors, still internal and cognitive—spatial memory is one of their favorites, or more generally dynamic memory, which would allocate resources across different objects as a function of the level of detail required (see also Bays & Husain, 2008). Yet, there is very good psychophysical evidence that unambiguously points to a perceptual function in predictive remapping. Melcher (2007) showed that even visual form adaptation migrates in advance relative to the next gaze position. Rolfs and colleagues (2011) provided evidence, with a double-step saccade task, that the detection of orientation changes to gratings improves at "the remapped location"— say, upper left if the task involves making an eye movement to the upper left in the second step. In this case, the percentage of correct responses to changes at the current upper left (an irrelevant location) increases even before the first step. In short, the receptive fields do really shift in advance, and they do really come with facilitated perception.

At this point, I would like to call back to mind the two pieces of the puzzle we received from Matin and colleagues (1982). (1) Structured visual fields abolish the perceptual illusions that are due to curare. (2) Even with structured visual fields, the troubles in linking sight with sound remain. The first piece of the puzzle suggests that corollary discharge and predictive remapping are not crucial for the perceived stability of the entire visual scene. The second piece suggests that the issues are focused on selective points in the environment where we need to integrate information. With Melcher (2007) and Rolfs and colleagues (2011) we take this to involve perception. Thus, we are compelled to think that corollary discharge and predictive remapping contribute to selective information processing, allowing us to integrate features and understand them as stable properties of the environment. This would happen for just one or a few hotspots in the visual environment. Our areas or objects of interest in the environment would be tracked virtually through a tight linkage with gaze control. Cavanagh and colleagues (2010) use the term "attention pointers."

Our sense of visual stability would require the remapping of such attention pointers. Even Lauwereyns (2010) might be comfortable with calling this a matter of "attention," seeing as the selective information processing in this case probably does match with the hardcore definition of attention, implying heightened sensitivity and improved signal-to-noise ratios. Even though the retina by itself can take care of much of the computational work needed to provide visual stability, and even though philosophy says we do not need to build detailed internal representations of everything, we do still see corollary discharge and predictive remapping playing an important role. They facilitate our sense of stability and our ability to process in detail a privileged subset of the information available to us. They contribute to our internal coding of some (selected, important, relevant) portion of what is in front of us. We need corollary discharge and predictive mapping here precisely *because* we are coding internally—holding on to some kind of information for longer than the duration of a single gaze fixation. The retina cannot help us in that case. But the internal sense *can*—with the help of all possible cues, including those about our movement intentions.

Dynamic Sensitivity

The story about corollary discharge and predictive remapping is not finished—far from it. I think it should be expanded by connecting it with another one, about dynamic visual sensitivity. Given that we now understand remapping to be done selectively, only for areas of visual interest, we are ready for the next step—to compare this form of remapping with the dynamic visual sensitivity that precedes the movement of the eyes to a target.

Twice already I have referred to Posner's (1980) location-cueing paradigm (in the section *Covert versus Overt Processing*, chapter 1, and in *The Orienting Response*, chapter 3). I must mention it one more time here. As soon as Posner (now more than thirty years ago) neatly proved that we are able to dissociate our selective visual information processing (covert visual attention) from the gaze fixation point, researchers started wondering about the correspondence between the two modes of orienting. The evidence of separable allocation was unambiguous, but did the covert and overt mechanisms of orienting complement each other? Did they compete or interact in any way? Rizzolatti (1983) argued that covert attention reflects the activity in the brain's pragmatic maps for the programming of eye movements. He called it the "premotor theory of attention" and went on to provide psychophysical evidence of a tight coupling between covert visual processing and oculomotor parameters (Sheliga, Riggio, & Rizzolatti, 1994). Most researchers agreed that, in one way or another, eye movements are typically preceded by selective visual processing (e.g., Deubel & Schneider, 1996; Henderson, 1993; Findlay, 2003, 2009).

The psychophysical studies converged on the notion of dynamic sensitivity in the service of saccade target selection. This would be the normal situation, the system's settings by default. An area in the visual field would be selected for further processing. This selection would happen covertly, inside the head, and call for the gaze to center on the selection. When a new region is selected, the eyes will follow. It is a form of predictive remapping—of the foveal field. The covert selection moves to a peripheral location, which will become the new focus point of the gaze.

The most parsimonious account posits that corollary discharge and predictive remapping happen only for selected regions of the visual field—this was our conclusion from the previous section. We can rephrase the predictive remapping as a form of dynamic sensitivity coupled to the gaze. Now I suggest this remapping may occur for both foveal and peripheral areas of the visual field. The examples discussed by Wurtz, Goldberg, and their associates all concentrated on situations in which the selected regions were peripheral ones, both before and after the eye movement. Those were all examples of predictive remapping of the periphery. However, structurally, functionally, that kind of remapping may be no different from predictive remapping of the fovea. Whether remapping the fovea or a selected region in the periphery, the point is that the selected area shifts in advance of the eye movement. In both cases, the sensitivity is dynamically linked to movements of the gaze.

Am I taking an unwarranted shortcut? Are both types of remapping really analogous, computationally, neurophysiologically? We might be inclined to say that, in the case of remapping the fovea, it is the eyes that follow our selection. The gaze moves to where the sensitivity went. The gaze shift is consequent on the remapping. However, in the case of remapping a selected region in the periphery, the order seems not quite the same. In that case, it is because our gaze will move somewhere that the remapping adapts in advance. The remapping, even though it is predictive, seems to be consequent on the gaze shift, even though that is as yet only intended, not actually carried out. Or, on second thought, is this maybe the same order after all? The gaze shift is really consequent on the remapping.

One thing to bear in mind here is the concurrent remapping of more than one selected region: It can be done in parallel for the future foveal field *plus* one or more peripheral regions. My best guess is that by default we engage in predictive remapping of the fovea. This is the essential one from which all further computations begin. Depending on the circumstances, the remapping can be conducted also for a few peripheral areas of interest—this is likely to involve capacity constraints and dynamics along the lines suggested by Bays and Husain (2008). By definition, corollary discharge and predictive remapping are in fact orchestrated by the mechanisms for saccade target selection. Does this mean we can speak of core predictive remapping (the fovea) and associate predictive remapping (the selected peripheral regions)? The first type of remapping would reflect the intended gaze shift. The second type would benefit from corollary discharge to synchronize its dynamics with the intended gaze shift.

In any event, we will only find out how the neural circuitry actually works by conducting the relevant experiments. As for the basic relation between dynamic sensitivity and the control of eye movements, many of the most fascinating studies have been carried out by Tirin Moore and his colleagues (see Moore, Armstrong, & Fallah, 2003, for an early review on "Visuomotor origins of covert spatial attention"). Moore and Fallah (2001) applied electrical stimulation to the FEF as the monkey performed a visual search task. The stimulation was subthreshold: not enough to elicit an eye movement. It improved the monkey's visual sensitivity in the "movement field" (the location where the eyes would always go if the stimulation was suprathreshold).

Moore and Armstrong (2003) also applied electrical stimulation in FEF and took the additional step of recording the activity of neurons in area V4 (in the posterior visual cortex); this time the monkey viewed line segments of different orientation. Subthreshold stimulation in FEF produced heightened visual sensitivity in the tuning of V4 neurons as long as the movement field of the FEF stimulation site matched with the receptive field of the V4 neuron. The effect size depended on whether there was a competing visual target in the neuron's receptive field. Without competition, and so without a need for visual selection, there was not much influence from the FEF stimulation. This crucial factor of selection will be elaborated on in the next chapter. But clearly, the set of two stimulation studies already provide a solid empirical link between FEF activation and improved visual sensitivity in V4 at the future foveal field (i.e., the target of the impending gaze shift as controlled by electrical stimulation).

Can we take the FEF activation here to mean *saccade target selection*? I think we can, and I bet most neuroscientists probably think so too, but it is not a trivial step. It means we take the FEF electrical stimulation to implant an intention to shift the gaze—in Hollywood language this would be categorized as an electromechanical case of "inception" (I am referring, of course, to the 2010 movie with Leonardo DiCaprio, written and directed by Christopher Nolan). The causal manipulations by Moore and Fallah (2001) and by Moore and Armstrong (2003) are exactly the kind that may win over skeptics like Alva Noë (2004)—toward thinking that the internal life of the mind really happens in the activity of neurons, whether activated by a spontaneous external process (an event in the world), a spontaneous internal process (say, imagination), or an artificial mechanism (not necessarily devious in character; I think of deep-brain stimulation for Parkinsonian patients).

This is not to say that artificial stimulation can replace the world or create a virtual reality as rich as the real one we live in (see Dennett, 1991, for a convincing argument against the feasibility of a "brain in a vat"—the sheer computational complexity very quickly leads to something practically impossible). The point is that the activation of neurons (no matter how) suffices to produce the workings of the mind. Less clear is whether we should understand the activation of neurons to be a necessary condition. In absolute, categorical terms, the answer should probably be "No," at least for certain cognitive functions. In line with Clark (2008), I recognize that we already make use of a variety of tools and devices that perform cognitive functions outside the mind/body—storing and processing information via automatic algorithms without any help from neurons. This raises the question of exactly which neural activity is indeed necessary (irreplaceable) for any given cognitive function. It sounds like an empirical question to me—one in which engineers are likely to play a leading role, pushing the active boundaries of the artificial mind/body. The answer, I believe, will go straight to the heart of elusive concepts like consciousness and experience. In the meantime, though, I propose we do well to learn more about the causal connections between neural activity and cognitive functions.

With pleasure I note that Moore and colleagues have gone further down the track of causal manipulations. Noudoost and Moore (2011) found that both the monkey's visual search performance and the sensitivity of V4 neurons were enhanced by injecting a dopamine-related drug (the selective D1R antagonist SCH 23390) into the FEF. This modulation occurred only when the receptive fields of the V4 neurons overlapped with the movement field of the FEF site. Conversely, injecting another dopamine-related drug (the D2R agonist quinpirole) influenced the monkey's behavioral performance but did not affect the sensitivity of V4 neurons. Such data help us on the way to characterizing the neural circuitry (including the neurochemistry) that underlies the dynamic sensitivity.

Schafer and Moore (2011) tried something different again, which may or may not fit the bill of a causal manipulation. When we voluntarily increase or decrease our own brain activity, do we control it in a way that counts as causal evidence? The rather controversial issue is that of bio-feedback (or "neurofeedback") in the tradition that traces back to Fetz (1969). Here, the trick is to get subjects, typically monkeys, to control their own neural activity to obtain a desired result, say, a food reward. The monkeys receive auditory or visual feedback of their own neural activity and are rewarded for either high or low firing rates. Of course, the monkeys catch on quickly; they listen to their own spikes, and they do indeed manage to make the neurons fire more than a minimum threshold or less than a maximum threshold to obtain a treat. Fetz (1969) called it "operant conditioning of cortical unit activity." Neurofeedback has never really taken off as field for mainstream neuroscience, but some researchers are becoming interested again (e.g., Kobayashi, Schultz, &

Sakagami, 2010). Schafer and Moore (2011) showed neurofeedback to work for FEF neurons as well. Critically, they found the neurofeedback training to facilitate the monkeys' performance on a separate visual search task. Particularly, the visual sensitivity increased; oculomotor parameters were not influenced. The effects pertained to the covert processing for target selection (Schafer and Moore do not hesitate to use the word "attention")—the predictive remapping of the fovea, not the actual eye movement.

Of course, the causal manipulations alone are not sufficient to establish the link between saccade target selection in FEF and improved sensitivity in V4. We still need the correlational studies in parallel, to convince ourselves that the effects under, say, electrical stimulation (artificial inception of intention) match with those seen under control conditions. In such an effort, Zhou and Desimone (2011) recorded simultaneously in V4 and FEF and were able to estimate the information flow between these two areas on the basis of latency analyses: V4 provides bottom-up sensory signals about visual features whereas FEF feeds back task-related biases, prioritizing the important bits. Han, Xian, and Moore (2009) gathered comprehensive data about the variety of dynamical changes in V4 during saccade preparation. They found a widespread decrease in sensitivity for nontarget areas of the visual field—not just a lack of predictive remapping for the unattended bits in the image but an active suppression starting shortly before the eye movement.

These data put another spin on the classic concept of saccadic suppression (see Matin, 1974, for a landmark review), which holds that visual perception shuts down during eye movements—possibly a wise tactic for the visual system, seeing as no useful sensory information can be registered while the eyes are in midflight; we would anyway get nothing but senseless streaks of light on the retina. However, active suppression would require energy and so imply a biological cost. The behavioral evidence for saccadic suppression had been mixed until Burr, Morrone, and Ross (1994) were able to demonstrate that the phenomenon is real, but not general. In many cases, we do not actively need to suppress visual noise during eye movements. Brooks, Yates, and Coleman (1980) provided compelling evidence that at least some kinds of visual analysis can take place during saccadic eye movement, indicating that active suppression certainly does not extend to all visual information (the paper also received an honorable citation by Dennett in *Consciousness Explained*, 1991, p. 362). Instead of expending precious molecular resources on suppression, the visual system can simply let the noise be. However, it turns out to be useful, and worth the effort, to filter out some of the low-spatial-frequency information during saccades to prevent a disturbing sense of background motion. Consistent with this proposal, Thiele and colleagues (2002) obtained neurophysiological evidence to demonstrate very real and active saccadic suppression of image motion in area MT.

Saccadic suppression has always seemed like another fine candidate for a derivative of corollary discharge. With the evidence from Han, Xian, and Moore (2009), we have reason to think that the suppression starts before the eye movement, in parallel with predictive remapping and equally (but differently) influenced by corollary discharge. Without a doubt, the phenomenon of saccadic suppression should be an excellent target for a research project à la Sommer and Wurtz (2002, 2006). Dynamic sensitivity may well prove to be the product of complex interplay between facilitation and suppression. Not all the irrelevant information in the visual field will require active suppression—only the competing information that poses a threat to our selective focus and/or our sense of stability. The good news for hungry researchers is that, at the moment, we know next to nothing about how such interplay unfolds.

The Self in the World

Still on the topic of dynamic sensitivity and predictive remapping, I believe we should also consider the type of coordinates used in the spatial map. Figure 4.6 represents data that urge me to think this thought. Olson and Gettner (1995) recorded from neurons in the SEF while the monkeys made eye movements either to a dot or to one side of a horizontal bar (as cued with a little icon at the start of a trial). In the given example, using single dots as saccade targets, we are tempted to conclude that the SEF neuron has a movement field to the upper left. Most researchers would naturally assume that such activity is based on an egocentric, retinotopic map. However, too often this assumption remains unchallenged and unchecked.

Carefully probed, the SEF neuron proves that it can adapt to the usage of an object-centered map. Here, the neuron exhibits a leftward movement field relative to the horizontal bar, not the retinotopic coordinates. If the actual movement is to the right, but left of the horizontal bar, the neuron increases its firing rate (though the saccade is to go "outside the retinotopic movement field"). The opposite is true for actual movement to the left, but right of the horizontal bar: The neuron does not respond (though the saccade is to go "inside the retinotopic movement field").

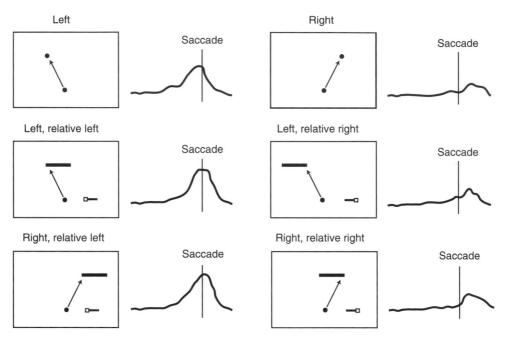

Figure 4.6
Object-centered direction coding (modeled after Olson & Gettner, 1995). Shown are six pairs of panel and graph. Each panel (left of the pair) indicates a required saccade, either to a target dot or to one end of a horizontal bar. For horizontal bars, the target side is cued by a small square superimposed on a sample bar at the beginning of the trial. (The sample bar is presented to the right of the initial fixation point.) Each graph shows the response of a prototypical neuron (always the same neuron) in the supplementary eye field. This neuron consistently increases its activity before an eye movement to the "relative" left, that is, to the left of the bar, regardless of whether the eye movement vector goes to the left or the right in absolute spatial terms. Thus, the neuron appears to code direction on the basis of an object-centered map.

The movement field is computed not on the basis of eye coordinates but using a map centered on the horizontal bar.

How does the object-centered map come about? Does it involve some sort of translation from egocentric coding? Or do we work with relations among object features very early on in our information processing? In chapter 3 we saw that already in the retina objects can be segregated from the background. It is theoretically feasible that much of the spatial coding in predictive remapping proceeds from structural relations that we extract from the scene in front of us—in short, allocentric coding (the preferred hypothesis in the literature on spatial mapping in the hippocampus). We often assume that predictive remapping with eye movements works on the basis of retinotopic coordinates, but we have no proof. Might it actually (computationally) be easier to remap on the basis of object- or world-centered coordinates? Or do we use a sequence, say from retinotopic (at the current fixation), to object-centered (where in the world to go next), and back to retinotopic (translating the worldly coordinates to specifications for bodily action)?

I would venture to say that, likely, we do work with several different kinds of spatial map during predictive remapping. Hippocampal researchers tend to overemphasize allocentric coding and forget that the subject is tracking *the self* in the world. Researchers studying saccade target selection go too far in the other direction, thinking too much in terms of retinotopic coding and forgetting that the subject is tracking the self *in the world*. Each level of processing, from sensory to motor and back, is naturally constrained to its own mode of spatial coding. We do well to heed the natural constraints of muscles and sensory organs, muscle fibers and receptors. But what gets coded in the dark middle, the covert and selective? Should it be "fuzzy," that is, compatible with multiplicity, plastic and dynamic—a sensitivity that can shift from egocentric to object-centered on demand?

Computational models would obviously identify the covert and selective activity with that of "hidden units"—seated in a layer (or rather, in several sets of layers) between sensory input and motor output, with multiple connections to the sensory and the motor. These hidden units must have access to several coordinate systems. It would not be a great leap to suggest that the traffic of information in those hidden layers can go in different directions; the spatial nature of the mapping may be biased this way or that, toward retinotopic, object-based, or effector-oriented coding, depending on the needs or inclinations of the visual system at a particular moment in time.

Flexibility would be dictated by task requirements. The sensorimotor interactions in vision naturally demand the ability to read sensory patterns in bodily coordinates, to extract features of the world, to plan actions and predict outcomes, all in a sequence that is not linear and has no predefined beginning or ending. The story about corollary discharge, predictive remapping, and dynamic sensitivity will not be complete until we understand the coordinate systems involved. This is, of course, a question about the nature of the underlying codes, the representation—it will take us to chapter 5.

The Costs and Benefits of Affordances

Before rushing to chapter 5, I would like to raise one final point relevant to the role of the observer in seeing and grasping—on the economics of perception. Let me start again from Posner's (1980) location-cueing para-digm. I guess it has that unbeatable elegance and simplicity which forever lends itself to being used as oxygen for an argument—much like Des-cartes's dictum about thinking (and therefore existing) never ceases to tickle us.

When Posner (1980) introduced his paradigm, he did so in the lan-guage of economics, referring to "costs and benefits of attention shifts" (p. 12). Covert selective information processing implied improvement for the visual items that were selected and disadvantage for those that were rejected. Posner provided an exact metric for the costs and benefits in his paradigm by comparing behavioral performance (as measured in reaction time and percentage of correct responses) across three cueing conditions: valid trials, neutral trials, and invalid trials. The validity referred to the relation between an attentional cue (e.g., an arrow, cen-trally presented) and the actual (peripheral) location of a subsequent target. In valid trials, the target appeared at the cued location; in invalid trials the target appeared elsewhere. In neutral trials, no location was cued.

The neutral trials served as the baseline against which to evaluate the effects of the cues (following the subtraction method pioneered by Donders, 1869, 1969; see chapter 1). The improved performance with valid cues relative to the baseline reflected "benefits"; the less efficient performance with invalid cues relative to the baseline reflected "costs." In its elegance and simplicity, Posner's (1980) paradigm established this one obvious and far-stretching point: that our selective information pro-cessing has indeed a measurable impact on perception. We cannot talk about vision without talking about selection. The active boundaries of vision are to a large extent determined by our covert states, our biases and interests, our selection criteria.

How do we set the selection criteria? Do we set them voluntarily, or are we bound by imperative influences from the environment as a func-tion of physically salient information? These questions can be asked from an economic perspective, treating our capacity for information process-ing as a limited resource. As observers, we can weigh the potential value of new (as yet unprocessed) information (e.g., "What do we stand to gain from it?") against the efforts required for processing (e.g., "How long would it take us to find out?"). In some cases we might consciously deliberate over such questions. More often, our preset biases and sensi-tivities will determine our visual selections implicitly. These biases and sensitivities in perception, I have suggested several times already, are aimed primarily at meaning—a rich form of structured information, something of intrinsic value.

Working with the proposals that selective information processing is a limited resource and that meaning is what we are after, we can now put the two together to explore the economy of perception. The critical currency would be information value, or meaning. Some information would have a high value, be it from a utilitarian or aesthetic perspective—it might be "interesting," "important," "funny," or "beautiful." The information may appeal to us for many different reasons, but it should be possible to rate the value in one dimension; indeed, I would argue that this is usually what our gaze does (unless there are specific social or visual sensory reasons to strategically aim our gaze elsewhere, in which case we rely on covert selective processing). The gaze picks one point to focus on: the point that promises the most valuable information. The critical currency—information value or meaningfulness—determines the ratings of potential gaze targets.

Our biases and sensitivities set the implicit priorities of different types of information; they modulate the valuation. The efforts required for processing, as well as the speed and accuracy, influence the information value of particular items, though not always in negative or easily predictable ways. Particularly in aesthetic judgments, the mysterious or "ungraspable" items may sometimes be the more valuable. Figure 4.7 suggests as much, to me at least, with face-like features in a stone underwater. In the (leisurely) context of a visit to Aoshima (having recently consumed liquids and foods; with no immediate danger from predators for anyone traveling with me), this stone was the most deserving of my gaze precisely *because* I could not figure it out right away. Of course, I would have lost interest immediately if suddenly one of my offspring had started screaming (for no good reason, probably; but still, my parental instincts would have ruled my gaze allocation). Information value will always be determined relatively—compared to the concurrent competition within reach for the gaze.

With the crucial role for observer-dependent biases and sensitivities, it will be obvious that the concrete gaze selections in given circumstances must show considerable variability among individuals. Nevertheless, we can aim to uncover general economic trends in the perceptual choices ("not the poem, but the poetics," I suggested in chapter 1; a similar thought applies here, "not every individual movement of the gaze, but the economic principles"). Meaning will be the intrinsic attractor of this economy. Many of the principles are waiting to

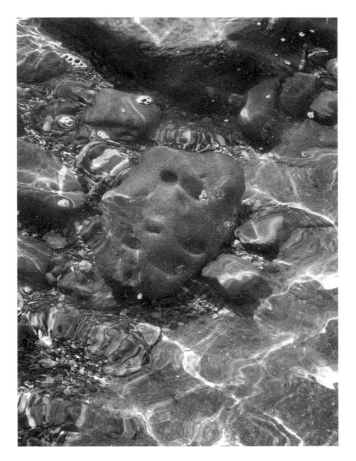

Figure 4.7
Rocks and stones underwater, near Aoshima, Miyazaki prefecture, Japan. Aoshima ("Blue Island") is famous for its ancient shrine (the one main building on the tiny island), its remarkable tropical climate (noticeably different from neighboring areas), and its surreal landscape. On December 27, 2010, my perception for perception got stuck on the curious object in the middle. My digital camera detected faces, and so did I, briefly at first, but not upon inspection.

be investigated—those hungry researchers have plenty of unknowns to rejoice about.

The ideas about visual economy and the role of meaning were raised by J. J. Gibson (1979|1986) in his ecological perception. "Perception is economical," Gibson decreed (p. 135), and his "radical hypothesis" was "that 'values' and 'meanings' of things in the environment can be directly perceived" (p. 127). These ideas naturally evolved from a view that aimed to place the observer in the most complete and situated sense in the world—it reflected the philosophy of the embodied mind before it was recognized as a school of thought. Gibson understood that the role of meaning, at its most fundamental, resides in the fact that we have limits, that our *res extensa* is finite.

Put positively, we might look at the limits of our being as that which allows us to be powerfully exclusive. We can liken it to a good scientific theory—it pays to be sharp and precise in our concentration rather than diffuse and boundless in a vague approximation of everything. A theory that predicts everything to be possible predicts nothing; epistemologically, the infinity of "everything" is meaningless. Our bodies, by being limited, give specific meanings to things in the world—meanings that are uniquely there for us. Objects and events become behaviorally relevant as a function of how they stimulate our limits, our homeostasis, our needs and wants, and our abilities to process information.

However, does Gibson (1979|1986) go too far when he claims that we perceive the values and meanings of things *directly*? The radical word sneaks in when he talks about affordances (p. 127):

The *affordances* of the environment are what it *offers* the animal, what it *provides* or *furnishes*, either for good or ill. The verb *to afford* is found in the dictionary, but the noun *affordance* is not. I have made it up. I mean by it something that refers to both the environment and the animal in a way that no existing term does. It implies the complementarity of the animal and the environment.

I think I understand "affordances" as "potential for interaction"—synonymous also with "behavioral meaning." Moving on from this less than ideally limited definition, Gibson speculates (still on p. 127) as follows:

Perhaps the composition and layout of surfaces *constitute* what they afford. If so, to perceive them is to perceive what they afford. This is a radical hypothesis, for it implies that "values" and "meanings" of things in the environment can be directly perceived. Moreover, it would explain the sense in which values and meanings are external to the perceiver.

As for the last sentence, I would disagree with the "external" in the same way as I disagree with Noë's (2004) notion of external virtual content. How we interact with objects or events in the world very much depends on our biases and sensitivities, shaped by nature, nurture, nature-via-nurture, and nurture-via-nature. The same stimulus excites different behavioral meanings in the heads of the observers (sometimes literally the eyes of the beholders). The potentials for interaction, I believe, are just as much part of the internal virtual content as the biases and sensitivities.

On p. 135, Gibson (1979|1986) adds that "[i]t is never necessary to distinguish *all* the features of an object and, in fact, it would be impossible to do so." It is right after this sentence that he observes, "Perception is economical." Then, interestingly, without getting any more specific about his own view, Gibson shifts the radical hypothesis to the past, to the Gestalt psychologists, who "recognized that the meaning or the value of a thing seems to be perceived just as immediately as its color" (p. 138). Of course, the Gestalt psychologists earned their name for the core concept that the organization (Gestalt, whole) operates as the principal attractor in perception. However, in much of their work (studying the structural impact of physical factors such as proximity, similarity, continuation, and closure), the focus was less on behavioral meaning than on mathematical regularities inherent in the visual scene—types of structures that are indeed external.

I would rather see the role of meaning as an attractor that goes beyond the sensory surface, beyond the organization of percepts as it is dictated by the physical properties of the visual environment. Meaning would pertain to the level of objects and events, requiring information integration and implying a more active role for the observer. This involves cognition and memory, construction and reconstruction of information. I agree with Gibson that the perception of meaning and values is economical; not all the features of an object or an event have to be processed for it to be perceived. This is exactly where bias comes in. By relying on prior expectations, we can take shortcuts to percepts on the basis of minimal information—perhaps just a handful of sensory features. The biases are aimed at the most valuable meanings. As observers, we are minimalist theorists, working with as little evidence as seems reasonable in given circumstances. "Reasonable" here means sufficiently likely to produce a positive outcome (a correct perceptual judgment). The criteria for perception are flexible and subject to reinforcement. If the criteria are too loose and we take too many wrong turns, we revise our perceptual strategies—we tighten our criteria.

The orientation to meaning beyond the sensory surface implies that the word "direct" is out of place for this kind of perception. The bias for meaning and our sensorimotor interactions with the visual environment would conspire to activate percepts. This activation happens inside our heads as a cognitive product that cannot be reached without sensory stimulation or without a context of priors (a set of internal references to meanings). The appropriate word for such a process would be "indirect" — even more appropriate would be the word "interactive." The process might have somewhat Kantian characteristics; I will touch on this in chapter 5, where we continue our inquiry into the cognitive functions of vision. With the visual system as a mind-machine for meaning, I will outline an intensive approach, in which the gaze serves to achieve maximal processing in a limited area—a matter of force and emphasis, of *in* (toward) + *tendere* (stretch, tend), that is, "tending toward" a particular purpose or plan.

5   The Intensive Approach

A Box.

Out of kindness comes redness and out of rudeness comes rapid same question, out of an eye comes research, out of selection comes painful cattle. So then the order is that a white way of being round is something suggesting a pin and is it disappointing, it is not, it is so rudimentary to be analysed and see a fine substance strangely, it is so earnest to have a green point not to red but to point again.

Reading this text by Gertrude Stein again (as I must have dozens of times already) I continue to be mystified by the strange leaps and casual grammar—in a positive way, full of wonder. The effect it has on me is somewhat similar to that of the rocks and stones of Aoshima (see figure 4.7 in the previous chapter). The text, one of my favorite poems, belongs to the section "Objects" in Stein's 1913 collection *Tender Buttons* (here quoted from Stein, 2008, p. 128). Even today it reads as a rather radical experiment, one that pushes, perhaps crosses, the boundaries of the comprehensible, but it does so in a way that invites us to play along, to stretch toward the other side.

Trying to make sense of the poem, I find myself exploring various sequences of vaguely visual images. Some of the successive images are easily traceable as semantic associations: from "eye" to "research" and from "research" to "selection" (we could read them as general statements about human cognition). Other leaps are less obvious. They cut crucial links or deliberately take a sharp turn: from "selection" to "painful cattle," for instance. We have to fill the gap or straighten the story. I can imagine cows being picked for slaughter, and in hindsight, this image colors my reading of the sequence *eye–research–selection*; at the same time, the adjective "painful" looks awkwardly placed even though it gives me the image of cows on the way to the slaughterhouse—does this mean the emphasis is on the observer who suffers when seeing the poor cattle?

Yet other leaps are clearly derived from formal language features: a vowel shift, for instance, moving from "redness" to "rudeness," and the breaking up of "pin" into "disappointing," with alliteration and rhyme. Meanwhile the poem seems to talk about its own poetics, giving us advice about how to read it; "it is so rudimentary to be analysed and see a fine substance strangely." Especially the word "rudimentary" works mysteriously here, linking back to the earlier "rudeness" and suggesting that the act of analysis is only the first, immature step; why not go one step further? Beyond mere practical understanding, looking for, and seeing, the wonder of strangeness, in accordance with one of Stein's famous dictums: "If you enjoy it you understand it" (Stein, 2008, p. 10).

The last sentence of the poem exploits a (not very obvious) grammatical ambiguity with "to have a green point," where "green" can be read as a noun and "point" as a verb in order to connect it with the final "to point again." Then we arrive at an interpretation that implies the same advice as that of the preceding sentence, that is, to keep looking; we should not be disappointed or give in to redness (the stern teacher's corrections?) or rudeness but let the green do its business of pointing again until it speaks to us. The grammatical ambiguity of "to have a green point" takes us, with the cognitive psychologists Frazier and Rayner (1982), to *The Garden of Forking Paths* (the famous story by Jorge Luis Borges, 1998, first published in 1941). Readers' eye movements typically derail at such forks in the garden paths; the ambiguities are looked at longer and revisited more frequently than other words in the sentences (see also Ferreira & Henderson, 1990; Staub, 2011). In Stein's poem, this phenomenon of looking again at a grammatical ambiguity occurs at the very point (literally the word "point") where the poem calls for us to look again—it is a remarkable instance of iconicity, or similarity between form and meaning in language (a cherished topic in linguistics and literary theory, the subject of an entire book series, edited by Olga Fischer and Christina Ljungberg; e.g., Conradie et al., 2010; De Cuypere, 2008).

The idea that form and meaning can reverberate and reinforce each other toward an expansion of meaning and a more captivating form is fundamental in poetics, but it also teaches us something about perception in general. The multiplicities work only when we give them time to sink in, when we allow ourselves to look again and to intensify our information processing. The orientation to meaning beyond the sensory surface is a matter of intensity. We can increase the amount of processing by limiting the area (making a selection, as in Stein's sequence *eye–research–selection*) and by forcefully tending toward, or stretching for, meaning within that area. This is an intensive process that creates active percepts from the interaction between what we believe about the world (our expectations and biases) and what we find out about local, current aspects of the world by engaging in sensorimotor activity.

I Presuppose Therefore

Between what we believe about the world and what we find out by looking we create active percepts in the field of thought. This intensive process cannot escape the Kantian notion that "neither concepts without an intuition in some way corresponding to them, nor intuition without concepts can yield knowledge" (Kant, 1781|2007, p. 85). The two fundamental sources of knowledge must somehow work together: In Kant's worldview, intuition receives impressions, and cognition derives objects of thought from the impressions. Cognitive psychologists recognize the same sources of knowledge by talking about bottom-up versus top-down information processing, a tradition that can be traced back, in spirit if not in exact words, to William James (1890|1950a, 1890|1950b). Bottom-up processing would be automatic, under exogenous control (driven by salient physical features), that is, intuition receiving its impressions. Top-down processing would be voluntary, under endogenous control (determined by our objectives), that is, cognition deriving objects of thought.

My own favored conception of information processing, in terms of bias and sensitivity, does not quite overlap with this worldview. Our biases set expectations and favor options (e.g., percepts of objects) as a function of positive or negative prospects, familiarity, and proximity. These can be voluntary or implicit, active or passive, and so are not exactly the type of cognitive faculty that Kant connected with concepts or that cognitive psychologists routinely classify under top-down processing. Sensitivity refers to the quality of information extraction (the signal-to-noise ratio, or the veridicality of percepts), and this can be enhanced exogenously or endogenously—again orthogonal to Kant's worldview. Yet, in other ways, my conception with bias and sensitivity does partially overlap with Kant's proposals, particularly with respect to the necessity (or inevitability) of interaction between intuitions and concepts.

Biases are like concepts in that they project virtual information; they set the likelihood of percepts. Sensitivity works synergistically with sensory input and so receives impressions like intuition does. And like Kant's concepts and intuitions, bias and sensitivity operate interactively in perception, as I have emphasized in chapter 2. Hunches (bias) are checked up by collecting new evidence (sensitivity), hypotheses are tested, and contextual cues guide our gaze. Conversely, unexpected data (clear evidence from sensitivity) require us to rethink our mental models of things as they are (a reevaluation, possibly an adjustment, of our biases).

Ludwig Wittgenstein, to visit another unavoidable classic, casually said something similar in a beautifully crisp way that makes my head spin. It comes in the form of a rhetorical question: "Doesn't a presupposition imply a doubt?" The remark begins a new paragraph in section V of part II of *Philosophical Investigations* (1953|2003, p. 154^e)—a strange paragraph that talks about the behavior of a moving point, the study of behavior, the approach of psychology, and the tacit presuppositions in such study. From there, Wittgenstein makes a sudden leap (nearly as big as some of the leaps by Gertrude Stein), generalizing to tacit presuppositions in all "language games."

Doesn't a presupposition imply a doubt? A bias would not be a bias if it implied certainty. A bias would be a decision if it had no doubt. However, bias does *not* make decisions by itself. It is only a tendency, a readiness (in *The Anatomy of Bias*, I have suggested that bias often works as a disinhibition mechanism, a temporary removal of an otherwise ever-present blockage; Lauwereyns, 2010). It needs some trigger, some tiny bit of stimulus or excitation (however noisy), before it can translate to a decision (an overt action or a covert commitment, such as recognition or activation of a percept). Thus, presupposition does indeed imply doubt. Bias calls for sensitivity, for sensory evidence or lucid logic; expectations need to be confirmed or disconfirmed, or principally shown to be false.

While I am busy visiting the Absolute Beginners (to speak with a delightful rock musical film; British, 1986, by Julien Temple, with David Bowie), I should probably include René Descartes (a rock star of a different variety, who aimed "to reject shifting ground in the search for rock," 1637|2006, p. 25). Did he not connect doubt with the act of thinking and the very basis of our being? *Dubito ergo cogito ergo sum* is the paraphrase most often given. Descartes spoke more fully (three pages after the search for rock in *A Discourse on the Method*):

I came to think that I should [...] reject as completely false everything in which I could detect the least doubt, in order to see if anything thereafter remained in my belief that was completely indubitable. And so, because our senses sometimes deceive us, I decided to suppose that nothing was such as they lead us to imagine it to be. [...] But immediately afterwards I noted that, while I was trying to think of all things being false in this way, it was necessarily the case that I, who was thinking them, had to be something; and observing this truth: *I am thinking therefore I exist*, was so secure and certain that it could not be shaken by any of the most extravagant suppositions of the sceptics, I judged that I could accept it without scruple, as the first principle of philosophy that I was seeking.

I have deleted some of the doubts expressed by Descartes before he moved on to his metacognitive observation, that he was occupied by the act of doubting. Doubt produced the first principle of philosophy. With Wittgenstein, we can put presupposition before doubt: *I presuppose therefore I doubt therefore I think therefore I am* (or following Maclean's translation, *I am presupposing therefore I am doubting therefore I am thinking therefore I exist*).

Coming back to that other rock star, Kant, I feel tempted to posit bias not only as the first principle of philosophy but also as a synthetic a priori judgment, namely, *there must be something*; there is more than randomness or nothingness—there is meaning. It makes sense to say "therefore." Causal relations exist. Sometimes we can go from *this* to *that* (with the word "because," with the symbol of an arrow, or with a lateral gaze shift). All of our thinking revolves around our intrinsic bias toward meaning. Our complete being is focused on causal relations, on the fact that there are things that make sense, that we can discover the meaning of things. Even as fetus in mother's womb, our neural circuits are shaped by nurture, by experience. Our neurons are tuned for us to expect outcomes, to connect things with things.

Learning, the role of experience, only makes sense if there is sense to be made, if there is not just randomness. The knowledge that meaning exists and can be learned is with us, innately, as a *synthetic a priori* judgment, in Kant's vocabulary (1781|2007, pp. 37–43): This knowledge is a priori because our bias toward meaning is given beforehand; it does not itself depend on learning. It is *synthetic* because the predicate "learnable" is not directly part of, but connected with, the concept "meaning."

I would like to summarize this synthetic a priori judgment, my first principle of philosophy, with Descartes plus Kant plus Wittgenstein, as follows:

I presuppose *therefore*.

Everything begins with our biases. We are intrinsically tending toward meaning, stretching toward purposes. This basic stance is perhaps a sibling, or at least a distant cousin, of Daniel C. Dennett's *intentional stance* (1987). Dennett's stance suggests we treat others as agents who have beliefs and desires; their actions are interpreted to be *meant* or

purposive. Dennett sees us apply this stance toward humans and sometimes other animals, even "lower animals" such as frogs (1991, footnote
10 on p. 194). Thus, we would be able to read intentions into others'
actions, and the extent to which we engage in this kind of reading would
be under voluntary control. My proposal of a basic bias toward meaning
goes further than that. It is not limited to the interpretation of agents'
behaviors but applies to *all* interpretation.

Everything is interpreted as if it might have some kind of meaning,
regardless of any agent's intentions (whether human, animal, or god)—
meaning, here, is primarily antithetical to randomness, and it starts with
expecting some kind of regularity. Beyond this, there are a whole slew
of biases (the entire network of positive and negative prospects, familiarity fallacies, and proximity traps, a pandemonium of biases, latent and
occurrent); these give direction to the interpretation, actually fill in the
meaning of the expected regularity. The intentions of things would
be relatively autonomous, in the sense that they operate within the
observer, often without voluntary control by the observer, and often
without assumption of a particular agency responsible for bringing things
about. These intentions would be more like Gibson's (1979|1986) affor-
dances or like the intentions that Merleau-Ponty (1945|2008, p. 281)
noticed everywhere: "From every point in the primordial field intentions
move outwards, vacant and yet determinate; in realizing these intentions,
analysis will arrive at the object of science, at sensation as a private
phenomenon, and at the pure subject which posits both."

Realizing these intentions, these biases toward meaning, is indeed what
we need to do to arrive at a proper study of perception. The biases characterize the observer; they define the observer's subjectivity. In this
sense, the intentions are not absolutely autonomous; they are bound to
the observer, they belong to the observer. They are a core element in
what I call "the intensive approach" in perception. I prefer the word
"intensive" over "intentional" because the latter connects too strongly
with purposeful, deliberate behavior. Both "intensive" and "intentional"
trace back to the same etymological roots, but the word "intensive"
carries more meanings that fit my conception: not just the tending toward
meaning but also the notion of concentration or force (as in agricul-
ture, according to the Oxford Dictionaries Online, "aiming to achieve
maximum production in a limited area") and the connotations from
physics, where "intensive" denotes measurement in terms of intensity
(with important nonlinear properties; see DeLanda, 2002|2004, for a
fascinating introduction on the role of intensive processes and dynamics

in physics and philosophy). I also prefer the word "approach" over "stance" because the latter sounds too static. "Approach" emphasizes the deeply interactive, sensorimotor nature of perception.

The intensive approach to perception, with a fundamental role for observer-dependent biases, ultimately urges us to look deeply inside our heads to examine how we gain access to things as they are. This is, of course, why I keep sparring with the stimulating challenges offered by Alva Noë's (2004) radical externalist project. The challenges are badly needed. They sharpen our senses and allow us to apply different perspectives as we look inside our heads. Thanks to the externalist project, we are acutely aware of the dynamic, sensorimotor processes that cannot be captured in a simple input–output structure. We remain very much on the alert about the power of the outside world, the one and only store of its entire being, often (naturally) the best reminder of itself. At the same time, we recognize the economic nature of perception, the issues of value, of costs and benefits in processing, and the advantages offered by minimalism (exactly the place where biases come in—they minimize the amount of sensory evidence required). But here is also where the externalist project and I part company. I want more; I feel we have not started explaining anything until we talk about the actual mechanisms that perform the "processing" in information processing. Those mechanisms live inside our heads.

To understand how perception works, we need to study the biases in action, the mechanisms of the intensive approach. This does require us to take a peek inside, to examine what happens in neural circuits during covert information processing when we focus on some portion of the information available in the world. Tracking eye movements and analyzing the observer's own reports (say button presses or verbal descriptions) gives us food for phenomenology and functional taxonomy, but not enough clues to explain the underlying mechanisms. We need the phenomenology and functional taxonomy in combination with the neural: brain *and* the gaze. This obvious truth does not translate to obvious practice. For all the lip service about interdisciplinary projects, the real deal remains a rare event. Many philosophers of mind continue to be complacent about their extremely sketchy readings in neuroscience. Most artificial intelligence researchers, cognitive scientists, psychophysicists, and cognitive psychologists stick to their familiar tricks. All of these people really think only about the gaze. Conversely, the vast majority of neuroscientists remain highly skeptical of phenomenology, philosophy, and anything that smells like it might involve speculative thought or that strange faculty of virtual experimentation: imagination. These neuroscientists have never read a page of Merleau-Ponty or Žižek nor even of Dennett or Noë. They do not read *Psychological Review*. They study the brain, and we are lucky if they record some behavioral parameters while they are at it.

My advice is simple and more a matter of creating habits than of making efforts. Philosophers: Pay more attention to neuroscience (actually *read* just one article a month from *Neuron* or *Journal of Neuroscience*). Neuroscientists: Practice reading (actually *read* even as little as four books a year, at least one of which should be fiction and one philosophical). If we cannot read each other, we may as well forget about studying perception. It is absurd to address the interactive processes of perception without exploring the agents in the interaction. No perception without brain. No perception without the gaze. Now then, having talked a good chunk of philosophy in this chapter, and having ranted about laziness in reading, we are more than ready (eager!) to enter the inner chamber, the brain.

Entering the Inner Chamber

I propose to aim straightaway for the inner chamber of the inner chamber: the thalamus (from the Greek *thalamos*, "inner chamber" or "bedroom," also "the receptacle of a flower," according to the Online Etymology Dictionary). The brain structure that we call "thalamus" apparently owes its name to Galen, the great anatomist of antiquity (the reference to Galen was made by E. G. Jones in his massive two-volume book about the thalamus, which I confess not to have read; I got the reference from Saalmann & Kastner, 2011). It is not a trivial inner chamber of the brain. We encountered it already in chapter 4, with the work by Wurtz and colleagues on internal monitoring, corollary discharge, and predictive remapping. There we focused on the medial dorsal nucleus and its function in the pathway from the superior colliculus (in the midbrain) to the FEF (in the cortex). This is just one of several thalamic structures that play heavily in the interactive processes of perception.

Already in 1932 Le Gros Clark proposed that the cortex critically depends on the thalamus, a statement vigorously reinforced by Saalmann and Kastner (2011) in their review of the cognitive and perceptual functions of the visual thalamus. The thalamus and the cortex are really one hybrid system, in which much of the input to the cortex comes via the thalamus, even a significant portion of the corticocortical information processing (i.e., projections from one part of the cortex to another; see Theyel, Llano, & Sherman, 2010, and Wróbel et al., 2007, for very different but equally compelling types of evidence). The relations between the thalamus and the cortex, and within thalamic structures, are extremely complex, with projections to multiple cortical areas from many of the thalamic structures. The thalamus and the cortex together create a host of parallel circuits that feed information back with reentrant connections in strange loops.

The thalamus, then, is perfectly placed to modulate what goes on in the cortex. Judging from its anatomical connections alone, the thalamus seems the ideal site to install tools for selective information processing — gain mechanisms, gating mechanisms, filters, switches, and so forth. Francis Crick (yes, of Crick and Watson, who taught us the structure of the DNA molecule) formulated this hypothesis in 1984 (see Singer, 1977, for a precedent) and offered it as a core element in his explanation of consciousness and the soul (*The Astonishing Hypothesis*, 1994|1995 — not a bad book but doomed from the start by the silly title). Scientific evidence that the thalamus does indeed process information selectively depending on task requirements emerged around the same time from monkey single-unit studies (e.g., Petersen, Robinson, & Keys, 1985; Robinson, Peterson, & Keys, 1986). An early human imaging study (using positron emission tomography) provided converging data (LaBerge & Buchsbaum, 1990).

These early studies focused on selective spatial processing in a visual thalamic structure called the "pulvinar." Among visual thalamic structures, the pulvinar is the largest and the one most extensively and reciprocally connected with the cortex. Other specifically visual thalamic structures are the LGN (further divided into magnocellular vs. parvocellular) and the thalamic reticular nucleus (TRN). The LGN gets input from the retina but also from the primary visual cortex and several subcortical structures — including inhibitory input from the TRN. McAlonan, Cavanaugh, and Wurtz (2008) found that these structures also exhibit correlates of selective spatial processing (see figure 5.1). The magnocellular LGN showed subtle enhancement with selective spatial processing in the first peak of activity in response to visual stimulation. The activity in the parvocellular LGN started later; here, the enhancement with selective spatial processing was stronger and more sustained. The response in the TRN went in the other direction, with suppression as a function of selective processing. Particularly for the first peak of activity, it looked very much like there was reciprocal modulation between the LGN and

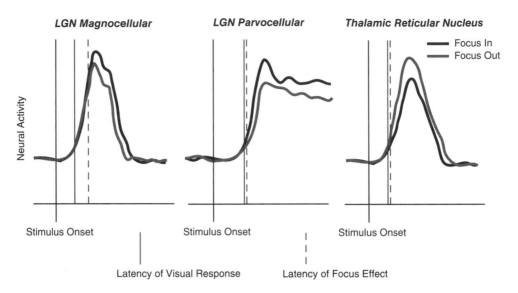

LGN Magnocellular   **LGN Parvocellular**   **Thalamic Reticular Nucleus**

Neural Activity

Focus In
Focus Out

Stimulus Onset   Stimulus Onset   Stimulus Onset

Latency of Visual Response   Latency of Focus Effect

Figure 5.1
Effects of selective spatial processing in the visual thalamus (based on McAlonan, Cavanaugh, & Wurtz, 2008). The main findings are presented for magnocellular lateral geniculate nucleus (LGN; left graph), parvocellular LGN (middle graph), and the thalamic
reticular nucleus (right panel). The three types of neurons show distinct patterns of modulation as a function of the focus of "attention," in terms of the onset and the duration of the
activity, as well as the direction of the effect (suppression vs. facilitation).

the TRN. This effect of selective processing happened on the first
pass from the retina to the cortex—there was no possibility of cortical
influence.

These are striking data, in line with Crick's (1984) predictions, which
received a prominent citation in the abstract (the name Crick appeared
in full, instead of the usual little superscript number). But before we run
too astonishingly far with the data, it is useful to describe the behavioral
procedure in detail so we get a concrete idea about just what kinds of
attention, consciousness, and soul-searching we are talking about. The
monkeys (sitting, head restrained) were required to fixate their gaze at
the center of the screen, where a cue appeared: either a vertical or horizontal bar. This cue served as the sample stimulus. A quarter of a second
later, two other stimuli were presented in the periphery, one inside and
one outside the receptive field of whichever neuron was being recorded.
One of these two stimuli matched the sample stimulus; the other did not.
These two stimuli always appeared at the same positions within a recording session; only the sample stimulus varied on a trial-by-trial basis,
sometimes a vertical bar, sometimes horizontal (given the fixed positions

of the peripheral stimuli, the sample stimulus at the center effectively served as a directional cue). The monkeys had to concentrate their visual processing on the target that matched the sample stimulus while maintaining their gaze fixated on the center (i.e., covert selective visual processing). After between half a second and one second, either the matching stimulus or the other stimulus might dim (around 40% reduction in luminance). The likelihood of dimming was 50% and independent for the two stimuli (so there was a 25% chance that both dimmed; 25% that neither dimmed). The monkeys had to move their eyes to the matching stimulus when it dimmed in order to obtain a reward. If there was no dimming, or if the other stimulus dimmed, the correct response was to maintain fixation at the center. The monkeys would do this for hundreds of trials in an afternoon.

This kind of procedure has all the hallmarks of an elegant Wurtz-like paradigm (this should not surprise us: Wurtz was the senior author of the paper). The types of processing involved are extremely lucid and straightforward: detecting a change in luminance at a specific position in space, selected as function of visual similarity among simple orientation stimuli. The task neatly controls for factors such as retinal eccentricity. It guarantees us that the monkey's performance can be no accident: If the monkey can reliably make correct responses, then he (or something inside him) must have done the right computational work (which is relatively easy to model). The behavior must be oriented to a reward, task dependent, and under voluntary control (if the monkey has had enough juice, he will stop working; he gets to go back to his cage).

However, what does the paradigm tell us about "attention" or "consciousness"? We may wish to be careful with those words. Once again—I cannot help harping on this point—I believe "attention" is too vague a concept in contemporary psychology and neuroscience. Worse, it is downright misleading if it comes with the tacit assumption that effects of selective information processing reflect improved visual discrimination, implying an increase in the signal-to-noise ratio (i.e., sensitivity, which is what most researchers associate with "attention"). Effects of selective processing often derive from *indiscriminate* increase in activity as a function of anticipation—not better information extraction but differentially weighted information (i.e., bias). The behavioral paradigm used in the study by McAlonan, Cavanaugh, and Wurtz (2008) in principle allowed the monkeys to orient their spatial selective processing to the target location before the target actually arrived; the monkeys could anticipate the target, and this could create biased information processing

(Downing, 1988; Lauwereyns, 2010): "virtual projection" instead of, or in addition to, "actual extraction."

Looking inside the monkeys' heads, the neural codes for the target region in the visual field might have been activated on the basis of internally generated information (anticipation) before, or independent of, any influences of sensory input. In this regard, the time window of 250 milliseconds between the onset of the sample stimulus and that of the peripheral stimuli is interesting because it is right around the length of time it usually takes for humans to orient "attention" from a central cue (e.g., Cheal & Lyon, 1991; Cheal, Lyon, & Gottlob, 1994; Eriksen & Collins, 1969). If anything, monkeys might be a bit faster than humans when it comes to this kind of simple visual spatial processing. So, are the effects in the study by McAlonan, Cavanaugh, and Wurtz (2008) due to bias or sensitivity?

We cannot tell for sure. It does look like the effects of selective processing emerge after, and are triggered by, the onset of the target stimulus; this would be suggestive of synergy with sensory input (a typical property of sensitivity). However, it does not rule out an additional role (or even a leading role) for bias. The authors offer no behavioral analysis, and the neural data cannot be interpreted in terms of additive or multiplicative effects (signatures of bias vs. sensitivity; Lauwereyns, 2010). Instead, the paper uncritically talks of measuring attention mechanisms and supporting Francis Crick's ideas. It is not necessarily wrong, but less precise than we would wish for, especially in the case of such a beautiful and important study.

As for "consciousness," that (even more) elusive concept may not apply at all. Often we perform very complex, task-dependent actions without being fully aware of them. You may not remember, but perhaps you parked your car, got out of your car, locked it, walked out of the garage, and nodded hello to one of your neighbors, all the while deeply absorbed by this chapter 5 of *Brain and the Gaze*. You may suddenly find yourself in front of the sliding doors to the entrance hall of your apartment block and realize with a start that you must have somehow navigated your way all the way here. But did you actually lock the car?

In one out of ten cases, when I ask myself a similar question, I did not lock the car. Often I can honestly not tell whether I performed the action, and that is why I do have to go back and check (that, plus the fact that I estimate there to be a certain usefulness to locking my car in the society where I live, even if it is Japan, and even if car theft is much less likely here than in other parts of the world). Yet, in the sequence from parking my car to arriving at the sliding doors, I would have successfully completed a set of complex sensorimotor processes that require a minimum of online, context-dependent control to adapt to the local metrics on a particular day. This might mean that some behavior—even if it is oriented to reward, task dependent, and under some amount of voluntary control—does not qualify as entailing "consciousness."

I am not implying that the monkeys in the study by McAlonan, Cavanaugh, and Wurtz (2008) were deeply absorbed by this chapter 5 of *Brain and the Gaze* (admittedly, that would logically be impossible; this chapter did not yet exist at the time the monkeys were making their eye movements). But we should at least acknowledge the possibility that consciousness played little or no part in the monkeys' task performance, either because their minds were elsewhere or because they did not have the kinds of minds that support the type of consciousness we think of as "consciousness." We are still lacking a solid operational definition of consciousness. This is not good news, nor necessarily bad news. Perhaps consciousness is simply one of those wishy-washy words like inspiration and imagination that we should entertain as language games—closer to poetry than to science. Perhaps these language games play with families of phenomena, which must be teased apart and broken up to particulars if we want operational definitions. In the meantime, let us continue playing the games in all their breadth *and* move on with Wurtz-like studies to address the phenomena one by one. The games give ideas; the Wurtz-like studies are the way to test which ideas hold up under what conditions.

Echo Variations

The study by MacAlonan, Cavanaugh, and Wurtz (2008) was a natural extension of the work by Wurtz and colleagues on internal monitoring and predictive remapping in the thalamus. This progression sets the right example. It is high noon for us, in the Fred Zinnemann/Gary Cooper sense of that expression, to deal with the old villains, the gang of killers, the artificial partitions of sensory versus motor processes. We must study the mechanisms of covert selective processing in conjunction with those of corollary discharge and all the so-called "motor" aspects of eye movements. Wurtz and colleagues (2011) made a first gesture toward outlining the full scope of active vision in the thalamus. In comparison, the review by Saalmann and Kastner (2011) offers a more comprehensive but also more restrictive view of active vision in *visual* thalamus, based on preconceived anatomical borders (still too soft on the old villains of input–output structure).

However, Saalmann and Kastner (2011) do a great job of chasing away another set of recurrent demons. Reading their review, even the most skeptical traditionalist will have to admit that the thalamus is most certainly not a mere relay station that passively transmits information to the cortex. Several important human fMRI studies from the Kastner lab (e.g., O'Connor et al., 2002; Schneider et al., 2004) contributed directly to the revival of interest in the thalamus, showing that task factors modulate the strength of the BOLD response to visual stimulation, sometimes even in advance of visual stimulation—a telltale sign of bias. Other studies show that not only does the response magnitude change but so do the firing mode (e.g., Bezdudnaya et al., 2006; Fanselow et al., 2001) and the synchrony (e.g., Wróbel et al., 2007). All of these studies together create the critical mass that will help us break bad habits in thinking about perception and consciousness as Dennett urged us two decades ago (1991, p. 316): "We must break the habit of positing ever-more-central observers."

We break the habit by realizing that information is not simply passed on from one neural structure to another—no relaying from observer to ever-more-central observer. Every neural projection changes the information, takes care of a portion of the perceptual work. There is no recursion of exact copies; every echo is a variation, an abstraction. As the thalamus contributes to perception, modulating information with the aim of completing a task, it does what Wallace Stevens decreed poetry must do in his great poem *Notes toward Supreme Fiction* (1954|1984): be abstract, change, give pleasure. In the supreme fiction of vision (which we call "the truth"), a part of the poetry happens in the inner chamber of the thalamus. Here poetry means the art of making ideas. It happens not in a Cartesian Theater, but through a complex network of parallel projections that transform, convert, integrate, and/or combine information, producing activity that competes, cooperates, or merely coincides with other activity. There is no single place, no precise point where all these projections come together to trigger perception or consciousness. Instead, perception lives in the distribution of the activity, in the intensities of different neural responses across various regions in the brain. The only observer is the whole person, with his or her entire brain. Consciousness is the nonlinear product of what lives in the brain at a given moment in time, with active boundaries for "in" and "out"—boundaries that resist being drawn and that change in the drawing.

The parallel activities of various echoes imply a multiplicity of coding, with distinct populations of neurons contributing to different representations, or even single neurons contributing to different representations as we already discussed for retinal ganglion cells in chapter 3. By "representation" I mean a correspondence to information, where the information is itself an abstraction of *something* (a "content-fixation" in the parlance of Dennett and the philosophy of intentionality; see *The Intentional Stance*, 1987). The abstraction varies in complexity and dimensions from simple visual features at a certain position at a certain moment (the color of a patch in the left upper quadrant of my visual field at this very moment) to complex combinations over a range of positions in a particular time window (a performance of *The Nutcracker* on a Sunday afternoon at my local community center or my lunch spread out in front of me). Some abstractions are so radically abstract we can probably declare them to be nonvisual (say, the figure of the Eternal Return in the writings of Nietzsche, or Cantor's concept of transfinite numbers). However, the extent to which certain representations relate to vision is not always clear. Obviously visual are the simple features, remaining close to traceable characteristics of light bouncing off surfaces. But very soon we move into territory where the objects of what we see by virtue of contact with visual information are in fact supreme fiction—real all right, but only organized as units in our perception (i.e., the tracing to patterns of light becomes ever more idiosyncratic; is this grain of rice that fell off my plate still part of my lunch or not anymore?).

The neural representations, then, are pieces (not digital bits) of information active in the brain. The intensity of the neural activity quite literally (linearly) determines the strength of the representation. The neural activity also contributes to the likelihood that the representation plays an active role in our perception (including attention and consciousness) and in our behavior—the relation between neural activity and its overt or covert selection can occasionally be linear but will in most situations be nonlinear, as a complex function of competition with alternative representations. I offer this proposal as a *hypothesis*—but one that already receives important preliminary support from a host of studies. These studies connect modulation in neural activity in response to visual features (whether relating to bias, sensitivity, or both) with modulation of behavioral performance in response to those visual features (I could probably cite dozens of papers here, but let me pick a nonrandom handful: Bisley & Goldberg, 2003; Cohen & Maunsell, 2010; Huddleston & DeYoe, 2008; Lauwereyns et al., 2002a; Nobre, Rao, & Chelazzi, 2006;

Polk et al., 2008). I am happy to note that, slowly but steadily, this empirical work is moving toward a more mathematically oriented treatment of the relationships between neural activity and behavior—the only way we will be able to get a handle on the complex dynamics. General topology is still a long way off, but some papers start talking about linear versus nonlinear mechanisms.

Most of the cited studies, however, are rather sketchy about the nature of the representation, or the actual content that is being fixed during content fixation. Researchers usually connect differences between stimulus features to differences in neural activity without any further concern about which information is effectively represented by the neural activity. The temptation is to say "the activity codes the stimulus" and then to take for granted that the activity codes the entire thing. This approach is particularly tricky for complex stimuli, which could be distinguished in any number of ways from alternative stimuli in the set. In such cases, we cannot really tell *what* the neural activity codes (how much information it takes in from the stimulus and how much it leaves out in the world) unless we systematically probe the various stimulus features involved. It is an issue that neuroscientists generally would do well to consider more carefully.

To represent information via activity in neural circuits is really a matter of laying down a trace that affords recombination with information elsewhere in the brain, for instance, derived from other sensory modalities. The representation becomes an element that can factor into various configurations. Such configurations imply hierarchical organization, with representations composed of other representations. The higher-order representation does not necessarily require the continued or complete activation of all elements that belong to the configuration. I insert this remark thinking of the Gestalt psychologists' take on holism but also Dennett's favorite topic of "filling in," to which I will turn in the next section.

The representations do not only lay down traces for recombination. They also afford activation or reactivation in their own right, presenting information again in a new context, or bringing it back from past to present. Such reactivation can be externally induced by (or in synergy with) what is physically going on in the world. This does not equal the concept of bottom-up processing in cognitive psychology nor that of intuition in Kant's worldview: The reactivation can be the result of voluntary control when we deliberately choose to revisit certain information in the world—in that case we guide our sensory receptors so as to enable externally induced reactivation. Some representations can also be internally generated without physical stimulation, via implicit associations or explicit recall, either to reconstruct a past episode ("memory"), to anticipate a future event ("prediction"), or to create a new object ("imagination"). Of course, there are limitations to how much information we can and do reactivate or represent.

The extent of the limitations and how we work with them is first and foremost an empirical question. On the topic of echo variations, one of the most often invoked phenomena relating to consciousness and vision is that of rivalry with ambiguous images—the famous Rubin vases, Necker cubes, rabbits that turn into ducks, and so on. In neuroscience the case of binocular rivalry has been studied most extensively: the competition that occurs when each eye gets a different image (taking the parallax to the extreme, so that there can be no integration or unifying interpretation; see Blake & Logothetis, 2001, for review). Sabine Kastner and her colleagues (Wunderlich, Schneider, & Kastner, 2005) have also for this phenomenon observed critical modulation in the LGN, which indicates that the activity in this part of the inner chamber tracks what we see (our percepts) rather than solely what the eye receives (the classic caricature of sensory input).

In general for all types of visual competition, when we make no specific effort to focus on either of two competing images, they will oscillate and take turns drifting in and out of consciousness. Even when we deliberately try to pick one rather than the other, it may be hard to do, especially in the case of binocular rivalry—unless we are primed with object cues (Mitchell, Stoner, & Reynolds, 2004). In the case of ambiguous figures that overlap in space (and across both eyes), the gaze may be instrumental in maintaining the continuity of a percept or in eliciting a reversal. The best studied example of this type is the Necker cube (the transparent cube with corners that look to be closer or farther away than other corners relative to the observer's viewpoint). Louis Albert Necker himself (a crystallographer, geographer, and mountaineer, interested in all kinds of strange optical effects and illusions) had hinted at a possible role of eye movements in the perception of his cube almost two centuries ago (Necker, 1832).

Contemporary psychophysics appears to agree, suggesting that gaze shifts serve to erase the prior percept and that the position of gaze fixation modulates the strength of the current percept (Einhäuser, Martin, & König, 2004; Ross & Ma-Wyatt, 2004). Thus, the gaze becomes a tool that benefits the higher-order aspects of perception beyond the initial acquisition of visual information. It works toward conscious processing, indexing objects, and keeping representations active long after patterns of light first impressed their forms upon our retinas.

Filling In

Patterns of light can, of course, also continue impressing upon our retinas to the point that we see afterimages—yet another variation in the echoing visual representations. Figure 5.2 provides the materials for a good demonstration. If you have the time and access, it would be worth your while to check the original paper by Shimojo, Kamitani, and Nishida (2001) from which I borrowed the concept for the figure. The authors offer not only a very detailed and considered explanation but also a set of figures in color, which makes for significantly more drama. However, even without color, you should be able to get curious afterimages from figure 5.2 if you follow the instructions (given in the figure caption). I would like to highlight three aspects of these afterimages.

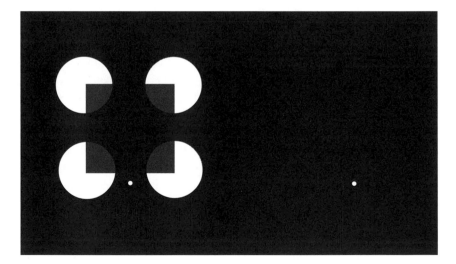

Figure 5.2
Stimulus display for strange afterimages (adapted from Shimojo, Kamitani, & Nishida, 2001). Please fixate your gaze at the small white dot on the left, surrounded by the four disks with gray patches. Hold your gaze strictly there for at least twenty seconds, fully concentrated on the display, and then shift to the small white dot on the right. Savor your wonderful visions. You might sometimes see the disks complete, sometimes partially occluded, sometimes nothing at all, and if you really look hard, perhaps occasionally you might even see a square surface entirely separated from the disks. The disks may come and go two or three times over the course of several seconds. Feel free to repeat this experiment a number of times (but perhaps not more than four or five, or you might start feeling a bit dizzy).

First, even though I gave you only a static figure, your afterimages are dynamic. You may see two or three different types (four complete disks, four partial disks with a square surface over them, perhaps even a square surface by itself). These different afterimages oscillate; it may happen that one moment you see the four disks, then no afterimage at all, next the return of the disks. The afterimages will drift in and out of your consciousness beyond your control. All you can do is look as intensely as possible and hope they keep coming.

Second, the afterimages are multiple. To be sure, this was implied already in my first point, but it is an important observation and neatly separable from the temporal dynamics. We get *different* afterimages, implying the existence of parallel and competing representations. The representations create a kind of rivalry that shares commonalities with binocular rivalry and other types of visual competition. Intriguingly, the competition between complete, isolated disks versus partially occluded disks indicates that we have parallel representations, constructed at different levels of visual analysis: before and after the segregation of surfaces. The partial disks plus a square surface are consistent with a simplistic view of afterimages as floating negatives due to the consumption of retinal resources. However, the complete disks, without the square surface, do not quite fit that old story. They imply a representation at a level after surface segregation.

Shimojo and colleagues (2001) attributed the surface segregation to the cortex, but given the smarts of the retina (as we discussed in chapter 3), I believe a second-order retinal representation is at least as likely, perhaps operating in concert with the LGN to prolong the competition with a first-order retinal representation. In this regard, it is also relevant to note that there was no interocular transfer of the afterimages—if you look at the figure with your left eye only, and then shift to the empty space, you can see the afterimages with your left eye, but not your right. Yet, interocular transfer is what we should expect if the surface segregation was done in cortex because visual projections from both eyes converge already in the LGN. Shimojo and colleagues struggled to marry the lack of interocular transfer with a cortical explanation, but it makes perfect sense if the surface segregation was already accomplished in the retina.

The dynamics and the multiplicity are fascinating. However, the fact that we can see complete disks, without the square surface, points to something more than just higher-order segregation of surfaces. It suggests a filled-in surface. Something made the partial disks look like complete disks. This is my third point: the filling in. With color figures, it is also possible (or much more easily possible) to get an afterimage of a complete square surface floating by itself—a considerably more impressive instance of filling in (I must admit I cannot see an afterimage of the square surface with figures in grayscale though my postdoc says he can; in color, however, even I get the filled-in square surface very clearly).

With this third point, I realize I am moving into very dangerous territory. "This idea of *filling in* is common in the thinking of even sophisticated theorists, and it is a dead giveaway of vestigial Cartesian materialism," warned Dennett (1991, p. 344). Noë added that "the quick inference to the existence of a process of filling in is fallacious; it commits the homunculus fallacy" (2004, pp. 46–47). The insertion of *quick inference* is critical here. We shall be careful not to commit that crime. Noë (2004, p. 238), however, did appreciate the study by Shimojo et al. (2001) and asked for direct evidence of a neural process of filling in. Just such evidence started emerging around the time, or even a bit before, Noë's landmark work (De Weerd et al., 1995; Huang & Paradiso, 2008; Komatsu, Kinoshita, & Murakami, 2000; Matsumoto & Komatsu, 2005). For instance, Matsumoto and Komatsu showed that V1 neurons with receptive fields embedded in the blind spot respond to line segments presented there.

Heavy-duty computational studies are now able to provide very reasonable algorithms that explain both the neural data and the perceptual phenomena of filling in (e.g., Supèr & Romeo, 2011). They do so without the help of magic but with the kind of systematic operations that circuits of flickering bits of electricity can achieve. This does not mean that we now are bringing in the Cartesian Theater. It simply means we have yet one more representation active among all the others in the complex circuitry of the brain, and this extra one happens to be filled in. Why should the brain bother filling in, instead of simply ignoring whatever is missing and thereby saving time and energy? This is the (very pertinent) question asked by Dennett (1991). "I don't want to prejudge the question," he writes (p. 353), but he ends up doing so anyway two pages later, without a single look at any empirical data ("So now we can answer our question about the blind spot. The brain doesn't have to 'fill in' for the blind spot," p. 355).

Admittedly, logically, at first sight, the brain should not have to fill in. However, in truth, the brain does fill in—in some cases. If we think a bit deeper about the issue, we might find reasons for filling in after all. Perhaps it facilitates the salience of representations that are useful for further visual and semantic analysis. If this sounds like putting up a show for a central observer, it really is not: It is simply bringing a good chunk of information into the complex dynamics of processing, ready to be changed, abstracted, and reutilized for other representations. Filling in might make for more stable elements in the hierarchical organization with second- or higher-order representations. There could be negative reasons as well: to prevent disruptions. A lack of firing in a particular neuron could hamper the generation of waves in a neural circuit. For brain waves to propagate information, it might sometimes be necessary that local elements "play along." If you are sitting in a packed football stadium where tens of thousands of people are doing the Mexican Wave (or *La Ola*), you might find yourself doing your part before you know it (see Farkas, Helbing, & Vicsek, 2002, for an interesting analysis of the dynamics underlying the Mexican Wave).

We do have reason to believe that filling in has an important role to play in building certain kinds of representation. This does not mean we fall prey to the homunculus fallacy or the Cartesian Theater. We need to be ready to consider where and when filling in makes sense if we wish to provide a complete explanation of how neurons represent information in the process of perception. I completely agree with Dennett (1991, pp. 354–355) that we do not fill in all the Marilyns when we walk into a room and notice that the wallpaper is full of her. I wholeheartedly endorse Dennett's explanation: "Having identified a single Marilyn, and having received no information to the effect that the other blobs are not Marilyns, [the brain] jumps to the conclusion that the rest are Marilyns, and labels the whole region 'more Marilyns' without any further rendering of Marilyn at all." I am particularly happy to note the role attributed to bias (the jumping to the conclusion). And it must be true that the representation of "more Marilyns" occurs at a different level than that of the visual detail that prompted the identification of the first.

For complex representations such as those of faces, it is safe to think we do not fill in, but for simple ones we do. Why? It must be due to particular characteristics of how the information is represented. We know that processing goes from simple to complex along the ventral stream. Importantly, the receptive field sizes change along with the complexity, from very small receptive fields for simple information in the primary visual cortex to very large receptive fields for complex information in the inferior temporal cortex (Desimone et al., 1984; Gattass, Sousa, & Gross, 1988; Gattass, Gross, & Sandell, 1981). Face processing occurs at a level in the visual system that has very wide receptive fields.

Presumably, face representations are activated by the combination (the converging projections) of lower-level representations.

The local spatial information is abstracted out by the time the analysis starts pertaining to face configurations. We need no filling in at such levels of abstraction and complexity—here the brain simply has no use for such detail, and it would only be a waste of valuable resources to implement the redundancy. However, for the simple features, the case is different. Receptive field sizes are small; gaps in the spatial resolution can hurt the representations. It may be useful for a neuron to fire spikes even if it receives no firsthand evidence, only excitation from its neighbors. This could reflect a lateral spread of activation, a bias effect within one module, not unlike the bias effect Dennett saw possible with the Marilyns in a vertical sense, from a lower-level module to a higher-level one.

"The fundamental flaw in the idea of "filling in" is that it suggests the brain is providing something when in fact the brain is ignoring something," writes Dennett (1991, p. 356), and in the next sentence he adds a rather ugly remark about "crashing mistakes" by even very sophisticated thinkers (Žižek, 2006|2009, p. 232, speaks of Dennett's "usual acerbic style"). I thought of the dog ridiculing the cat for being hairy (a Vietnamese idiom) or (the Greek counterpart of the same phrase) the donkey saying to the rooster, "Your head is too big." The fundamental flaw would be to think that there is always and necessarily a fundamental flaw in the idea of "filling in." We must avoid making those crashing mistakes by keeping our eyes wide open and carefully collecting data, looking to see when and how filling in *does* happen.

Magnitude and Duration

From the empirical work on filling in, we learn that the visual system makes representations of information at different levels of abstraction. These representations can coexist, with lower levels remaining active even when higher levels have already emerged. The brain does not necessarily discard first-order representations once they have served for second-order analysis. The continued life of first-order representations may serve a purpose in some cases, enabling not just one but several divergent types of higher-order analysis. The lifetime of first-order representations, you might suspect, depends on context and task demands. Your suspicion is correct, as demonstrated by Supèr, Spekreijse, and Lamme (2001) with

Sequence of Events

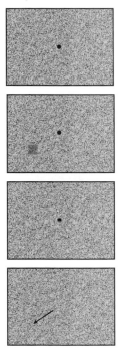

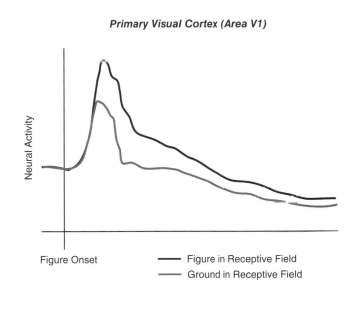

Figure 5.3
Working memory in primary visual cortex (after Supèr, Spekreijse, & Lamme, 2001). The left panels give the sequence of events (from top to bottom) in the behavioral task. The monkeys had to maintain their gaze at the fixation spot, embedded in a display with random dots ("the ground"). Then, the dots within a small area briefly moved ("the figure"). The monkeys had to keep the target area in mind ("working memory") and delay doing anything about it until the fixation spot disappeared. At this time, the monkeys had to make a saccade to the target area. The graph on the right shows that the neural activity in primary visual cortex maintained a higher level of activity for figure over ground throughout the waiting period.

task-dependent sustained activity in primary visual cortex even when the original stimulus has long gone (see figure 5.3).

The authors of the work in question suggested that the sustained activity reflects "working memory." The monkeys had to remember the position of a briefly presented motion stimulus (a set of moving random dots in a small window in the periphery) so that they could make a saccade to it after a delay period of maybe one second or more. The stimulus itself was flashed for only two video frames (28 milliseconds), but neurons in primary visual cortex whose receptive field overlapped with the stimulus showed a stronger response than neurons with receptive fields elsewhere. This enhanced response lasted for the entire delay period while the monkey fixated his gaze at the center. For old-school thinkers, the data must have been mindboggling: a sustained response in primary visual cortex to something that simply was no longer there to be sensed. Was this a case of "seeing things," or if not, then what? At the very least, no one could escape the conclusion that some kind of representation was being kept active.

The most likely mechanism would be a feedback loop, involving the thalamus and cortical structures upstream in the dorsal pathway (likely candidates include lateral intraparietal cortex and the FEF). What we do not know is the exact nature (or the level of abstraction) of the information contained in the representation. It could be a fairly detailed description of the motion stimulus, including information about direction, speed, texture, and so on. However, it could also be nothing more than a position index, that is, the minimal information required for a correct behavioral response. The latter interpretation would be consistent with the view of Awh and Jonides (2001) on a similar behavioral paradigm: They propose a role for "spatial attention," operating as a subroutine of working memory to maintain information active without performing any computations on it. Suggestions such as these allow us to move to the desirable middle ground, somewhere between the categorical denial of information representation and the unchecked assumption that the representation captures all the information carried by the stimulus.

That middle ground is extremely important. We need to explore it empirically. The construction and continued existence of representations at different levels of abstraction is *the* core question according to the intensive approach. It is a question about what happens in the brain while we are focused, overtly or covertly, on stimuli in the world. The intensive approach works from the hypothesis that the length of time and the amount of effort we spend gazing at information matters, well beyond the acquisition of sensory features and well after all the line orientations, textures, and colors have been detected and discriminated at a particular point of fixation.

The hypothesis calls for us to consider factors such as the magnitude and duration of neural activity that codes sensory and higher-level features. This is an important point that often slips through the cracks. For instance, Dennett (1991) repeatedly claims "that the brain only has to make its discriminations once; a feature identified doesn't have to be redisplayed for the benefit of a master appreciator in the Cartesian

Theater" (these exact words are from p. 292, but similar remarks recur in the book). Of course, Dennett is right to defend us against our worst nightmare of a master appreciator in a Cartesian Theater. However, the brain does not make its discriminations just once, without passing on information.

The magnitude and duration of neural activity crucially determines the accessibility of sensory features for further processing (not by a master appreciator but by the rest of the brain). This does not rhyme with the suggestion that "the brain only has to make its discriminations once"—a suggestion that, at least to my ears, sounds too much like a digital, all-or-none state transition. That is how a serial Von Neumann machine (our contemporary concept of a computer) may operate, but not the brain with its chaotic, nonlinear processes, with all kinds of things happening in various places, where timing and coincident input is of the essence and information processing cannot be translated to a linear sequence by knitting back and forth (contrary to what Dennett, 1991, pp. 217–218, suggested).

When we keep information in active vision, we increase our opportunities to analyze it, to see it in the context of what we know and what we remember, and to read new meanings into it. We can do this by holding the stimulus in our gaze or by maintaining whichever representations we have of it as best we can, especially in case the stimulus is no longer there to be gazed at. In the usual order of things, we would prefer to aim our gaze at the object of our interest. This gives the higher-order analysis a push. It provides us with a constant supply of sensory detail pertaining to the relevant stimulus, and this facilitates the maintenance of lower-level representations. It also means we have to spend less effort guarding the information against competing stimuli. It is much easier for us to think about a painting by Magritte when we are looking at that very painting in an art book than when we are watching the evening news on TV. Thinking and looking naturally reinforce each other. When they converge on the same thing, we devote the maximum amount of resources to analyzing the object of our interest.

Put differently, there is more to the gaze than its spatial coordinates—not just where we look (gaze position) but how long (gaze duration) and how hard (gaze magnitude). If "gaze magnitude" sounds slightly depressing from an eye-tracking perspective, I would like to suggest that it may actually be expressed metrically in the gaze, via pupil size. This notion has had a turbulent history in science ever since it was first presented by Hess and Polt (1960) in famous work (rife with prejudices) about women's increasing their pupil sizes for pictures of mothers with babies, but not for pictures of nude women (the four male subjects in the tiny sample produced the reverse pattern of data). The follow-up article by Hess and Polt (1964) linked pupil size with mental effort in a problem-solving task. Kahneman (1973) even suggested that pupil size was *the* best measure for effort.

The basic idea is that pupil size reflects a physiological response. An increase in arousal, fear, attention, interest, or mental effort—in one word: intensity—would activate the adrenergic sympathetic nervous system, leading to pupil dilation (whereas pupil constriction depends on the cholinergic parasympathetic nervous system; Barbur, 2004). Nobody really knows whether this physiological response is a by-product of our anatomy or whether evolution favored us for having this function installed in our visual system. The dilation gives more light, and that may help in certain conditions. But pupil size also matters for visual acuity; sudden dilation might come at the expense of acuity. In any case, even if the pupil response is just a by-product, the idea that pupil size effectively correlates with intensity in vision should already suffice for good behaviorist analysis.

However, a major issue with pupil size is that it also varies as a function of light conditions (an increase in light leads to pupil constriction). For this reason, phobic as we are of confounds in data, mainstream psychology turned away from measuring pupil size altogether. A few brave souls are now trying to regenerate interest (e.g., Porter, Troscianko, & Gilchrist, 2007; Takeuchi et al., 2011). I think they are on the right track. It is technically feasible to add measures of light conditions and pupil size to any eye-tracking paradigm. With these data we can aim to separate effects of luminance from other (intensive) factors in pupil size variation. This is certainly not a lot of work compared to issues of noise reduction that neuroscientists routinely have to face in electrophysiological or fMRI studies. We need to up the ante in psychology and psychophysics as well, particularly in the more cognitively oriented studies that have tended to rely on low-tech methods—we have very good reasons to engage in more intensive research on the intensive processes of perception. The topic is worth the effort, and the twenty-first century offers us the technology. The only reason for not using these tools would be acedia (negligence, including sloth), deadly sin number four according to Dante, seven centuries ago in *The Divine Comedy* (Alighieri, 1995).

Critique of Pure Vision

The intensity of our gaze matters. The length of time we focus on particular information is crucial for our powers of association and synthesis (what Kant called "the imagination"—"a blind but indispensable function of the soul without which we should have no knowledge whatsoever, but of which we are scarcely ever conscious," 1781|2007, p. 104). The associations and efforts of synthesis are processes of active vision that happen inside our heads—they are acts of inner vision, to quote a title by Semir Zeki (2000; very appropriate for a book about visual art and neuroscience). Creative, active processes of valuation and interpretation are the hallmark of what the brain does. No externalist philosophy can dance its way around this. Much of what we do inside our heads when we engage in active vision amounts to traveling back and forth between memory and imagination, between sensation and imagination. If some theorists would object that all this higher-order activity leads us away from pure vision (after all, even Kant said the imagination was *blind*), then I would like to ask them where they draw the line. What is pure vision and what is not?

Any such line would be suspicious—just as problematic as any categorical divide between consciousness and the unconscious, as convincingly argued by Dennett (1991). Perhaps the "blindness" of imagination that Kant talked about is something like an attractor for vision; I would think of it as the ultimate abstraction of language (a place of negativity; see Agamben, 1991). In any case, the crux about vision is that it has active, nonlinear, chaotic boundaries. These pertain to the construction and continued presence of representations inside our heads. Our task is to characterize vision by understanding how the boundaries work, how we construct and maintain representations of objects and features. Once more, for scientists this means we need to measure brain activity as well as behavioral parameters. Sometimes neurons can tell us about nonsensory, associative representations triggered by visual stimulation even when the subject's behavior is controlled by other factors (see Messinger et al., 2005, for an elegant demonstration).

As we construct internal representations of objects and features, we continue noticing different aspects and new connections to things we have experienced before. At this point I would like to invite you to remind yourself of how this works with a concrete set of visual stimuli. Please look in turn at figures 5.4, 5.5, and 5.6, carefully reading the

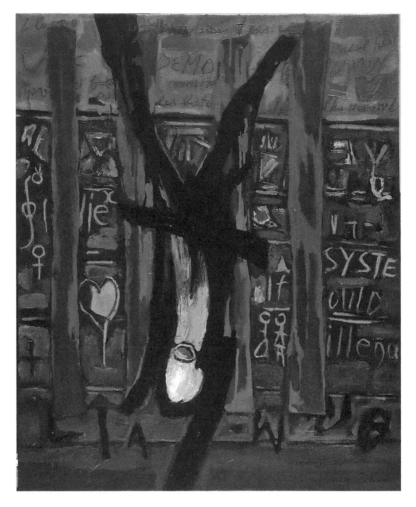

Figure 5.4
An as yet untitled painting by the artist and neuroscientist Minoru Tsukada, first displayed at the Tamagawa Dynamic Brain Forum in Atami, Shizuoka prefecture, Japan, March 2009. Please let your gaze roam over this image for at least twenty seconds, then visit figures 5.5 and 5.6 and come back here.

captions. Then come back to figure 5.4 in the end. Take your time. Magnitude and duration are crucial. Do not read on until you have given yourself at least a few minutes with these figures.

When I first saw the painting by Minoru Tsukada (figure 5.4), it reminded me of the other two images. If I had not known the other two images, I might have been less affected (or less disturbed) by the intriguing, tantalizingly readable painting, midway between figurative

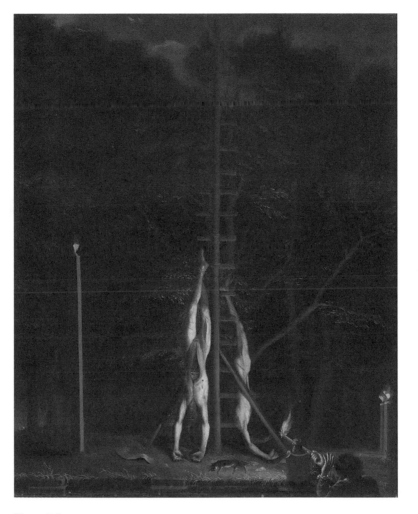

Figure 5.5
The Corpses of the Brothers De Witt, on the Groene Zoodje at the Lange Vijverberg, The Hague, 20 August 1672, by Jan de Baen (collection of the Rijksmuseum in Amsterdam, The Netherlands). Johan and Cornelis de Witt, important politicians of the Dutch Republic, were lynched by a mob, their corpses mutilated—one of the most shameful events in Dutch history, presumably orchestrated by monarchists. Johan de Witt was a gifted mathematician and a good friend of Spinoza, who lived in the same city. Johan is the one "*met sijn eijgen hair*" (with his own hair), says the inscription on the back, but that does not help me with this reproduction (from memory, viewing the actual painting in Amsterdam, I believe I decided Johan was the one on the right).

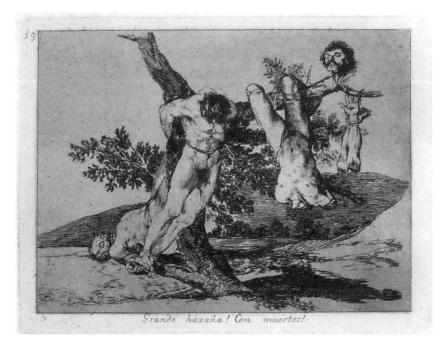

Grande   hazaña ! Con   muertos!

Figure 5.6
Plate 39 of *The Disasters of War* by Francisco Goya, a series of prints secretly made between
1810 and 1820, while the painter continued painting portraits for his masters at Court, trying
to stay out of trouble and think free thoughts privately. Plate 39 is one among several
that most clearly depict what Goya called "the dismemberment of Spain" by Napoleon
Bonaparte. "*Grande hazaña! Con muertos*" can be translated as "A heroic feat! With dead
men!" The prints were first published in 1863, many decades after the death of their maker.
It is quite possible we would never have seen *The Disasters of War* if Goya had tried to
show them to his contemporaries.

and abstract (even literally teasing our compulsive habits of reading by
including deliberately occluded and distorted bits of graffiti). The memo-
ries of the other images colored my mood, but also controlled my gaze—
it made me focus on particular details as I wondered about their meaning,
comparing or associating them with thoughts that were playing in my
head. I saw a creature hanging upside down, perhaps human, partly
burned, partially dismembered (at least one arm missing), with open
mouth or slit throat.

Did I see that creature or did I imagine it? Seeing it *was* imagining
it. Active vision performed the Kantian synthesis. The comparison with
remembered images—famous works of art that silently exposed and
denounced the horrific nature of war—also allowed me to read the
context (the graffiti in the background) in dialogue with the painful

central figure (I am using the word "painful" here in the way it fit in Gertrude Stein's poem at the beginning of this chapter). I focused, in turn, on the heart (on the left) and the words "lie" (above the heart) and "system" (on the right). This dialogue involved ideas about the intrinsic danger of violence in systems and the heart's (or love's) power to transcend. These thoughts were further removed from the visual stimuli than my seeing of the central figure as a victim of violence hanging upside down. However, did these thoughts no longer belong to the domain of active vision?

They still coincided with my gaze. I would look straight at the heart, see the painful figure in parafoveal vision, and think about love's power to transcend. What shall we call this, if not perception?

Wittgenstein writes (1953|2003, p. 165) as follows: "I contemplate a face, and then suddenly notice its likeness to another. I see that it has not changed; and yet I see it differently. I call this experience 'noticing an aspect.'" And a bit later (pp. 180–181), "[W]hat I perceive in the dawning of an aspect is not a property of the object, but an internal relation between it and other objects." This comes down to inner vision, where the re-cognizing happens, bringing the past to bear on the present, using our knowledge of the world to make sense of visual impressions.

This is perhaps the biggest difference between the intensive approach and Noë's (2004) enactive view of perception: The intensive approach concentrates on the construction and maintenance of representations in relation to our knowledge of the world (our biases, our memory); the enactive view wishes to deny the inner life of vision and so chooses to remain silent about the role of memory and the mechanisms of recognition. My impression is that the enactive view implies a strict separation between perception and cognition. In my opinion such separation is artificial; it runs counter to the core notion of active boundaries in vision.

According to the intensive approach, the active boundaries of vision move from not-seeing to seeing with the aid of memory and imagination. It often involves the transition from bias to sensitivity, from anticipation to recognition, from virtual to actual. Also in this sense, the approach is adequately called "intensive," in accordance with Kant's principle for "the anticipations of perception" (1781|2007, p. 196): "In all appearances the real, which is an object of sensation, has intensive magnitude, that is, a degree." In comparison, Kant states: "I call an extensive magnitude that in which the representation of the whole is rendered possible (and is therefore necessarily preceded) by the representation of its parts" (p. 193). This distinction matches with that between extensive and intensive properties in physics (see DeLanda, 2002|2004, pp. 24–25). The extensive is intrinsically divisible (the whole equals the sum of its parts); in contrast, dividing the intensive may lead to a change in kind (the whole does not equal the sum of its parts).

The real becomes visible through its appearances. More specifically, the real has intensive magnitude in its appearances. This intensive magnitude allows us to anticipate the rest (what is virtual) and thus to construct a representation of an entire object, a whole that is greater than the sum of its parts. Here I would like to suggest with Gilles Deleuze (1968|1994, p. 208) that "[t]he virtual is opposed not to the real but to the actual" (p. 209). The indivisible object stretches from actual (what can be sensed, what gives "appearance") to virtual (what we anticipate to be there through the intensive approach). DeLanda, our favorite interpreter of Deleuze, observes poetically (2002|2004, p. 40): "The virtual, in a sense, leaves behind traces of itself in the intensive processes it animates, and the philosopher's task may be seen as that of a detective who follows these tracks or connects these clues."

It is not just the philosopher's task. It is what we all routinely do in perception. We gain access to things as they are through the intensive approach, working from actual sensations to obtain virtual information (anticipations, biases). We combine the actual and the virtual into wholes that are greater than the sums of their parts: objects of thought, internal representations that do not always have to fill everything in. These representations in turn can guide our sensorimotor exploration; they become instrumental in eliciting and accessing further appearances (intensive magnitudes) of things as they are.

True Colors

In the intensive approach we interact with appearances to increase our understanding of what is present around us. From the interaction we glean true colors, "shining through," as according to the pop song written by Billy Steinberg and Bob Kelly, forever linked with the strangely textured, roughish voice of Cyndi Lauper. The effects the appearances have on us coevolve with our interaction; they are at once deeply subjective (dependent on our biases and sensitivities) and thoroughly objective (present in the world, as measurable phenomena, physical processes inside and outside our bodies). Here I feel justified to claim Johann Wolfgang von Goethe's *Theory of Colors* (1810|2006) as an ancestor of the intensive approach as well as (or even rather than) the enactive view.

Alva Noë (2004) gave Goethe a prominent place at the beginning of his book, using a motto lifted from the first page of the preface to Goethe's first edition (here I give the same quote in a different translation, older, clumsier, but more accurate—by Charles Lock Eastlake; Goethe, 1810|2006, p. xvii):

Indeed, strictly speaking, it is useless to attempt to express the nature of a thing abstractedly. Effects we can perceive, and a complete history of those effects would, in fact, sufficiently define the nature of the thing itself. We should try in vain to describe a man's character, but let his acts be collected and an idea of the character will be presented to us.

Goethe's theory of colors was a vigorous response to Newton and uniquely physical explanations—a wonderful poetic *and* scientific enterprise that, in a way, invented phenomenology as well as behaviorism. It offered an empirically oriented investigation of subjective experience at a time when psychology had not yet grown into a scientific discipline of its own. Noë (2004) did not tell us why he picked the quote, but it must have something to do with the apparent rejection of abstraction and the preferred focus on effects, on happenings in the world that constitute the entirety of what can be characterized. For Goethe (1810|2006), however, this did not mean that we can do without abstraction altogether (p. xix):

Every act of seeing leads to consideration, consideration to reflection, reflection to combination, and thus it may be said that in every attentive look on nature we already theorise. But in order to guard against the possible abuse of this abstract view, in order that the practical deductions we look to should be really useful, we should theorise without forgetting that we are so doing, we should theorise with mental self-possession, and, to use a bold word, with irony.

Inevitably, naturally, every act of seeing involves abstraction, "theorizing," or the construction of internal representations. Goethe's plea is for us not to deny, but to exploit the multiplicity (Žižek's parallax), toward a dialectics of internal representation and sensorimotor exploration. The bold word "irony" takes us to metacognition, to the necessity of evaluation and revision. We should constantly retune our biases and sensitivities, our ideas and internal representations, in light of new evidence, following the implications of effects and appearances. "[W]e should theorise with mental self-possession" to fully understand what is real in what we see. This means we have to factor our own perspective into the equation.

Goethe was the first theorist, scientist, and poet to think systematically about the differences between "objective" and "subjective" experiments

Objective   *Subjective*

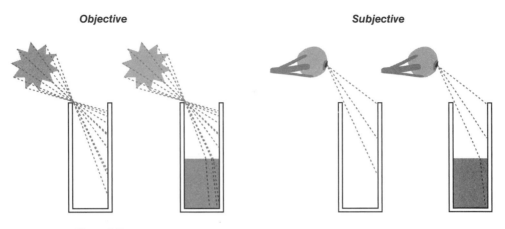

Figure 5.7
Objective versus subjective points of view, as described by Goethe in his daring, anti-Newtonian treatise on colors (1810|2006, pp. 42–43). Left: "At the point where the light enters the thicker medium it deviates from its rectilinear direction, and appears broken […] Thus much of the objective experiment." Right: "We arrive at the subjective fact in the following mode:—Let the eye be substituted for the sun[…] On pouring in water the eye will perceive a part of the bottom; and this takes place without our being aware that we do not see in a straight line; for the bottom appears to us raised."

(see figure 5.7 for a detailed example). Physics can capture light-reflecting properties of surfaces, but to understand the effects of these properties, we need to consider the perspective of the observer, the subject. The light-reflecting properties "cause creatures to go into various discriminative states, scattered about in their brains, and underlying a host of innate dispositions and learned habits of varying complexity," as Dennett put it (1991, p. 372) in his deconstruction of the slippery notion of qualia (the subjective features of conscious mental processes).

Today, color perception is fully understood to be bound to the subject. It is considered "a model system for understanding how information is processed by neural circuits, and for investigating the relationships among genes, neural circuits, and perception" (Conway et al., 2010, p. 14955). We are trichromatic animals because we have three different types of cone photoreceptors: L, M, and S, for long-, middle-, and short-wavelength regions of the visual spectrum (not quite the same as but somehow subjectively related to "red," "green," and "blue"). The relative activation of the cone types already gives a complex value for each point in the visual field at a particular moment in time, but the color that we see critically depends on the relation of this value to other values, as a function of the spatial and temporal context. Seeing colors is therefore — perhaps somewhat surprisingly, against habits of speech in neuroscience

—a *spatial* process. It is a matter of exploring contrasts and engaging in sensorimotor interaction as correctly emphasized by Noë (2004).

Goethe (1810|2006) was already aware of a role for eye movements in color perception. With a compilation of his words (on p. 13):

It has been stated that certain flowers, towards evening in summer, coruscate, become phosphorescent, or emit a momentary light ... as I was walking up and down a garden with a friend, we very distinctly observed a flame-like appearance near the oriental poppy ... the apparent coruscation was nothing but the spectrum of the flower in the compensatory blue–green colour. In looking directly at a flower the image is not produced, but it appears immediately as the direction of the eye is altered.

How we compute the contrasts, the way in which we engage in the sensorimotor interaction, depends on experience, culture, and even language (see Winawer et al., 2007, for striking category effects in the speed of discrimination among different types of blue by Russian speakers, but not English speakers). However, the sensorimotor interaction does not tell the entire story. Qualia like those of colors come with an "idiosyncratic complex of dispositions" (Dennett, 1991, p. 389), a pandemonium of associations, weaker and stronger, sometimes even heartaches, thrills, and waves of nostalgia. For Goethe, these effects were aesthetic— "belonging to taste as mere internal sense" (Eastlake's note; Goethe, 1810|2006, p. xxxi). The study of aesthetic effects formed an integral part of his theory. Goethe went quite far in his phenomenological observations—a brief sample: "The effect of this colour is as peculiar as its nature. It conveys an impression of gravity and dignity, and at the same time of grace and attractiveness. The first in its dark deep state, the latter in its light attenuated tint; and thus the dignity of age and the amiableness of youth may adorn itself with degrees of the same hue" (p. 173). Test: Which color was he talking about? Answer: If you are not sure, then you are right—you are not Goethe. If you are sure, then either you are Goethe or you are mistaken.

At which point did Goethe move outside the realm of science? Will we ever be able to study the aesthetic effects of colors scientifically? Conventional answers would be "No" to the second question, and "From very early on in his project" to the first. Those are old thoughts, and they deserve to be revised. The answer to the second question should be "Yes"—we already have evidence of feasibility (see Mehta & Zhu, 2009, for data showing that red induces avoidance motivation whereas blue enhances performance in a creative task). The answer to the first question must be "Never." Goethe's work on colors *was* science from the beginning to the end—not mainstream, to be sure, but science nonetheless—one of a kind, the stuff of inspiration, for choosing mottos, pushing boundaries, and rethinking our heritage.

Perhaps the one-line take-home message from Goethe is that subjective experiments produce important data, compatible and convergent with objective experiments. The meaning of the world lives in our subjective experience. Goethe urges us to explore this experience with "irony," moving between our theories and the effects in the world. The meaning of the world, as we find it in our subjective experience, does not stay confined within us. It goes out into the world. In the near-poetry of Merleau-Ponty (1945|2008, p. 498),

At the heart of the subject himself we discovered, then, the presence of the world, so that the subject was no longer to be understood as a synthetic activity, but as *ek-stase*, and that every active process of signification or *Sinn-gebung* appeared as derivative and secondary in relation to that pregnancy of meaning within signs which could serve to define the world.

Merleau-Ponty borrows the word *"ek-stase"* from Heidegger to speak of stepping outside our temporality, toward pure selflessness. In doing so, our subjective experience is no longer merely a matter of internal processing but the first basis, the principle that underscores every process of signification. Meaning moves beyond the personal perspective. The way we make sense of things becomes part of the interaction with the world. This interaction is how we shape and define the world: always in negotiation with others—with the gaze of others.

My gentle-hearted Charles! when the last Rook
Beat its straight path along the dusky air
Homewards, I blest it! deeming, its black wing
(Now a dim speck, now vanishing in light)
Had cross'd the mighty Orb's dilated glory,
While thou stood'st gazing; or when all was still,
Flew creeking o'er thy head, and had a charm
For thee, my gentle-hearted Charles, to whom
No Sound is dissonant which tells of Life.

Samuel Taylor Coleridge composed these lines inspired by a little hiking trip that he was unable to join. They are lines 69 to 77 of *This Lime-tree Bower my Prison*, a poem that found its near-final form in July 1797 (here reproduced from Coleridge, 2001, pp. 353–354). His wife, Sara, née Fricker, had "accidentally emptied a skillet of boiling milk" on his foot, according to the poor man himself (as I gather from a quote by Harper, 1928|1969, p. 12). Samuel Taylor Coleridge had to sit out the walk his friends were up to. We have no reason to believe that Coleridge did not deserve to have the skillet emptied on his foot, nor do we have reason to believe that he did. Perhaps it really was just an accident, but whatever happened, it was good that it did because it gave us one of Coleridge's finest poems, which is tantamount to saying it gave us one of the finest poems in the English language.

The literary critic George McLean Harper (1928|1969) identified it as a "conversation poem," one of a group of eight, including *The Nightingale*, for which Coleridge had coined the term. "These are his Poems of Friendship," decided Harper (p. 4), and they are characterized by their "[p]oignancy of feeling, intimacy of address, and ease of expression" (p. 8). Harper also claimed, "They cannot even vaguely be understood unless the reader knows what persons Coleridge has in mind" (pp. 4–5).

I plead guilty to complete lack of such knowledge. However, I take heart in the fact that Coleridge probably was in a fog about it as well. *This Lime-tree Bower my Prison* was originally addressed to "you, my Sister & my Friends" (including Dorothy and William Wordsworth among others) but later revised so that Charles Lamb became the sole target of the apostrophe ("My gentle-hearted Charles!")

Yet even in complete ignorance and a great fog, I believe the poem has the power to speak for itself, to us—indeed, any good poem speaks to its readers and deserves to be considered a conversation poem. By this definition, I am the addressee of any poem that I read, and so I feel justified to keep reading what I read and to reject Harper's conclusion that my understanding will be worse than vague. My stance as addressee, however, puts me in direct conflict with the apostrophe, the poet's appeal to that gentle-hearted Charles. This basic conflict underlies the strange effects of apostrophes in general—they violate the gaze control (see Culler, 1981|2001, pp. 149–171, for a sharp-minded exploration of the topic). Instead of looking at me when it speaks, the poem looks at somebody (or even some*thing*) else.

The poem does this deliberately, perhaps to urge me to look where the poem is looking, to share my attention with that of the poem. Most rhetoricians would argue that apostrophes serve as intensifiers, to signal a deep commitment. That does not explain the awkwardness or the sense of (vicarious) embarrassment we feel when reading sudden invocations of "O…" and "Thou…" Some of the awkwardness must be due to idiosyncrasies of fashion; we simply have outgrown certain habits. However, contemporary poetry still uses apostrophes—more subtle ones, with open forms, say, addressing an unidentified "you" that could be us or somebody else, an unnamed, but very specific individual, a lover, a friend, or perhaps even the writer himself or herself. In this way, contemporary poetry might achieve the desired intensification and personal investment without creating an explicit conflict of gaze control (the poem looks at "you" as if you could really be the "you" it had in mind).

Coleridge chooses the way of the radical artifice, to borrow a phrase from Marjorie Perloff (1991|1994)—he goes for the extreme as vanguard poets still do in our age of boundless media, if not with the same devices. Coleridge's fictive address to "My gentle-hearted Charles!" maximally emphasizes the direction of his thought and challenges us to play along and look in the same direction (as if we were in Coleridge's shoes). Curiously, this thought, directed at another, is unmistakably *visual*: The poet focuses on the last rook's straight path in the dusky air, across the mighty orb's dilated glory until the bird is completely out of sight. We see it, too, with the poet's eyes, in our own imagination (not in any Cartesian Theater but with our intensive approach, building the relevant representations). But how is such focus compatible with Coleridge's call to his friend?

"While thou stood'st gazing" are the crucial words. Coleridge connects with his friend through the visual imagery. He imagines Charles gazing at the very same last rook, and it is this connection that allows Coleridge to bless the bird (a member of the species *Corvus frugilegus*, in our collective unconscious often associated with bad luck and imminent death). Gentle-hearted Charles would have considered the bird charming (even a paradoxical portent of Life), and so Coleridge manages to conjure up a positive sentiment for it too. The gaze of the other reverberates and moves in many ways in these wonderful lines. We look with Coleridge's eyes, who sees what Charles Lamb sees, to create the most intense connection between the poet and his friend, the friend and the poor black bird, the poor black bird and the mighty orb's dilated glory, imminent death and a message of Life, and between all of this and the poet's readers.

Emission

The gaze of others moves us. We could call it "The Moving Gaze" with the understanding that the moving here is of a different variety than that of "The Moving Retina" in chapter 3. Here, the gaze actively produces effects outside the body of the gazer, in the world, and more specifically in the minds of others, who gaze at the gaze — an act that becomes reciprocal when the two gazes fixate on one another. The effects of the gaze on others, or of the gaze of others on us, can be thought of as a form of emission. The effects involve the emission of signals; the gaze of others contains information that influences us. Thinking about it this way, the ancient battle between intromission and emission theories of perception deserves to be looked at again from a new perspective.

In Ancient Greece, some of the leading figures in speculative thought about perception (notably Euclid and Ptolemy) favored the idea that light travels from the eye outward to make visual contact with objects in the world — this is the emission theory of perception (Howard, 1996). The theory made an analogy with the sense of touch; vision would be an active form of perception quite literally along the lines of Noë's (2004) image of a blind person tapping her way around to get a sense of the proper size of things in the world. By beaming out our inner light, we would spray our visual powers all over the physical presences around us. Things that throw themselves in the way of our beams would become the objects of vision, in perfect harmony with the etymology of the word "object."

Almost exactly a millennium ago, the great Arab scientist Alhazen gave the emission theory a blow it never recovered from. ("Alhazen" is how his name is conventionally written in English; his actual name, limited to the 26 letters of our alphabet, was Abu Ali al-Hasan ibn al-Hasan ibn al-Haytham.) Alhazen simply asked observers to take a look at the sun. Could they keep their gaze fixated? Did they feel their eyes being burned? It took no further theorizing or speculating about geometric and other problems. The fact was plainly there for anyone to see: Light had to be traveling from the sun into the eye to do its damage there—the intromission theory prevailed. Alhazen managed to settle the issue with a straightforward bit of very easy empirical observation. This single appeal to data was picked by the novelist Richard Powers (1999) as his choice for Best Idea of the Millennium in a series in *The New York Times*.

Of course, Powers referred to the general idea of relying on data, not the specific suggestion of staring at the sun to prove that the intromission theory was right. Empirical observation yielded knowledge that could topple false beliefs, traditions, even gods. I could not think of a better idea for the past (or any other) millennium (Richard Powers very often gets it very right; he is one of those writers whose books neuroscientists should put on their wish lists, perhaps beginning with his 2006 neurological exploration *The Echo Maker*). This appeal to observation also underscores the huge importance of our present topic of brain and the gaze. If "eyes wide open" is the best idea of the millennium, then we have very good reason to be interested in how that works.

However, was the emission theory buried alive? With Alhazen and our eyes wide open, we see that light travels from outside (in the world) to inside (in the eye). Yet with Goethe we realize that perception goes beyond the physics of electromagnetic waves. In the study of perception we should also have our eyes wide open for the subjective experience. Taking another look at the last figure in the previous chapter (figure 5.7; the one that draws what was described by Goethe, 1810|2006), we see that the objective perspective follows the laws of physics as they were already known to Alhazen. Yet, the subjective perspective looks suspiciously like a return of the living dead, with beams of brightness traveling out of the observer's eye, with no sun or other light source around.

Goethe—observing and writing more than eight hundred years after Alhazen—may have ignored the works of the great Arab scientist, but he could not have escaped indirect influence via such luminaries as Roger Bacon, Franciscus Aguilonius, or René Descartes.

There can be no doubt that Goethe, like every sane scientist, accepted the intromission theory—of light, if not of perception. However, when it comes to the subjective perspective, there still seems to be some validity for a conceptualization in terms of emission effects. Figure 6.1 shows a contemporary example of how we intuitively rely on the idea that "something" can beam out of our eyes. The sign, embedded in vigorous vegetation, is quite explicit about its attempt at persuasive communication, threatening potential garbage dumpers with heavy punishments and urging good citizens to spy on their criminal neighbors. Here, the glare of the authority figure reinforces the message. The artist who designed this sign must have implicitly made a connection between the gaze and the power to influence.

The point is that the gaze actively causes perception, creating signals and changing the value of stimuli in the world. In the example of figure 6.1 the gaze of the police officer carries information. The gaze becomes itself an object of perception; it tells something about what the other is looking at. It might even suggest more; combined with facial expression, the gaze contributes to emotional expression. Before developing this theme, I would like to point to another way in which the gaze has a formative influence on information processing for the one who is gazing in the first place (i.e., a formative influence of my own gaze on my own information processing). At the most general level, there is an intrinsic connection between gaze fixation and choice. Fixation naturally implies a choice: A stimulus is selected for fixation. This choice might tempt us into thinking it is *our* choice in a broader sense—not simply an object for fixation but an object of preference. As Keith Waldrop (2009, p. 100) wrote in the poem *Silk* (the very same poem that I mentioned in relation to stargazing in chapter 1): "The longer I look, the / stronger the enchantment."

Choice by Association

With the intensive approach, I posited that the gaze allows us to continue information processing beyond the primary task of identifying the objects in our vision. By locking our gaze onto particular objects, we facilitate the further cognitive work, giving longer duration and greater magnitude

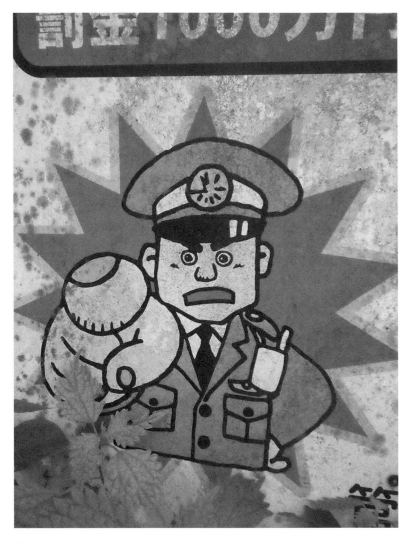

Figure 6.1
The gaze of another in full emission. This unhappy police officer stopped me in my tracks in the luscious green of a Kyushu forest on June 13, 2010. The weatherworn sign appeared to be surrounded by stinging nettle (though I might overgeneralize the shape of the leaf, still hurting from many stings in childhood). There was to be no dumping of garbage, or else a choice between two hyperboles (a five-year prison sentence or a fine of ten million yen, which converts to more than a hundred thousand U.S. dollars). Note the dangerous glare as well as the dramatic emphasis of proximity in the size of the tip of the officer's right index finger.

to the relevant neural representations. The work after the initial perceptual description would be of a higher order, in connection with items in memory, to create new associations and revise old ones, to evaluate the objects and potential courses of action, and so on. The gaze here works as a "deictic pointer," to borrow an important concept from Dana Ballard and colleagues (1997; see also Yu, Ballard, & Aslin, 2005)—the gaze indexes the object of thought during complex task performance. Such deictic pointing is an efficient cognitive strategy that reduces the load for working memory. By holding things in vision, we can free up resources that would otherwise be needed to hold things in mind. It is one of the most pertinent lessons we learn from the philosophy of embodied cognition (see Clark, 2008, for an excellent exposition). We can let the world be its own memory store and use the gaze to look up whichever information we currently need.

However, the intensive approach goes one step further. It suggests that the deictic pointing does something in addition to maximizing the memory capacity as we engage in our interactions with the visual world. It *changes* the quality and the strength of the representation of the indexed object. The poet Keith Waldrop even suggested a direction for the change. The gaze would increase the value of its object. Shinsuke Shimojo and colleagues (2003) provided corroborating evidence, specifically in case the subject has to express a personal preference. When choosing the most attractive of a pair of faces, the subject's gaze gradually develops a bias toward the face that will turn out to be the favorite. When performing a shape discrimination task with the faces, the gaze bias appears less pronounced. The authors made the strong claim that the gaze actively contributes to the preference formation—an emission effect of sorts, as if the gaze endows the object with likeableness, a sprinkling of favorable light particles.

This strong claim might not be all that crazy. In one sense, it even sounds like an extremely basic mechanism of approach, a hardwired form of heading toward the attractant. In the literature on behavioral processes, this type of approach is associated with the genius of Ivan Petrovich Pavlov (for a comprehensive introduction to his legacy, see Bouton, 2007; Dickinson, 1980). We can see Pavlovian approach in action in organisms as simple as the nematode, particularly the species *Caenorhabditis elegans* (or "*C. elegans*," for short; made famous by Sydney Brenner, 1974). The one-millimeter worms move their elegant way to attractive odorants like diacetyl—a reflexive behavioral process we call "chemotaxis," the worm being pulled toward the stimulus. It involves no conscious liking of any kind but might be considered a precursor of neural and physiological mechanisms underlying emotion in vertebrates. The little worms may even find themselves in a bind—turning and squirming, embodying the conflict—when faced with an aversive cupper barrier on the way to the attractive odorant (e.g., Shinkai et al., 2011).

Looking at striking video clips of the little worms squirming during the conflict, some of us might find it hard not to anthropomorphize and read a mental struggle into the behavior. To some extent, the data actually do suggest an internal conflict at a very elementary level, in the sense that the outcome of the push–pull contest depends on the protein profile of interneurons (Ishihara et al., 2002; Shinkai et al., 2011). The principal investigator, my friend and colleague Takeshi Ishihara, even admitted he had named the critical secretory protein HEN-1 after "hesitation." Somewhere along the line, we may suspect, things are different for worms as compared to humans, but the research with these and other invertebrates serves as a welcome challenge to investigators of behavior in "higher animals." We need to come up with paradigms and models that point to critical computational differences among the different species.

As it is, the output of the most detailed model of human gaze and preference formation—developed by Krajbich, Armel, and Rangel (2010)—looks remarkably like the trajectories of worms undergoing the push and pull of different stimuli (see figure 6.2). The model assumes

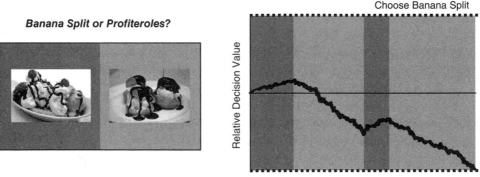

Figure 6.2
The relation between gaze fixation and decision value (modeled after Krajbich, Armel, & Rangel, 2010). Subjects are presented with a choice between two desserts (left panel; backgrounds in different shades of gray to represent the two options). The right panel depicts a so-called "accumulator" decision-making model that links gaze fixation with an increase in the value of the item being looked at. Once the relative decision value reaches either of the decision boundaries, the subject picks the associated option (in this example, a clear violation of her diet).

that gaze fixation directly leads to an increase of the value of the associated object. The gaze produces a virtual approach to an attractant in a way that is computationally indistinguishable from Pavlovian approach. The virtual approach here is formulated as the accumulation of a relative decision value. When this value reaches a threshold, the subject makes a choice. The accumulator model aims to explain both the choice made and the time taken to do so. As such, it is inspired by reaction time models that address the stochastic processes underlying decision making (e.g., Ratcliff & Smith, 2004). It is also compatible with neural data that suggest a growth of the strength of representations toward a decision threshold (e.g., Churchland, Kiani, & Shadlen, 2008; Hanes & Schall, 1996).

I am a great fan of this kind of accumulator model. It is a powerful tool to correlate behavioral parameters of decision making (rates of choice, reaction times) with neural dynamics. However, I would place my bet against a direct connection between gaze and increase of value. Anecdotal observation convinces me that humans and other species like monkeys and rats deviate—occasionally quite dramatically—from Pavlovian-like approach in their relation between gaze and choice. Sometimes we look intensely at an option only to decide against it at the very last instant. We may hold a book in our hands at a bookstore and contemplate buying it, even decide to go ahead with the purchase. Sometimes we make a U-turn before arriving at the cash register, prey to second thoughts, coming up with more and more reasons against the choice. Rats in a double-T-maze may try to figure out which way to go for the biggest reward. They pause at the junction, have their head pointing in one direction for a good while, and then suddenly shoot into action in the other direction.

Humans and other animals with complex brains have the power to disconnect their choices from Pavlovian approach. The gaze can index the object of thought, but the actual thinking happens inside the head. When we look at an option, we compile a rich object file about it; we imagine the outcomes, explore the meanings, and gradually develop a more comprehensive basis for evaluation. The intensive approach implies that we gain a deeper understanding about the options, aided by the gaze, by the magnitude and duration of relevant neural representations. However, the direction of the evaluation is not determined. More often than not, we end up accumulating evidence against the object we are gazing at. The gaze alone cannot tell us what happens inside the brain.

To understand the dynamics of decision making, we do need to investigate the goings-on in neural circuits in parallel with the behavioral parameters. The Antonio Rangel laboratory (the same that developed the model of gaze and choice) is on to it already (Lim, O'Doherty, & Rangel, 2011). They recorded BOLD signals as human subjects viewed and picked their choice of cookies or potato chips. This time subjects were asked to control their gaze in compliance with color cues (consisting of frames, presented around the visual targets). Under these conditions, the activity in ventromedial prefrontal cortex and ventral striatum correlates with the relative decision value of the item in the gaze. Put differently, the brain computes the likeableness of the fixated object in the given choice context. Sometimes the object being looked at does not get a high valuation, and looking at it longer does not increase the enchantment. The gaze's power of emission appears to be limited after all.

However, we should bear in mind that the gaze was not allowed to move freely in this fMRI study. Forced gaze fixation might disrupt the natural flow from gazing to liking. Though the gaze does not necessarily produce enchantment, I think there is a *favored* relation between the gaze and choice—not a fixed behavioral pattern but a bias (exactly the word used by Shimojo et al., 2003). We know that the gaze naturally connects with approach; Johansson and colleagues (2001) even spoke of obligatory looking toward an object before grasping it as mentioned in chapter 4. To grasp, we must look (or "grasping therefore begin-with-looking"), and so we are tempted to reverse the relation even if logic does not warrant the move ("begin-with-looking therefore grasping"). We can take the model by Krajbich and colleagues (2010) to represent the default settings of the relation between gaze fixation and relative decision value. Under normal circumstances, internal credit tends to accumulate in favor of the object we gaze at, but there is room for influence of context and for seemingly inexplicable idiosyncratic behavior, perhaps even creativity and some kind of free will.

Gaze Following

The gaze as a deictic pointer facilitates the observer's intensive approach to particular information in the visual field. This overt pointing, the embodiment of interest, reduces the cognitive workload of the observer and so proves to be a profitable function. However, the overt nature of the behavior elicits a slew of secondary effects. The gaze can be read as a cue by others. It effectively signals what is of interest to the observer at a given moment in time in a particular setting. The gaze attaches ratings of informativeness to items in the visual environment. If you show great interest in a certain object, there is a good chance that it is actually deserving of interest in general. I had better take a look as well.

Given the systematic bias relating gaze to choice, our eye movements must be predictive of reward. The gaze should be a perfect stimulus for operant conditioning, for learning to use the information strategically to obtain reward, even if the subject does not read anything "mental" into the other's gaze direction and simply acquires an association between a visual stimulus (the relative position of the pupil) and an opportunity to obtain a reward. A classic in this vein is the object-choice task: We hide food in one of two cups and give the subject a hint by looking at the baited cup. Capuchin monkeys can learn to follow our gaze (Vick & Anderson, 2000), rooks can do it too (Schmidt et al., 2011), but South African fur seals need more than the eye alone, say, head direction or finger pointing (Scheumann & Call, 2004).

Is there more to gaze following than operant conditioning? Dogs seem to be particularly good at using social communicative signals, including gaze direction (Hare et al., 2002). Puppies less than three months old, even the ones who had limited experience with humans, performed better than chimpanzees and wolves on the object-choice task (though most needed a manual pointing cue along with the gaze). Michael Tomasello, the senior author, is well-known for his healthy skepticism when it comes to interpreting the cognitive abilities of animals. However, in this case he did not hesitate joining his coauthors in concluding that the dogs had a fairly sophisticated faculty of social cognition bred into them.

Gaze following in dogs and in humans would be a hardwired function, an instinct. Actually, chimpanzees, macaques, and other primates may also have basic aspects of gaze following in their innate repertoire even if they need training on the object-choice task (but see Emery et al., 1997, for data to suggest that rhesus monkeys follow the gaze of conspecifics in something resembling an implicit object-choice task). Beyond any doubt, and without operant conditioning, the great apes and little monkeys follow the gaze of conspecifics to look at food (Tomasello, Call, & Hare, 1998). Chimpanzees display abilities in gaze following that imply the usage of abstract spatial maps to locate visual targets and to take into account the perspectives of others. They track targets past distractors (Tomasello, Hare, & Agnetta, 1999), and, in competitive situations, they prove they know what other chimpanzees can and cannot see (Hare et al., 2000).

If gaze following is hardwired and innate, we may expect it to produce reflexive orienting in Posner's (1980) spatial-cueing paradigm. Sure enough, two decades after the invention of the paradigm, several human psychophysics labs more or less simultaneously came up with a variant in which the "exogenous cue" was the gaze of another. All the data agreed: We automatically follow the gaze (Driver et al., 1999; Friesen & Kingstone, 1998; Langton & Bruce, 1999). Deaner and Platt (2003) applied the same logic for behavioral experiments with rhesus monkeys looking at the gaze of conspecifics and obtained remarkably similar data, both in the magnitude and in the temporal dynamics of the effects of gaze following. This study opened the door to neurophysiological investigation, targeting single-unit activity that could shed light on the underlying brain mechanisms.

Such work is incredibly labor-intensive. We may sometimes rather nimbly fantasize about what the data would look like if we did this or that experiment, recorded here or there in the brain. It often takes two or three years' full-time work for two monkeys and one or two researchers (who, of course, need the occasional support and strategic interventions of other team members and the principal investigator) to do the surgery, perform the recording sessions, analyze the data, and go through the various rounds of writing and rewriting to get the study finally in publishable format. If it takes four or five years, then that would not be unusual. There is a huge economic and personal cost on top of the inherent ethical issues. Yet these studies, when properly designed and carefully carried out, do live up to the considerable expectations we must place on them.

Michael Platt and his student Robert Deaner joined up with two other volunteers and together worked six years to get from the behavioral data to the activity of single neurons in the LIP. Stephen Shepherd presumably performed the lion's share of the actual recordings and analyses (Shepherd et al., 2009). Was it worth the effort? Yes, indeed, very much so. We see the brain in action and find an internal signature of gaze following. We have a first clue in hand about how the brain constructs a representation of spatial priority as a function of the gaze of another.

Figure 6.3 reconstructs the main findings. Particularly the activity during the delay period between the onset of the cue (the gaze of another) and the onset of the saccade target deserves to be carved into our conception of brain and the gaze. When the gaze of the conspecific points in the direction of the LIP neuron's receptive field, the spiking rate settles at an elevated baseline as compared to when the gaze points

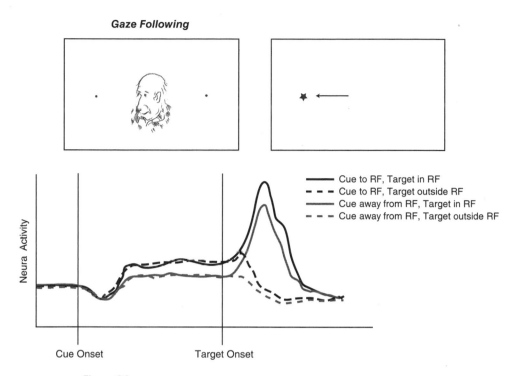

Figure 6.3
A neural correlate of gaze following (adapted from Shepherd et al., 2009). The upper panels represent the task design. The subjects (monkeys) are presented with a social cue (the face of another looking in one direction; in the actual experiment the stimuli were faces of monkeys). Then the subjects are asked to make a saccadic eye movement to a target (the star in the panel on the right). The graph sketches the gist of data from neurons in the lateral intraparietal area (LIP). When the social cue points to the receptive field (RF) of the neuron, the spiking rate remains sustained at a higher level than when the social cue points in the opposite direction. This difference persists until well into the neural response to the target.

in the alternative direction. This activity implies an increase in spatial priority of one direction over another as a function of the conspecific's gaze. More specifically, the priority is expressed as a sustained higher magnitude for the neural representation of the relevant spatial direction (in a way similar to other neural correlates of spatial priority; e.g., Lauwereyns et al., 2002b; Platt & Glimcher, 1999). The prioritization occurs in advance of target onset and leads to an additive increase in the LIP neuron's response to the actual visual information carried by the target — these are all hallmarks of a bias effect (Lauwereyns, 2010).

Gaze following, then, is implemented as a gaze bias favoring the target that the other is looking at. I copy your visual choice. When you look at something, my LIP neurons and their connections will make me naturally inclined to look at the same thing too. Copying, mimicking, following the lead—such actions and skills have enormous implications, far beyond "Monkey see, monkey do," toward the most intricate social and cultural processes. What and who do we copy? Whose gaze would I follow? In figure 6.3 I took the liberty of modifying the social image, wishing to move back to humans, as seems to be warranted by Deaner and Platt's (2003) initial behavioral study.

I wondered which human gaze I would like to follow most of all—"I" being all of my selves as according to Damasio's famous trio of proto-, core, and autobiographical (for the most recent update, see *Self Comes to Mind*; Damasio, 2010). I concluded my favorite gaze had to be that of the Dutch poet and biologist Leo Vroman, a living legend, war survivor, expat, successful investigator (interested in the mechanisms of blood clotting; e.g., Vroman, 1965), and tireless observer—now well into his nineties (closing in on his century), he is still amazingly sharp of mind and curious about everything around him (as evidenced by his massive, most recent volume of poetry; Vroman, 2011). The grand old scientist–poet has a keen eye, likes to take photographs, and makes wonderful drawings. Indeed, the drawing in figure 6.3 is a self-portrait, or actually half of a portrait, the other half (omitted here) being Vroman's portrait of me (in the original drawing Leo is looking straight into my eyes).

So by following Vroman's gaze I come back to me, a tricky return—it is not inspired by narcissism; it elicits self-criticism. The gaze of another, focused on me, appeals to my conscience and asks the confrontational question: What do I see in the mirror? Do I deserve Leo Vroman's gentle-hearted appraisal?

Mirror Neurons

The image or metaphor of a mirror runs deep, from neuroscience to psychoanalysis and cultural studies. The LIP neurons involved in gaze following might actually be instances of a more general and increasingly famous type, called "mirror neurons." In fact, Shepherd and colleagues (2009) presented their important data under the somewhat adventurous title "Mirroring of Attention." The word *attention* here is used in exactly the way I have repeatedly warned against in the foregoing chapters as well as in *The Anatomy of Bias* (Lauwereyns, 2010). The actual underlying neural mechanism looks like a prioritization through bias, yet it is labeled "attention," at the risk of confusion with the conventional notion, with us since William James (1890|1950a), that attention improves visual sensitivity. The usage of the tricky word in the title is acceptable only if we are willing to explicitly include both bias and sensitivity effects in our concept of "attention." The adventure of the title does not end there. It also leaps to the mirror—or splashes right into it if we can think of the mirror as a liquid surface, in accordance with Greek mythology (Narcissus, of course) and the imagery of Jean Cocteau's gorgeous *Orphée* (already mentioned in my Prelude; the 1950 movie links the splashing into the mirror with the radical, death-defying curiosity of the poet).

Gaze following would be one of the functions performed by "the mirror system," a complex, hybrid collection of neural structures that in one way or another code what others are doing or undergoing. Marco Iacoboni (the great expert of human fMRI work on the topic) introduced this system to a wide audience in his highly enjoyable and very well-documented *Mirroring People* (2008|2009). The mirror system would form the basis of a variety of critical social skills such as imitation and empathy, with implications that seem to expand boundlessly, all the way to morality and ideological issues. At times, Iacoboni appears a bit over-awed by the immensity of his topic (e.g., p. 8: "Decades in the future, will everything in neuroscience be seen as coming back to mirror neurons?" and p. 272: "We have evolved to connect deeply with other human beings. Our awareness of this fact can and should bring us even closer to one another"). However, even if we think in less grandiose terms about the role and the power of the mirror system, we must admit there are some very interesting things to learn from it.

To begin with, when Vittorio Gallese, Giacomo Rizzolatti, and colleagues first noticed neurons that we now call "mirror neurons," the game changed. We had to adjust our ideas about sensory and motor systems. The neurons in area F5 of premotor cortex (recorded in monkeys performing manual grasping tasks) were supposed to be "motor cells," but they showed strange visual responses. Slowly it dawned on the researchers that the visual responses code the actions of others and that this form of coding establishes a connection with the same actions as they are performed by the subject. At first, the researchers spoke carefully of "action recognition" (Gallese et al., 1996; Rizzolatti et al., 1996), but within two years, Gallese moved on to a radical concept of mind-reading "mirror neurons" (Gallese & Goldman, 1998), and Rizzolatti saw a connection between these neurons and the origin of language (Rizzolatti & Arbib, 1998).

Over the course of further empirical investigations it became clear that mirror neurons contribute to coding "in a fairly complex, multimodal, and rather abstract way," to use Iacoboni's exact words (2008|2009, p. 36). Mirror neurons are activated in similar ways by visual and auditory stimuli associated with others' actions (Kohler et al., 2002). They even fire their spikes when crucial visual information about others' actions is hidden from view but can be inferred from the previous sequence of events (Umiltà et al., 2001). Other evidence indicates that mirror neurons in the inferior parietal lobule code particular actions as a function of context (Fogassi et al., 2005). For instance, the neurons may fire more strongly when the observed actor grasps a food item to eat it than when the actor performs the same action to place an identical food item in a container (here the presence or absence of a container serves as a cue from which the monkey can predict the sequence of events). Put simply, these neurons link actions with their purpose.

All of this research leads to the obvious conclusion that mirror neurons do not simply "mirror" anything. They play a role in interpretation and the construction of abstract internal representations (see Nelissen et al., 2005, for monkey fMRI data on the multiplicity of coding in the mirror system). The coding is done in a format compatible with further intensive analyses. The information changes in the processing by mirror neurons. In fact, the mirror may not be the ideal metaphor for these neurons at all. "Mirror neurons help us reenact in our brain the intentions of other people," suggests Iacoboni (2008|2009, p. 78). This statement sounds more appealing to me. It reminds me of a passage by Merleau-Ponty (1945|2008, p. 410):

When I turn towards perception, and pass from direct perception to thinking about that perception, I reenact it, and find at work in my organs of perception a thinking older than myself of which those organs are merely the trace. In the same way I understand the existence of other people. Here again I have only the trace of a consciousness which evades me in its actuality and, when my gaze meets another gaze, I re-enact the alien existence in a sort of reflection.

The writings of Merleau-Ponty are apparently a great stimulus to Vittorio Gallese as well, and Marco Iacoboni even calls the French philosopher "[o]ur esteemed friend" (2008|2009, p. 115). Thus I feel entitled to zoom in on the word "re-enact" in both the Iacoboni and the Merleau-Ponty quote. I would remove the prefix from the word (or actually the first of two prefixes) since the activity of mirror neurons does not itself constitute a repeat, but a new, adaptive coding of something observed. I believe we should rename mirror neurons: Let us call them "enactive neurons."

I will admit right away that this renaming is not a very innocent proposal. It is aimed straight at the heart of Noë's (2004) enactive view of perception. Unfortunately, Noë completely ignored the work of Rizzolatti, Gallese, and associates, though it provided textbook examples of sensorimotor interaction and action in perception. Of course, the work did not fit in Noë's view, with his explicit resistance against internal representations. However, his mentor Susan Hurley (2008) forcefully and convincingly made the connection between active perception and the mirror system in her last article, on the shared circuits model. True enactive neurons are all about making abstracted information available internally, so that it can be used in a variety of cognitive endeavors, some of which may be uniquely human and supremely cultural.

Iacoboni (2008|2009) favors the view that the mirror/enactive system is a fairly autonomous operation that "reflects an experience-based, prereflective, and automatic form of understanding other minds" (p. 265), a claim well supported by the evidence (see Wagner et al., 2011, for an intriguing example with smokers watching movie characters smoke). Leslie (1994) called it a Theory-of-Mind-Mechanism, with emphasis on the mechanistic nature of the "theory." The notion is consistent also with the data on gaze following, discussed in the previous section (Deaner & Platt, 2003; Shepherd et al., 2009). However, this raises a problem of selection. How does the mirror/enactive system select which observers to follow, which actions to enact? This is the problem of gaze control, entirely overlooked by Iacoboni. I went to red alert on the issue when reading Iacoboni's description of the 2006 World Cup final of soccer (*real* football).

"A key episode in the Italian triumph was the sudden ejection of Zinédine Zidane, France's world-class player," writes Iacoboni (2008|2009, p. 106). "The cause was his savage head-butting of Marco Materazzi, an Italian player, in the chest." Even after multiple viewings of the images, Iacoboni reports (p. 107), "Still, I find myself experiencing strong emotions when Zidane head-butts Materazzi. I wince at Materazzi's pain," and "I also feel enraged all over again at Zidane for his act of aggression." Iacoboni does not mention or consider the possibility of provocation. He clearly chooses sides, for Materazzi, against Zidane, and his mirror/enactive system seems to work only for Materazzi, not for Zidane.

My own feelings were more complex. I was, and to some extent still am, a fan of Zidane, a true genius of the game. Perhaps dominant in my initial response to the violence was incomprehension, "Why does he do that?" This was immediately followed by suspicion, "Zidane must have been provoked." I was angry with Zidane for his aggression, and disappointed with his lack of self-control. But I was also not happy with Materazzi, and though I did wince, especially at the first moment of impact from the head butt, I also found myself unable to tell after multiple viewings how much of the emotional expression reflected real pain and how much of it reflected a desire for response from the referee. Materazzi later admitted to provoking Zidane with a lewd insult invoking Zidane's sister, an offense for which the Italian player was given a fine of five thousand Swiss francs and a two-match ban by the FIFA (a French acronym that translates to the "International Federation of Association Football," the relevant governing body and organizer of the World Cup). It was the first time a player received such punishment for a verbal offense. Zidane, on the other hand, received a fine of seven thousand five hundred Swiss francs and a three-match ban, which became irrelevant because he had decided to retire from the game; instead, Zidane agreed to three days of community service with children as a part of FIFA's humanitarian projects. All of these facts are very well-known and widely published but do not feature in Iacoboni's otherwise rich description long after the event.

The crucial issue is that of *bias*. Iacoboni, of Italian descent, with the same first name as that of Materazzi, views the events in a way that favors Materazzi over Zidane. His gaze sides with Materazzi, and the mirror/enactive system does its prereflective, automatic work within the constraints of this selection. Our enactive neurons process information contingent on the gaze—our gaze as well as the gaze of others on us (see Wang, Ramsey, & Hamilton, 2011, for an excellent demonstration). To gain a complete understanding of the mirror/enactive system, we must first of all address the issue of selection (by examining the role of the gaze, by investigating the bias mechanisms in neural circuits). Without it, we cannot begin to think about Iacoboni's (2008|2009, p. 272) beautiful words: "We have evolved to connect deeply with other human beings. Our awareness of this fact can and should bring us even closer to one another."

In the real world, bias operates, sometimes to disastrous effect as when it excludes certain people from other people's benevolent empathy. Tragically, newspapers are full every day of the lethal failures of the mirror/enactive systems of humans. To achieve Iacoboni's laudable goals, we need to learn to direct our gaze in more inclusive ways. In fact, given the prereflective, automatic nature of the mirror/enactive function, I see only two routes to more fairness in the distribution of gentle-hearted feeling for others. We can train (or condition) ourselves so that we acquire better implicit gaze biases, which allow us to automatically make the right choice (but note that this type of project is structurally similar to brain-washing and propaganda—a risky path of which we know very little). And, my preferred option, we can aim to direct our gaze strategically, potentially to counteract ugly biases lurking in our subconscious. For this, we need to learn about, and explicitly confront, our biases (see chapter 7 of *The Anatomy of Bias*, Lauwereyns, 2010).

Window to the Theory of Mind

When cognitive neuroscientists embraced the metaphor of the mirror, this was done under the rubric of mimicry, imitation, and understanding others. We agreed that the mirror/enactive system gives us something of a window to the minds of others, whether through implicit coupling or explicit theorizing. In thinking about this window, most researchers worked from a blank slate, ignoring the overtures from psychoanalysis and literary theory, where the concepts of mimesis and the mirror had been linked for many decades with the core dynamics underlying the human experience. During a career spanning more than fifty years, the French literary theorist René Girard (2008) has written extensively on mimesis and its impact on desire, developing the themes time and again in essays on the masterpieces by iconic authors such as Shakespeare, Proust, and Dostoevsky. The central observation is that mirroring goes beyond the copying for learning and generates intense emotions and motivations ("the true passions of the soul"), often becoming the source of personal conflict. We have yet to explore the notion of mimetic desire with respect to the mirror/enactive system.

Likewise, assuming poor scholarship poses no problem at all for good science, we failed to incorporate the perspective of Jacques Lacan (1966|2004) in our conceptualization of the mirror in the functioning of neural circuits. Yet, in one of his classic lectures (first given in Marienbad in 1936, then revised for Zurich, 1949) Lacan claimed a critical role for the mirror in the emergence of the self. He saw the mirror stage as formative of the function of the I: "This jubilant assumption of his specular image by the child at the *infans* stage, still sunk in his motor incapacity and nursling dependence, would seem to exhibit in an exemplary situation the symbolic matrix in which the I is precipitated in a primordial form" (Lacan, 1966|2004, p. 2).

This is not a crazy, obscure, or trivial idea. It points to the crucial grammar of seeing—the question of object and subject in vision. When I report "I see you," this involves two entities, "I" and "you," one of which is assigned agency in the act of observation (the subject "I") and one of which is designated as the content of the observation (the object "you"). Lacan pulls the moment of the mirror to the foreground as the first instance of self-*cognition* (before there can ever be self-*re*cognition). It marks the original encounter with a special visual object, one that cuts through boundaries and causes a crisis in the category of "objects" in order to become "subject." By Lacan's thesis, we need this mirror stage to realize that there exists such a special object, which constitutes "me"— the object that in this precise act of cognition transforms into subject. It would be a prelinguistic event that "situates the agency of the ego (…) in a fictional direction" (Lacan, 1966|2004, pp. 2–3). The object out there, in the mirror, shifts virtually to "in here," inside me.

This scheme is nicely compatible with Dennett's (1991) concept of the self as the Center of Narrative Gravity. With Lacan, we can think that the self starts developing its gravitational force even before it is able to spin proper stories, before the ego becomes structured enough to turn autobiographical. First, we need to construct a fictive center to see, and only *then* can this fictive center start creating stories about "me." Lacan (1966|2004, p. 3) suggests specifically, "[T]he mirror-image would seem to be the threshold of the visible world." It is through the encounter in the mirror that the subject comes into being and starts deploying his or her powers of agency as an independent observer. By this account, seeing is only possible once the subject has emerged from the mirror stage.

We do not literally need to think of this stage as an event that involves a mirror or a reflection in water or any other surface, even if Lacan seemed somewhat fixated on this point. The emergent self requires a basic understanding of agency, however implicit—a perception of causality between motor actions and sensory stimulation. I think it should essentially be a matter of contingency learning, for infants to develop the sensorimotor skills to grasp the connections between their own actions and the visual and other sensory outcomes they generate (e.g., Bushnell & Boudreau, 1993; Schmuckler & Jewell, 2007). Without contingency learning there would be no true seeing, no ability to detect cross-modal patterns in the complex sensory information. We know about the crucial role of contingency learning from congenitally blind individuals who get a first opportunity to "see" things after their cataracts have been removed. These newly sighted people initially suffer from "experiential blindness," to borrow Noë's phrase (2004, pp. 4–7). The naive observers need to go through a stage of contingency learning before they can make sense of their visual impressions.

To see, we need to learn, "This is what it looks like when I do *this*" and "That is what I get if I do *that*." We have to explore and construct our subjectivity. By the same token, we will encounter visual patterns that seem to adhere to some kind of contingency rules (they exhibit causality and agency) but are not actually controlled by us—"That is like me, but different." We learn to explore and construct the other. *That which is like me* is actually not just another object, but *somebody*, a subject with potentially a mind like mine. This other subject functions as a kind of mirror as well, not a duplicate of me, but an agency, a special being whose similarity-yet-difference becomes a crucial source for comparison and differentiation—perhaps even a crucial source of signification (as according to the philosophy of Emmanuel Lévinas, 1972|2003).

In this way, the mirror stage may precipitate the ego as well as the other, both the "I" and the "you," or multiple mutually reinforcing agencies. In *Theory of the Subject* the French philosopher Alain Badiou (an avid reader of Lacan) proclaims (1982|2009, p. 256) the following: "That subject that I come to be in certainty is something I could only anticipate, based on its supposedly being already there, through the evaluation of the other. And I can ground that subject retroactively only insofar as, through the effects of haste, it gains mastery, in its very place, over the contradiction of forces." In Plain (or at least plainer) English: The emergent "I" only fully becomes "me" through the gaze of the other. This process is a matter of "gaining mastery over the contradiction of forces," that is, contingency learning, learning who controls what.

Through the gaze of the other I gain my identity. Badiou suggests that it involves anticipation and presuppositions—essentially, the imaginary nature of the subject, consistent again with Dennett's (1991) Center of Narrative Gravity. We can understand this anticipatory fiction of the self as a collection of biases—biases that go from the very implicit (our sensorimotor skills, our strengths and weaknesses in perception, our expectations of how our actions relate to percepts) to the highly abstract and explicit (the autobiographical stories we tell ourselves and others).

In a suitably psychodynamic follow-up, Žižek connects the constitutive and interactive dynamics between the subject ("I") and the object ("you") with Lacan's famous *Objet petit a*—"the paradoxical object which directly 'is' the subject" (Žižek, 2006|2009, p. 213). This brings desire into the picture (I daresay, *into the mirror*), in a way that resonates with Girard's (2008) notion of mimetic desire. Speaking in slogans, we would get the following: "I want what you want" and "I am I because I desire this"—a fundamental mirroring that gives us passion as well as identity, or a Lacanian pastiche on Descartes, with *Desidero ergo sum* (never actually stated by the French psychoanalyst).

I suspect the last few paragraphs might sound a bit dense to fiercely empirical neuroscientists, so let me quickly draw two statements of possible pragmatic merit. First, we should study the mirror/enactive system from the perspective of subjectivity—how does this system coevolve with the self, with the understanding of our own perspective? I know of at least one fascinating study in this vein (Perner, Mauer, & Hildebrand, 2011), but at the moment most researchers seem to address the relevant components in isolation, focusing either on the developmental aspects of the mirror/enactive system without considering the factor of identity (e.g., Greimel et al., 2010) or on the differences in the mirror/enactive systems of normal subjects versus those with deficient self-awareness without considering the dynamics (e.g., Moriguchi et al., 2009). Lacan's hypothesis goes deeper. The self and the mirror/enactive system would shape each other. It is a hypothesis worth investigating.

Here is a second statement of pragmatic merit: We should study the mirror/enactive system also from the perspective of mimetic desire. We must be ready to consider the mirroring of others' emotions and intentions not just in terms of ("altruistic") empathy but also in terms of ("self-centered" or even "selfish") emulation. One intriguing behavioral study reports a type of mate-choice copying in humans that could be reflective of such "self-centered" mirroring of desire (Yorzinski & Platt, 2010). Other research addresses the dynamics behind our selective investment of empathy for others (e.g., Singer et al., 2006). Clearly, there is more room here for checking the optimistic assumptions in research on the mirror/enactive system. There may be less altruistic feeling and more selfishness (with Lacan, 1966|2004, p. 8, "we place no trust in altruistic feeling, we who lay bare the aggressivity that underlies the activity of the philanthropist, the idealist, the pedagogue, and even the reformer").

We can read Lacan's concern as a call for more care in formulating our operational definitions and in investigating the systematic variation with respect to the mirroring/enacting of others' mental states. In the cognitive neuroscience literature, "empathy" generally (often implicitly) refers to feeling what others feel in a way that promotes bonding between the self and others. This represents one, very appealing and desirable function. We may even wish to treat it as a standard—arguably a healthy approach, as long as we come forward, clearly and explicitly, with our normative judgments. To understand this function we must chart exactly how it differs from related, possibly "deviant" processes. For instance, feeling what others feel sometimes promotes the exact opposite of bonding as when I look at you, become jealous, and start feeling the same romantic desire you feel for a third person (in this case my mimetic desire turns you and me into love rivals). Another example, understanding (if not quite feeling) what others feel affords exploitation in the worst kinds of behavior our species is capable of (perhaps the most skilled torturers are endowed with exquisite mirror/enactive systems that allow them to precisely predict which horrible technique produces maximum effect).

In a way, the call for a more structured framework in the study of the mirror/enactive system reiterates my earlier point in response to Iacoboni's (2008|2009) presentation. We need to study the active boundaries of the mirror/enactive system, its constraints and conditions, when it works and to what end. In this effort, I expect we will learn a great deal by focusing on the role of the gaze. How do we engage in processing *this* bit rather than *that* bit of visual information? Our patterns of choice are likely governed by implicit associations, biases, and tendencies—mechanisms of inclusion and exclusion.

Let us indulge in a little (visual) thought experiment. Figure 6.4 raises the question of inclusion as concretely as possible. Can you return the gaze? Can you read the deer's mind? If not, why not? Would it be different for a monkey or a human? Would the human have to have—or *not* have—certain features (e.g., a particular color of skin, a certain type of headwear)? I am sure that factors such as proximity, similarity, and familiarity influence the probability of inclusion, but can we try harder? More technically, toward empirical inquiry: What kinds of emotions and intentions are we capable of mirroring/enacting in which conditions? What are the pitfalls? How far can we push Dennett's (1991) "heterophenomenological" approach (investigating the experiences of others through third-person accounts)? We hardly know the contours of this task. It involves neutralizing (objectifying) our own perspective and gathering all the possible data on the sensorimotor and cognitive skills of others (whether human or animal) in their context. It is an awesome challenge.

Yet we cannot ever give up on the task, for moral as well as scientific reasons. The entire enterprise of neuroscience, as it tries to connect the biology of humans with that of monkeys, rats, mice, fruit flies, and nematodes, critically depends on successful heterophenomenology. "We know

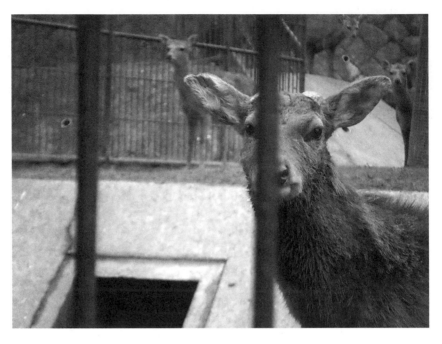

Figure 6.4
Do we extend the courtesy of mind reading? Four deer behind bars return our gaze. Especially the big eyes at the center of the image appear to demand some kind of interpretation, but we may lack the enactive neurons to properly assume the deer's perspective. This photograph was taken by an eight-year-old female observer upon her first visit to the Fukuoka Municipal Zoo and Botanical Garden, February 13, 2010.

what is really out there only from / the animal's gaze," offered Rainer Maria Rilke in the eighth of his Duino Elegies (Rilke, 1995, p. 377). That gaze would look out "into the Open," "free from death," and the animal, "when it moves, it moves / already in eternity, like a fountain." Rilke's eloquent and virtually ungraspable mysticism may paradoxically inspire us to concrete investigation. For Rilke, human consciousness is set apart from everything else in nature by language and awareness of death (a combination we already briefly encountered in chapter 5, in the guise of abstraction as the ultimate place of negativity; see Agamben, 1991). Our gaze would be turned inward, focusing on the recognition of objects, in an internal conversation with memory and meaning—perhaps not entirely unlike what I have dubbed "the intensive approach." In the eighth Duino elegy of Rilke, the implication is that animals would not have access to it.

Good and demanding poetry may serve as our secret well of scientific hypotheses (or it may simply tickle our curiosity). From Rilke we harvest the hypothesis that the human gaze employs the intensive approach and the animal gaze does not (but see Gertrude Stein, for the opposite hypothesis, "I am I because my little dog knows me," from "Identity a Poem," Stein, 2008, p. 301). If Rilke is right and Stein ironic, we may try to read the mind of the deer, but whatever we discover will be nonsense, and the deer does not bother to get the slightest bit from our eyes. To provide evidence in favor of this proposal, we should work from the null hypothesis that human and animal gazes do in fact share the same functions. Our task is to show exactly where and how things diverge—not to prove that humans are special or "higher" or "worthier" but to understand and to appreciate the similarities and the differences and, hopefully, to incorporate this knowledge in decision making and policies (including those with respect to animal welfare). The multiple meanings of the deer's gaze will be somewhere in the middle of a nonlinear process (a cloud of wily data). It is up to science to characterize the dynamics.

Gaze as a Love Object

Looking into the eyes of the other, the lyricist sighs, "These lovely lamps, these windows of the soul." This particular line of verse would be due to the French sixteenth-century poet Guillaume de Salluste, seigneur du Bartas, according to Hess and Polt (1960, p. 349). The quote received a prominent place (but no bibliographic reference) in Hess and Polt's groundbreaking *Science* article on pupillary responses to the content of pictures. The researchers did not actually pursue the topic of gaze perception (our reading of another's gaze), but the quote suggests they intuited a connection with their own work. If pupil size varies systematically, it should provide one of the most critical cues in another's eyes.

Figure 6.5 illustrates the point. Here, the gaze of the little girl (my daughter) attempts to gain control over the observer, with the very specific objective of obtaining candy from her parent (me). The emissive power of her gaze appears to be amplified by a remarkable widening of the pupils. Indeed, the corollary to the notion of pupil size as an index of gaze magnitude (introduced in chapter 5) is that observers may discriminate this information to deduce something about the internal states of others (their level of arousal or interest). Of course, this is not to say that Nanami in figure 6.5 deliberately tried to signal something with the size of her pupils. The physiological marker would be beyond our voluntary control unless we resort to indirect techniques such as Lee Strasberg's method acting or more direct interventions via pharmacology—particularly with extracts from Deadly Nightshade, that is, the

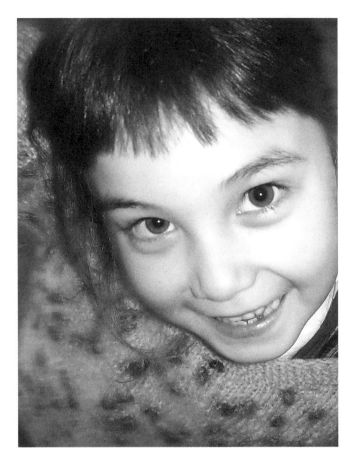

Figure 6.5
The art of begging for sweets. The portrayed subject, nearly six years of age at the time, failed to extract chocolate from her parent–photographer on this occasion, August 19, 2007, despite the positive facial expression and the widening of the pupils. The ensuing tantrum was not recorded.

perennial herbaceous plant *Atropa belladonna*, used as a cosmetic at least as far back as the Italian Renaissance (Schultes, Hofman, & Rätsch, 2001), though not an advisable product given the plant's hallucinogenic powers.

Perhaps it is fair to say that, by and large, pupil size represents an implicit factor, both in the person who owns the pupils and in the person who observes them. Processing the pupil sizes of others would be automatic and autonomous, one of the ways in which we read emotional expressions in others. Accordingly, Demos and colleagues (2008) found in an fMRI study that the activity in the amygdala is sensitive to pupil size. The researchers presented male subjects with photos of women in which the eyes had been digitally manipulated to create either large or small pupils. The BOLD responses in the amygdala increased for large pupils, even though the subjects, during debriefing after the experiment, reported not being aware of the size manipulation.

Interestingly, the pupil size did not affect the subjects' ratings of attractiveness. Pupil size alone does not do the trick and presumably plays a subtler role in complex dynamics that we have barely begun to explore. Looking a person in the eye, we integrate various types of information in our implicit readings, not just pupil size but also eye whites (Whalen et al., 2004) and myriad other aspects of facial expression. In figure 6.5 the smile is at least as dominant as the gaze in my daughter's ruthless attempt at persuasion. Only from the combination of the various features can we derive an interpretation—what kind of smile it is, what it tries to say. Niedenthal and colleagues (2010) proposed the simulation-of-smiles model, with a detailed architecture of potential routes among several modules: for the detection of smiles, the making of eye contact, the activation of reward circuitry, and the engagement of the mirror/enactive system. The gaze would function as a trigger for embodied simulation— without eye contact, the smile does not move us. Avoiding eye contact would have been the only way I managed resisting Nanami's plea.

The combination of gaze and smile strongly stimulates positive approach. The gaze seals a link, as in James Cameron's 2009 science-fiction movie *Avatar*, with the graceful blue creatures, the Na'vi, who say "I see you" to express the deepest possible connection between two individuals. Salecl and Žižek identified gaze and voice as "love objects par excellence—not in the sense that we fall in love with a voice or a gaze, but rather in the sense that they are a medium, a catalyst that sets off love" (1996, p. 3). This was for an edited volume in the SIC series (no K missing; SIC stands for psychoanalytic interpretation at its most elementary). In the same volume, Dolar finds overwhelming evidence in our legends, novels, and movies that "the hand of fate seems to operate primarily by the gaze" (1996, p. 134). The gaze "emerges as the firm rock of positivity on which to build one's existence, the authoritative and commanding presence by which to rule one's life, the steadfast support of one's being against all odds" (p. 135).

This gaze comes back to Lacan's mirror and insists on the narcissistic nature of love. The great myths seem to offer us no hope of escape. Of course, *any* love can be called narcissistic if it makes us feel good. Thus pulling an ancient tragic figure out of the closet does not necessarily help us forward in the search for explanations. As for more literal interpretations of narcissism and love, we could examine the role of similarity in various aspects of our being. However, tastes are notoriously tricky to discuss (in Latin it would be a *non est*), and many people bought Paula Abdul's wisdom, "Opposites Attract" (song released in 1989, written by Oliver Leiber; certified gold within a half year).

I will not dispute that the gaze has potential as a love object. Even monkeys will pay per view to get access to the eyes of others they look up to (Deaner, Khera, & Platt, 2005) or wish to mount (Oomura, Yoshimatsu, & Aou, 1983), though of course there exist other visual pleasures than merely the eyes — both studies also involved a monkey version of "the male gaze," with brutally sexist bias, in very much the sense given to the term by Laura Mulvey (1989|2009); juice was sacrificed, or manual labor performed, in exchange for pictures of female perinea, or even access to the real thing (the latter experiment, a legendary pioneering study, was performed at my very own Kyushu University, though the researchers have in the meantime found other destinations in life, if not in research).

With the male gaze we encounter a type of looking behavior that is anything but agreeable to perceive. Some gazes become objects that induce pain, fear, disgust, or hate. Mulvey, one of the earliest proponents of feminist thought in film and media studies, introduced the concept of the male gaze to discuss the dominance of heterosexual male perspectives in the way the camera is positioned and choices are made about what to show. We note that the job of movie director has remained extremely gender biased to this day. The male gaze implies unbalanced power between the observer and what, or who, is observed. To be subjected to the male gaze by force may be experienced as a form of violation that comes very close to an actual emission effect, as if gazing amounted to groping.

In fact, the ancient debate on intromission versus emission of light during visual perception might have been fueled to some extent by superstitions about the destructive power of "the evil eye" — among the most pervasive and persistent folk beliefs in the Indo-European and Semitic world (see Dundes, 1981|1992, for a cross-cultural set of investigations). Cinema has further offered us indelible images of powerful gazes. I am thinking specifically of Sergio Leone's widescreen close-ups of eyes, his signature technique to capture what I would call "the macho gaze" in spaghetti westerns. We see the Man with No Name (Clint Eastwood) stare down his opponent in a gunfight (the music of Ennio Morricone ringing in our ears) and know already from the stranger's eyes alone that the duel is decided before the shooting begins (see the 1964 movie *Per un pugno di dollari*, released in the United States in 1967 as *A Fistful of Dollars*).

Such display of power through the eyes may very well reflect a basic feature of nonverbal communication we share with many animal species —a thesis formulated close to a century and a half ago by Charles Darwin (1872|1965) in his still very rewarding *The Expression of the Emotions in Man and Animals*. The face-off via the gaze, with the strong staying put and the weak scampering away, would save all parties a good amount of energy, or even injury. The gaze in these instances, as it remains fixated on others, marks a challenge, a readiness to process to the very end—any kind of information, even if it involves the most physical and proximate, such as claws reaching for the jugular or fangs aiming for flesh.

As noted earlier with respect to the relation between gaze and choice, the spatial coordinates of fixation tell us nothing about the valuation, whether good or bad, positive or negative. The gaze is a tool for intensive processing, and as such we know that the gaze of others, as it remains fixated on us, implies special interest, but we need contextual information to color that interest (what we know about the others and the situation we are in; all kinds of nonverbal cues, smile or frown, body posture, etc.). Conversely, the gaze of others, when directed elsewhere, can imply a lack of interest or intensive processing and may be colored very differently from one situation to the next.

The animal that averts its gaze and scampers away signals submission. Figure 6.6 shows an instance from the opposite end of the power spectrum with gaze avoidance. Here, the Nazi scientist Dr. Ritter denies a middle-aged Sinti or Roma woman the privilege of his gaze as he goes over his notes. The denial of access to the eyes in this case seems to function as an instrument of control, imposing distance and signaling a lack of esteem. In a provocative study on "Dehumanizing the Lowest of the Low," Harris and Fiske (2006) obtained fMRI evidence pointing to a critical difference in the activation of medial prefrontal cortex when subjects observe images from various social groups. The BOLD data showed activation in this brain structure for all social groups, as we should expect, given the putative role of the medial prefrontal cortex in social cognition (Amodio & Frith, 2006). However, there was one marked exception: the extreme out-group of the homeless and drug addicts,

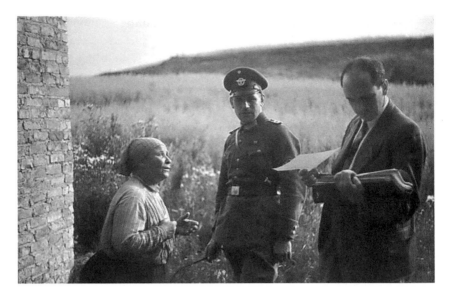

Figure 6.6
"Dr. Robert Ritter with an old woman and a police officer," dated 1936, by an unknown photographer (German Federal Archives: Bundesarchiv, R 165 Bild-244–71 / CC-BY-SA). Dr. Ritter worked as a scientist investigating the "biology of criminality" for the Nazi regime (Browning & Matthäus, 2004). His research on the Roma people contributed to the *Porajmos* (Romani word for "the devouring," referring to the genocide). Here, the unidentified Sinti or Roma woman vainly searches for the gaze of Dr. Ritter, who keeps his eyes locked on his papers.

which in a separate survey had been associated coldly with incompetence. For this extreme out-group the subjects cannot get their medial prefrontal cortices active; instead, blood flow increases in the amygdala and insula, consistent with the reported feelings of disgust.

How does the "dehumanizing effect" come about? Unfortunately Harris and Fiske (2006) did not consider gaze parameters in their study. Even though the subjects had their eyes open and showed visual activation in response to all images, it seems quite likely that their intensive processing worked differently for the extreme out-group. It would be interesting to know whether this is achieved by strategically aiming the gaze away from sensitive regions (e.g., the eyes and faces of the homeless and drug addicts) in a move similar to that of Dr. Ritter. Alternatively, subjects might have processed the images *more* intensively for the extreme out-group, checking the eyes and faces of the homeless and drug addicts with extreme care. In support of this proposal, negative gossip has been shown to produce prolonged perceptual dominance of faces in a binocular rivalry paradigm (Anderson et al., 2011). Our vigilance is aroused by people that seem suspicious.

I suspect that the gaze and intensive processing adapt to behavioral contexts. When we interact directly with others, we sometimes resort to using covert visual strategies, disconnecting the focus of the gaze and the locus of intensive processing. We may strategically look away to avoid expressing interest for a variety of reasons, not only those of Dr. Ritter; we might be worried that our gaze signals a challenge or an approach. The situation changes significantly if our gaze cannot be seen. We can relish our visual pleasures from a hidden vantage point (the voyeur's tactic and also, more innocently, that of the amateur ornithologist). Similarly, we can give way, overtly and shamelessly, to our curiosity or vigilance when we look at photographs (as in the studies by Harris & Fiske, 2006, and Anderson et al., 2011). In all of these cases, we are aware that the gaze is a natural index of interest. It pays to be careful about how we use it.

Optimally Interacting

The gaze is an instrument of social cognition, a communicative device with which we express signals and from which we acquire information—there is sending as well as receiving. From a utilitarian perspective we can ask the practical question of how we use this device most efficiently. In any given situation, there may be constraints to gaze distribution (by all individuals involved) suited for optimal interaction with others. Where do we look so that it promotes optimal interaction? The issue is that of sharing (see figure 6.7), a topic that also takes us back (lyrically, if not practically) to Samuel Taylor Coleridge's conversation poem at the beginning of this chapter. By looking at and thinking about the same things as others have in mind, we forge a connection not just with the objects of vision but with our fellow observers, whether competitively or cooperatively.

At the outset, the optimality of interaction—whether we join hands or lock into battle—can be a thorny issue, a headache and heartache with social, cultural, and even religious reverberations. Most of us will easily (and not sentimentally) agree that the joining of hands is by far the preferable strategy. We do well to look for win–win situations and non-zero-sum games. In practice this is not always possible and not always up to us to decide, but if and when we *are* set for positive interaction, sharing the focus of intensive processing is the obvious path to cohesive

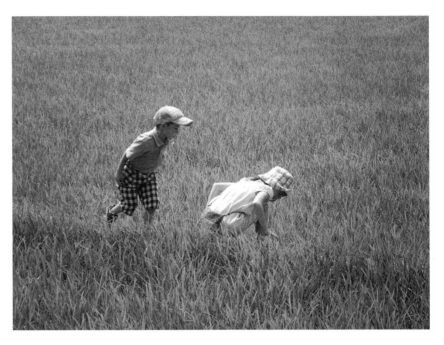

Figure 6.7
Wonder, shared by siblings in a rice paddy, on July 26, 2011, near Takeo, Saga prefecture, Japan. The idyllic scene with two gazes converging on a single point calls to mind Romantic verse ("The poetry of earth is never dead: / When all the birds are faint with the hot sun, / And hide in cooling trees, a voice will run / From hedge to hedge about the new-mown mead; That is the Grasshopper's—he takes the lead / In summer luxury," by John Keats, 1978|2003, p. 54, written on December 30, 1816). What, though, will the siblings do when they catch sight of the grasshopper?

group dynamics. It is a path that comes naturally to us, according to Michael Tomasello and his colleagues. This group of researchers proposed the cultural intelligence hypothesis (Herrmann et al., 2007), backed by data showing that human children, two and a half years old, reach levels of performance similar to those of chimpanzees and orangutans in the physical domain (tasks involving spatial memory, numerical cognition, tool use, etc.) but win hands down in the social domain (tasks involving social learning, gaze following, reading intentions, etc.).

Kovács, Téglás, and Endress (2010) went one step further, recognizing our social sense already in infants, barely seven months of age, who are influenced by others in ways analogous to what occurs in adults. Babies understand others' beliefs and are even willing to adopt these alternative views in case of conflict with their own. This makes for optimal interaction when others are in a better position to know than we are; they may have access to a wider perspective. Optimal interaction in this case means accepting the other's report as the more reliable. Accordingly, Bahrami and colleagues (2010) found in a low-level visual discrimination task that two heads are better than one only if they are clear about who knows best.

Bahrami et al. asked two observers to make a simple perceptual decision (decide whether the first or the second image includes an oddball with slightly higher contrast among six vertically oriented Gabor patches). The two observers made their individual decisions and then also a joint decision. If the two observers have similar sensitivities, their joint decisions are better than their individual responses (the merging of the two perspectives improves the signal-to-noise ratio with twice as many data). However, if the two observers have very different sensitivities, their joint decision making is actually worse than their individual performance (the two perspectives cannot easily be merged, and the process ends up confusing both observers in turn).

Optimal interaction requires more than gaze following to compute the same fixation point. We need to generate some kind of understanding of the other's intensive processing by taking contextual information into account. Through the application of the mirror/enactive system, we can try to put ourselves in the other's perspective and glean some information from that virtual stance. This can be a useful strategy, despite the inherent logical flaws. Sometimes we arrive at a good practical understanding of a situation by applying our projections about intensive processing even if these projections are principally *wrong*. Donald Hebb concluded as much after a two-year study with chimpanzees, in which the experimenters had carefully tried to avoid anthropomorphic description (1946, p. 88; italics as per original):

All that resulted was an almost endless series of specific acts in which no order or meaning could be found. On the other hand, by the use of frankly anthropomorphic concepts of emotion and attitude one could quickly and easily describe the peculiarities of the individual animals, and with this information a newcomer to the staff could handle the animals as he could not safely otherwise. Whatever the anthropomorphic terminology may seem to imply about conscious states in the chimpanzee, it provides *an intelligible and practical guide to behavior.*

I encountered this quote in Daniel Wegner's *The Illusion of Conscious Will* (2002, p. 24). Wegner adds, almost criminally vividly, "You have to think about the animals' minds in order to keep from getting mugged by them." The point will be clear enough. Even if the intensive readings are illusory, they have practical benefit. They allow observers to predict what will happen next. At the end of the day, this is the only measure for any theory of mind. How well does it allow us to understand what is going on, to what level of optimality does it let us interact with others? Pitched in the opposite direction, we know that without the ability to read (even illusory) intentions in others we function less efficiently. According to Baron-Cohen (1995), this is the root of many problems in some forms of autism. Normally we rely on "intentionality detectors" to gather who does what and why. Without such detectors, we suffer from "mind-blindness" and have to make do with unwieldy physical or mechanistic explanations.

We are lucky to have our intentionality detectors and even luckier if we can forge deep connections with them the way Coleridge did as he imagined how his friend, the gentle-hearted Charles, stood gazing. Or in the words of Hans Faverey (1994|2004, p. 142) from *Sequence against Death*, sighing lyrically, some four hundred years after Guillaume de Salluste, seigneur du Bartas (I cite only up to the first semicolon, which I read as a wink of the eye),

The eyes which grant
my eyes her eyes,
because this is how

the light in them goes between;

7 Seeing and Nothingness

extract
from the shadow of the object
which does not exist
from polar space
from the stern reveries of the inner eye
a chair

beautiful and useless
like a cathedral in the wilderness

place on the chair
a crumpled tablecloth
add to the idea of order
the idea of adventure

This fragment belongs to "Study of the Object" in Zbigniew Herbert's 1961 collection by the same name (the quoted lines are from Herbert, 2007, pp. 195–196). The Polish master of lyrical investigation wrote the poem several years before coming up with the unforgettable character of Mr Cogito, but the tone and the logic already announce Herbert's later invention. This is the ghost of Descartes speaking in confident elliptic verse, aware of the past (Wallace Stevens, "the idea of order") and ready to go beyond the present (adding "the idea of adventure" and a little irony, beauty inviting uselessness to join with an "and," not a "but"). The adventure we should risk and enjoy is that of the imagination.

The poem started with the apodictic assertion that "The most beautiful is the object / which does not exist" (p. 193). To see it, the mind must imagine, and "when it imagines, it turns towards the body and looks at something in the body which conforms to an idea understood by the mind or perceived by the senses" (Descartes, 1641|1996, p. 51). In accordance with this Cartesian definition of the imagination, Zbigniew Herbert

(2007) sets us going on the impossible approach to the most beautiful object with a sequence of strategic instructions. The first, to extract a chair from the inner eye, is a bit too vague for my mind to begin embodying that object. However, the bizarre, unpredictable appeal to a cathedral in the wilderness gives the right spark. I see the roofless San Galgano Abbey with grass and mud where there once was a stone floor—the ruins in the province of Siena, Italy, where Andrei Tarkovsky shot the final scene of his 1983 movie *Nostalghia*. I remember walking there many years ago; more images return as I continue with the adventure.

Then again, the San Galgano Abbey ruins are not really in the wilderness. I must combine it with another memory, that of the Bridge to Nowhere in Wanganui National Park, New Zealand. This conjunction almost works for me, in a tantalizing, near-visual way. Now, my imaginative powers warmed up, I am ready to place that crumpled tablecloth on the chair. I think I can see it, and Herbert was right; this plain, everyday scene, which does not exist, is the most beautiful crumpled-tablecloth-on-a-chair I have ever seen—useless, wonderful, a true adventure. Or does this not count as seeing?

The Horopter

What counts as seeing? Does the imagination give us virtual vision or something categorically different? Noë's (2004) enactive view of perception must firmly reject the idea of imagination as a visual faculty, given its inherent internal nature. Here is Noë insisting on a fundamental divide between true vision and another form of seeing things that are not there, very familiar to all of us (this quote is from his more recent book, *Out of Our Heads*, 2009, p. 179):

The fluidity and shifting grounds of dream experience reflect precisely that in dreams, but not in normal perceptual experience, we are decoupled from the world around us. What determines content in a dream is precisely not what is there in front of us. We can see what we want to see, or what we are afraid to see, or what we wonder what it might be like to see. Which is just another way of saying that dream seeing is not really seeing at all.

Of course, Noë is right in putting his finger on the decoupling. But this does not explain away the similarities between true seeing and dreaming. As scientists we should like to understand the underlying mechanisms and trace the extent of the commonalities. Our experience does not support a fundamental divide between true seeing and various forms of illusory seeing. The fact is we do sometimes get confused; there are moments we wonder whether what we thought we saw is really there. With the intensive approach we immediately realize that the confusion comes about when we cannot trace what triggered the activation of internal representations—errors and illusions are a natural by-product of the fact that perception constructs internal representations. For the enactive view of perception, such errors are an awkward problem. How can there be confusion between a thing in the head and one out of the head? Where does the confusion take place, by what mechanism? Noë offers no suggestions.

Yet, this is not a trivial matter. Error is intrinsic to the daily enterprise of being human. Sometimes we do not know what we see. Descartes (1637|2006, p. 28) famously took our confusions in the perceptual domain as a reason to reject vision in his search for a rock-solid first principle: "[B]ecause our senses sometimes deceive us, I decided to suppose that nothing was such as they lead us to imagine it to be." This radical rejection (only for the sake of argument on the way to a beginning) occurred on the very same page where Descartes arrived at his *Cogito ergo sum*.

Occasionally we really believe we see things that are not, or cannot be. Perceptual illusions, hallucinations, dreams, and false alarms are part of the territory of perception; no theory will be complete without an explanation of how our errors come about. Indeed signal detection theory (Green & Swets, 1966|1988) and with it all Bayesian accounts of perception and decision making make a compelling case for careful investigation of different types of error; again the pivotal concept is that of bias (Lauwereyns, 2010). The proper approach to virtual vision is to try to chart it as precisely as we can.

On this note I would like to visit Aguilonius (1613) one last time, our seventeenth-century predecessor, vision scientist, architect, mathematician, Jesuit priest, citizen of Antwerp, and collaborator of Rubens. Figure 7.1 presents an intriguing effort at measuring virtual visual projections in minute fashion. This image by Rubens was for book IV of *Opticorum Libri Sex*, "De Fallaciis Aspectus." If my high-school Latin is not mistaken, this translates to "On Vision from Deceptions." The image shows an experimental apparatus designed by Aguilonius to pinpoint the positions of double images from a single object on a projection wall.

The observer, presumably the same thinker assisted by the same putti as in figures 2.1 and 4.3, leans on one end of what vaguely looks like a baroque table tennis table (with conspicuous chimeras for legs), folded to afford solitary play (if we disregard the imaginary creatures). The observer focuses his eyes on a point on the vertical line in the middle of

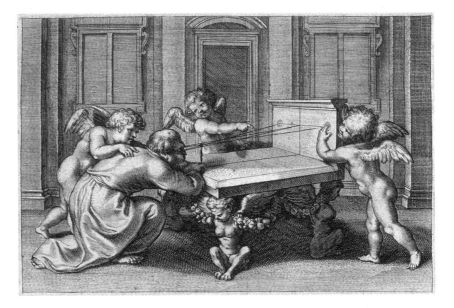

Figure 7.1
Experimental setup to investigate the horopter. An illustration by Peter Paul Rubens for
book IV of Franciscus Aguilonius's *Opticorum Libri Sex* (1613). The observer, with a little
help from his putti, aims to locate the virtual projections of a near object (a small sphere
close to his eyes) as he focuses on a point in the distance on the vertical line in the middle
of a projection wall. The virtual projections are diplopic images due to binocular disparity
(in Plain English: they are what he sees double because his two eyes have slightly different
perspectives).

the back half of the table tennis table (let me call this back half "the
projection wall"). On the way there, his focus must pass through the little
ball on a stick right in front of his nose. As a result, he sees double—
according to Aguilonius the optic radii (the observer's lines of sight)
carry the image of the object to the projection wall. The putti can point
to exactly where the virtual objects are. Thus we have a metric for these
strange impossible duplicates in our vision.

You can easily try something similar at home or in your office even
without the table tennis table; just focus on a point in the distance, preferably on a wall, hold your left thumb close to your nose straight in front
of that point in the distance, and note that you now have two half-
transparent left thumbs whose positions you can situate precisely on that
wall in the distance. The double images are another instance of the parallax due to the fact that our eyes have slightly different outlooks on the
world. In this sense, the demonstration is merely a metric variation of
Aguilonius's previous discussion (his treatment of binocular disparity in

book III of *Opticorum Libri Sex*; see figure 4.3). However, the metric variation makes an explicit move beyond the discussion of parallax by focusing on the virtual projections. To capture these, Aguilonius introduced the concept of the "horopter." He coined the word from the combination of the Greek words *horos* ("boundary") and *opter* ("observer")—the observer's boundary.

For Aguilonius, the horopter was exactly the projection wall: the horizontal plane through the focus point, which runs parallel to the plane between the left eye and the right eye (we can think of it as the line we draw between the two points we get when we abstract each eye to a single point). On this plane there would be fused ("real") as well as diplopic ("virtual") images. This is different from the term "horopter" in contemporary usage, where it refers to the spatial boundaries for fused images (the Vieth–Müller circle, approximately a circle that passes through the point of convergence and the two eyes; Vieth, 1818). Alhazen got closer to the contemporary horopter than Aguilonius did (see Howard, 1996, for comprehensive discussion, including English translations of excerpts from Aguilonius's text).

Did Aguilonius's work on this point mean a step backward from Alhazen? Strictly speaking, yes, with respect to our understanding of where in space images are fused. However, that was not what Aguilonius was after with his horopter, in a chapter on the act of seeing from deceptions. His attempt was to gather truth from and about perceptual illusions—with the horopter he tried to work out the optics of diplopic as well as fused images. His approach in this case turned out to be of limited practical value. But Aguilonius showed that the virtual projections involve forms of seeing that afford objective, scientific measurement. Moreover, these virtual projections can be explained as the product of the same visual powers that give us true perception. These are still relevant thoughts for any student of perception.

I also like Aguilonius's idea of optic radii carrying virtual images of objects to a projection wall. Connecting to our discussions in chapter 6, it is another instance of an imaginary emission effect, as if our eyes are searchlights that leave duplicate shadows of things on a distant wall. Like Goethe, Aguilonius knew better in terms of physics. The issue was not the physics; it was the sense we make of things. With Merleau-Ponty (1945|2008, p. 157), who thought the analogy of the searchlight was inadequate, let us say that the projection is one of intentionality—a matter of virtual meaning, living inside our heads, toward things in the world:

[T]he life of consciousness—cognitive life, the life of desire or perceptual life—is subtended by an "intentional arc" which projects round about us our past, our future, our human setting, our physical, ideological and moral situation, or rather which results in our being situated in all these respects.

For Merleau-Ponty, the intentional arc reflects the meaning-giving operation of consciousness. It is a virtual projection of meaning, which gives power of presence to things that are not there. This impossible presence (of the past, of the future) lives inside our heads, not physically in the world. Yet, indirectly the projected intentionality can make contact and interact with physical processes in the world, for instance, through creativity, when we use our projections of the future to shape our current surroundings. We can address our fantasies in engineering and art—it is the ancient Orphic project of singing the loved one into being, beyond death, beyond nothingness, through some kind of change or transformation (perhaps a matter of exploration rather than expression).

Powers of Presence

Presence is what counts, not just materially, but for the mind. "Out of sight, out of mind," the English idiom says. The Dutch formulate the idea more extremely, with *Uit het oog, uit het hart* ("Out of the eye, out of the heart"), specifying the anatomic organ that receives the visual sensory stimulation and connecting the reception there with the passionate movements of the mind, particularly those with which we text eternal messages like "I *heart* U." Interestingly, the German version represents the exact midpoint, *Aus den Augen, aus dem Sinn,* "Out of the eye, out of mind." I am not sure whether we can read cross-cultural differences in temperament into these variations. Things do get lost in translation. Via Chinese whispers and translation machines we move from "Out of sight, out of mind" to the terse truth "Invisible insane" (Lederer, 1987|2006, p. 105).

In English, matters are further complicated by an idiom that posits the opposite wisdom, "Absence makes the heart grow fonder." Perhaps English, the lingua franca, seeks maximum openness, accepting that sometimes we get *this*, sometimes *that*. In chapter 3 we concluded that sight is really part of the mind anyway, so we can also rewrite "Out of sight, out of mind" as the somewhat Zen-like observation (or reverberation), "Out of mind, out of mind." Put differently, this comes down to emphasizing the difference between inside and outside, between what is in the mind/sight and what is not. The idioms, consistent with the intensive approach, know that the essential issue is *selection*. The selection is straightforward when it regards things that are in front of us. For absent things, we have to work harder, via faculties such as that of the imagination, to let them enter our minds (perhaps the growth of fondness has something to do with the willingness or commitment needed for this extra work).

From the basic issue of selection we can zoom out to the more general proposal that vision and consciousness necessarily exhibit intentionality (Brentano, 1874|1995), or "aboutness" (Dennett, 1987, 1991). The act of seeing by definition takes an object. There is no vision, unless we see *something*. There is no consciousness, unless we are conscious of *something*. In the words of Badiou (1988|2007, p. 34), "All thought supposes a situation of the thinkable, which is to say a structure, a count-as-one, in which the presented multiple is consistent and numerable." The thinker thinks a thought; the object taken by vision or consciousness is a count-as-one. The study of perception focuses on *what* and *how*—the structure and how it is constructed. For psychologists and neuroscientists this means we must study the nature of the selected representation (the features included in the selection, or the content of the object file) and the determinants of the selection (e.g., whether under voluntary control or automatic, whether actively imagined or passively received).

Some of these questions can be asked in very direct ways in neurophysiological studies, even with humans. Particularly Itzhak Fried and Christoph Koch have pioneered this approach with patients who suffer from epilepsy and cannot be helped with medicine. In cases in which the seizure focus in the brain (the weak spot that generates epileptic seizures) cannot be determined through noninvasive neuroimaging, the patients are implanted with chronic depth electrodes for one or two weeks to determine the critical spot (so that the connections to this spot can be strategically cut with minimal loss of brain function). Since the patients have to have the electrodes implanted anyway, the researchers might as well take it as a positive opportunity to conduct experiments and obtain data they should otherwise never dream of obtaining (unless the dream is a nightmare). Most patients actually enjoy the mind/brain games and are pleased to know that they are contributing to cutting-edge science.

Through this approach, Kreiman, Koch, and Fried (2000) recorded what they called "imagery neurons" in the human medial temporal lobe. The researchers presented one of two possible images in a random sequence of, say, ten trials and then asked the patients to imagine the same objects when cued with auditory tones (e.g., high tone means "Imagine the same lady's face"; low tone means "Imagine the very same baseball"). Some neurons fired spikes selectively in response to particular images (e.g., only *this* face) and did so both for a visual image presented on a monitor and for the reconstructed or reactivated version in the mind (the authors did not hesitate in invoking "the mind's eye," a problematic metaphor). From such data we cannot conclude exactly *what* is represented in the count-as-one, but we do get existence proof of a shared level of representation, accessible via imagination as well as via direct visual perception.

Cerf and colleagues (2010) implemented a feedback loop between the human brain, the computer screen, and the signal decoder to study the voluntary control of imagery in a different way. In this neurofeedback study (with a rationale like that encountered in chapter 4; Fetz, 1969; Schafer & Moore, 2011) patients were presented with hybrid, superimposed images. The feedback system was organized so that the activity of neurons in the medial temporal lobe determined the actual (external) dominance of different patterns in the hybrid image. By selectively focusing on a particular pattern, the patients were able to increase its dominance in the image. This implies that, by selectively focusing on visual patterns, we exert voluntary control over the activity level of neurons in the medial temporal lobe. It is a natural way of increasing the power of presence of whatever it is that we are thinking about. Indeed, the patients were often able to get the desired neurofeedback results from the first trial, without any training.

These studies on imagery and voluntary control lend weight to the argument that vision and consciousness operate on the basis of internal representations that can be activated in several ways. The challenge for neuroscience is to decode these hidden information structures and to study how the internal representations are employed in various behavioral contexts (Gilbert & Wilson, 2007). One fine example of such a research effort is that by A. David Redish and colleagues (Johnson & Redish, 2007; Van der Meer et al., 2010) on the coding of future possibilities (travel paths) in rats running on T-based decision tasks. These codes are read on the basis of neural ensemble recordings by comparing the normal spatial coding while the rat is moving with transient, subtle signals while the rat is pausing at decision points. Similarities in the code suggest that the rat projects a virtual position. The data (particularly in hippocampal area CA3 and ventral striatum, but not dorsal striatum) clearly show that the transient, subtle signals are prospective and systematic, as if the rat plays a virtual scenario of itself moving forward in one direction or the other.

The ability to project the position of the self somewhere outside the body takes a more extreme form in the ever-popular stories about out-of-body experiences—with dying patients looking down on themselves lying on the operating table. Already halfway to heaven, they suddenly crash back into their bodies to resume the rest of their biological lives. In these stories, the projection amounts to a very convincing perceptual illusion. In a wonderfully creative study with the teasing title "Video Ergo Sum," Lenggenhager and colleagues (2007) were able to make something akin to an out-of-body illusion tractable in the lab. They had subjects look at a virtual video projection of their own bodies, filmed from the back. The virtual dummy was placed at a two-meter distance in front of the subject. The subject's back was stroked, and this appeared either synchronously or asynchronously on the virtual video projection. It was as if the virtual body underwent the same thing in real time or something else, disconnected from the subject. After the stroking, the subject (blindfolded) was led to a different position and asked to return to the original position. In the synchronous condition the subjects' return position tended to deviate toward that of the virtual video projection. There was no drift in the asynchronous condition.

Somehow, the virtual video projection influenced the subjects' sense of their own position in space, but only when the feeling of being stroked coincided with what the dummy underwent. The concurrent visual and somatosensory information forced "a connection" with the other body, strong enough to challenge the subject's own bodily boundaries. This is not to say that the subject felt they were one with the virtual dummy in the ecstatic way of Walt Whitman or the completely enlightened way of Zen Buddhism. Rather more mundanely, our active boundaries of self in vision are sensitive to the powers of presence of various stimuli. When what looks more or less like us matches with what we feel, our automatic pattern analyzers tempt us into believing that the coincidence is no coincidence. If it walks like a duck and talks like a duck... If it looks like me and feels like me... By thinking things through, we discover the logical errors, but by that time the coordinates of our original position will be lost irretrievably.

The study with the virtual dummies tells us how the powers of presence distort our perception. We can also recruit these powers in a positive sense, to enhance the vividness of symbols or abstract thought. Figure 7.2 gives an elaborate example from a Japanese cultural festival,

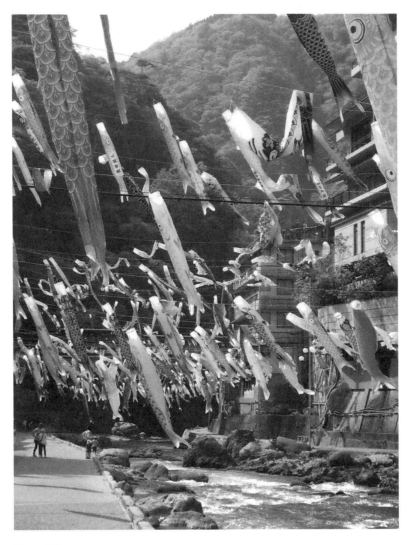

Figure 7.2
Carp fluttering above a river in Tsuetate, Kumamoto prefecture, Japan, on May 8, 2011.
Koinobori, or the "carp-shaped streamers" festival, takes place on Children's Day, on the
5th of May. Carp are famous for their powerful swimming upstream, a perfect model that
parents hope their children will emulate. Here the symbols are projected back onto a
natural scene to increase their powers of presence. Three days after the festival, the streamers are lazily floating with the wind—their heads in the downstream direction.

with symbolic artifacts reintroduced to the environment in which their biological models naturally appear (though the streamers are flying whereas the carp normally swim). The powers of presence may have multiple functions, but increasing the vividness of information would certainly be one of them, according to William James (1890|1950b, p. 305):

The opinion so stoutly professed by many, that language is essential to thought, seems to have this much of truth in it, that all our inward images tend invincibly to attach themselves to something sensible, so as to gain in corporeity and life. Words serve this purpose, gestures serve it, stones, straws, chalk-marks, anything will do. As soon as anyone of these things stands for the idea, the latter seems more real. Some persons, the present writer among the number, can hardly lecture without a black-board: the abstract conceptions must be symbolized by letters, squares or circles, and the relations between them by lines. All this symbolism, linguistic, graphic, and dramatic, has other uses too, for it abridges thought and fixes terms. But one of its uses is surely to rouse the believing reaction and give to the ideas a more living reality.

The quote comes from chapter XXI on "The Perception of Reality." We embody the things we think about not only with our own bodies but also by giving the things a material form our minds can latch on to. In doing so, Clark (2008) would argue, we extend our minds. I can understand this proposal metaphorically speaking, not literally—the carp-shaped streamers activate content-bearing mechanisms in our minds, but the actual nylon wind socks *are* external objects. When we talk about embodying in embodied cognition, I would like to think of it as giving a bodily form to a thought—a form of material indexing that always involves at least one process in the brain and one process outside the brain.

The brain process associates a sensory pattern with semantic features; it attaches meaning to something material. Outside the brain, we shape or identify a structure that serves to elicit a sensory pattern. This material process can pertain to our own bodies—this corresponds to the conventional notion of embodied cognition, by which we use our own bodies to index, represent, or otherwise process information. However, we can also "embody" our thought through external objects or even other people, as when I ask you to remember the second half of a string of digits or an address while I rehearse the first half in my mind (a division of mental labor that now seems ridiculously archaic to most of my undergraduate students). The out-of-body route to embodied cognition supports the same cognitive functions and engages similar brain mechanisms as that via our own bodies.

This concept of embodiment should not confuse us about the boundaries between internal and external with respect to brain or body. Those boundaries are studied in biology and biomedical engineering; in most cases it is fairly straightforward to determine what is in or out. Usually there is little doubt over lifeless artifacts versus processes that are fully integrated in the body's plasticity. If the concept of embodiment confuses us about the boundaries of our minds, I suggest that these are the active boundaries of my subtitle—between what is in the mind or in vision and what is not. These boundaries are concerned with the intentionality, the content of thought. As I have confessed a number of times throughout the previous chapters, my hypothesis in this respect remains both firmly classic and very contemporary, perhaps even boringly mainstream, completely in line with Spinoza (1677|2001), Damasio (2010), and Žižek (2006|2009): For anything to be in the mind there has to be something happening in the brain.

Blindness

The corollary of my Spinozan position is that where brain activity is lacking, there can be no mind. If the brain is dead, the mind must be too. The negative considered from one perspective (the brain) leads, across the dialectical gap and via the parallax, to a negative considered from the alternative perspective (the mind). Thinking from the negative, some of the most interesting questions about vision and consciousness are raised by the phenomena of blindness. Philosophers have pondered particularly "Molyneux's problem" of whether a person blind from birth, whose sight is suddenly restored later in life, will be able to distinguish objects (with which he or she is familiar from touch) simply by looking at them. The question was first formulated by William Molyneux (whose wife was blind) for John Locke (1689|1975) and later considered by just about everybody interested in vision (Noë, 2004, p. 242, lists fifteen names, including such luminaries as Gottfried Wilhelm Leibniz and Denis Diderot, and several others who already appeared elsewhere in our story).

Most thinkers agree that the answer must be "No," at least in the very first instant before the newly-sighted person has had the opportunity to develop the proper sensorimotor skills for vision. Once the skills are in place, we can assume that he or she will be able, through vision alone, to access internal representations previously acquired on the basis of touch. There would be no need to repeat the learning of how haptic information maps on to visual information for every single object in this person's semantic system. At some point the skills should kick in and make the translation automatically.

The underlying assumption is that sensory patterns afford flexible rewiring. Through neural plasticity, it should be possible for new sensory patterns to activate extant neural mechanisms that support the more abstract dimensions of thought—the content of what is re-cognized, together with the access it gives to secondary associations. Today, this is no longer a conjecture. From the pioneering work by Paul Bach-y-Rita (1972) in particular we know that sensory substitution is a very real phenomenon, of which we have yet to chart the limits. With the combined efforts of inventive engineering and intensive training people are often able to gain (or regain) an amazing amount of behavioral and cognitive functioning that initially looked to be forever unattainable (or incontrovertibly lost).

Bach-y-Rita developed tools that allowed the blind to "see" with their skin (these inventions seem destined to be linked with Molyneux's problem in all future philosophical treatises; see also Dennett, 1991; Noë, 2004; Clark, 2008). My favorite would be the chair that has a video camera mounted on it, with which light is transduced to somatosensory patterns on a bank of four hundred vibrating plates. The plates stimulate the skin on the chair user's back. Of course, visual perception via this chair is not quite as impressive as it is for most of us via our eyes, but it does enable somatosensory viewers (no longer truly "blind") to distinguish among the types of objects William Molyneux had in mind when he put his question to John Locke.

The richness of visual detail is lost without the retina, and this richness—the immediacy with which it overtakes our minds—must be crucial in the aesthetic pleasures we derive from vision. Jorge Luis Borges (1999, p. 357) missed them badly when he turned blind as he seems to confess in the poem "A Blind Man" (translated by Alastar Reid) from his 1975 volume *La rosa profunda* (*The Unending Rose*): "I say again that I have lost no more / than the inconsequential skin of things. / These wise words come from Milton, and are noble, / but then I think of letters and of roses." Yet Borges berated himself for it in the prologue to the same volume: "Going over the proofs of this book, I notice with some distaste that blindness plays a mournful role, which it does not play in my life. Blindness is a confinement, but it is also a liberation, a solitude propitious to invention, a key and an algebra" (p. 345).

By losing the retina, the cortical mechanisms of abstraction and association gain degrees of freedom. The liberating confinement facilitates, says Borges. It creates the natural space for complex computations that unlock William Blake's proverbial doors of perception, which have more to do with vatic vision than mundane visual processing. With the highest of the moderns and the finest of the Romantics, poets would have us think that these internal computations deliver supreme fiction, a thing of beauty and a joy forever—not the transient sensory pleasures, but the lasting objects of thought that command a different, more elusive concept of beauty. Interestingly, to explore the Romantic tradition a little further, John Keats also intuited a paradoxical key function for not-seeing in the contemplation of beauty. He did not call it "blindness" but "negative capability" in a famous letter to his brothers, George and Tom Keats, in December 1817. To convey the curiously casual nature of this intuition, with the wonderful giant leaps it makes, let me quote a longish fragment from the letter (Keats, 2002, pp. 60–61):

> I had not a dispute but a disquisition with Dilke on various subjects; several things dovetailed in my mind, and at once it struck me, what quality went to form a Man of Achievement, especially in Literature and which Shakespeare possessed so enormously—I mean *Negative Capability*, that is when man is capable of being in uncertainties, Mysteries, doubts, without any irritable reaching after fact and reason. Coleridge, for instance, would let go by a fine isolated verisimilitude caught from the Penetralium of mystery, from being incapable of remaining content with half knowledge. This pursued through Volumes would perhaps take us no further than this, that with a great poet the sense of Beauty overcomes every other consideration, or rather obliterates all consideration.

Negative capability would be the ability to stay undecided, to resist immediate judgment. Keats thought Shakespeare had it but appeared to find the capability lacking in Coleridge—an evaluation we might disagree with, given Coleridge's call for deliberate "suspension of disbelief" as a critical condition to make room for fantastic elements in fiction and poetry (Coleridge used this term in his *Biographia Literaria*, 1817|1984; the same year as Keats's letter). The genius of Keats piles twisted logic on suspicious judgment. After possibly misreading Coleridge, he jumps to the conclusion that negative capability "perhaps" connects to the great poet's sense of beauty. Does Keats lack the patience to pursue the issue through volumes? Or does negative capability in fact *prevent* such pursuit once the connection has been intuited—should we abandon the pursuit for fear that it destroys the mystery? Or would it merely be a waste of time? For whatever reason, Keats does not engage in the pursuit. My questions illustrate Keats's inherently ambivalent position, simultaneously attracted by the wonders of science and averse to its methods and reductive schemas. Positively simple: Keats possessed the negative capability no less enormously than Shakespeare did.

Though Keats never mentioned the words again, the concept of negative capability started leading a life of its own. Dozens of scholarly works spin a title from it; the pursuit through volumes is being carried out anyway. In Mobile, Alabama, there is even a Negative Capability Press. If the concept appeals to thinkers and researchers in various disciplines, it must be that it manages in a single brilliant stroke to teach and to tease. From the outset we have said that the problem in visual perception revolves around how to get access to things as they are. The active boundaries, we would naturally think, reflect our abilities to discriminate, to see differences among things. However, negative capability suggests something more complex. An important part of perception would be to resist discrimination, to try to remain in doubt or to accommodate multiple possibilities. Sometimes we need to keep options open, consider alternatives. On occasion we need to keep looking where there appears to be nothing at first. This requires an active blindness, an effortful, sustained not-seeing. If our basic visual biases are compulsively oriented to objects (whether wished for, familiar, or feared), then negative capability argues that these have to be kept in check to attain the highest achievement in perception.

Again the English language already has the truth in an idiom, positing there is often more to something than meets the eye. However, combined with all the other idiomatic wisdoms, we find ourselves in a bind, not obviously knowing when to see and when not to see or where to turn our efforts. If we work too hard at negative capability and accommodation of multiple possibilities, our active not-seeing will properly blind us. With a romantic image, our eyes are scorched by the light of beauty's sun. It is no accident that our neural circuits are compulsively oriented toward recognizing objects. Through evolution and learning the visual system is shaped to move forward and make efficient decisions about things as they are. Positive capability pays off. For negative capability to increase the payoff, we must master the art of choice and improve our direction of the gaze.

By this reading, negative capability becomes a matter of voluntary control, down-regulating the perceptual salience of certain items in order to increase the powers of presence of subtler information. This translation of Keats's concept should work for neuroscience. For instance, using the combined techniques of fMRI and transcranial magnetic stimulation, Mevorach and colleagues (2010) implicated the intraparietal sulcus in

"Ignoring the Elephant in the Room." Low-salient stimuli were selected thanks to suppressive influence from the intraparietal sulcus on visual cortical mechanisms that would normally propagate information about the more salient but presently task-irrelevant stimuli.

In other situations, we seem to have no trouble at all ignoring the elephant in the room—or rather the gorilla, as in the well-known study by Simons and Chabris (1999), which replicated and expanded a classic of cognitive psychology by Neisser and Becklen (1975). Subjects watch a video showing two teams of three players passing basketballs around, one team in white t-shirts, the other in black. The subjects are asked to focus on one team (preferably the white) and count the number of passes. As the players are doing their thing, an actor dressed in a gorilla suit slowly makes her way from one side of the room to the other, stopping midway to beat her chest. About half the subjects fail to notice the gorilla, and all of these are shocked to see what they had missed when the video is played again.

It is a dramatic demonstration of inattentional blindness, as defined by Mack and Rock (1998). Our selective looking blocks out salient information that does not match with the task or context—we are blind to things from beyond the "horizon of expectations," to borrow a concept from Karl Popper (quoted by Culler, 1981|2001, p. 59). Like many teachers anywhere I use the video in my first lecture when I try to convince a new generation of undergraduate students that psychology really deserves to be in their curriculum. It raises the right questions most vividly: What do we see? Why? How do we select and what do we expect?

The questions afford scientific investigation, with respect to neural mechanisms as well as psychological phenomena. Thakral (2011) conducted an fMRI study with an inattentional blindness paradigm that showed activity in prefrontal cortex for strange, unexpected items that went unnoticed. This activity profile overlapped with that obtained when the subjects became aware of the oddities. The data seem to capture Dennett's (1991) pandemonium in action, with different information elements (or competing stories) active in prefrontal cortex. The different representations vie for intensive processing and consciousness. Sometimes they gain in strength and rule the reporting, and sometimes they do not.

Figure 7.3 presents another case of sustained inattentional blindness, one that lasted several centuries even though the invisible item takes up a large portion in the center of the painting and surely elicits levels of

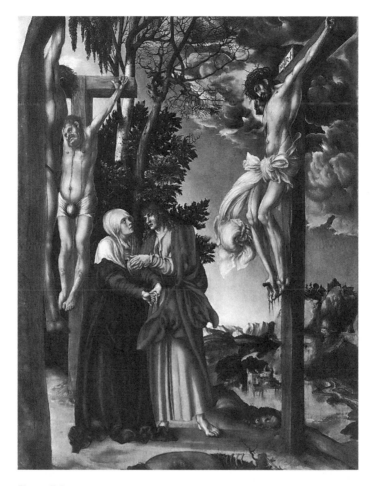

Figure 7.3
Klage unter dem Kreuz (Lament under the Cross), painted in 1503 by Lucas Cranach the Elder (collection of the Alte Pinakothek, Munich, Germany). Art historians would have us note the somewhat curious arrangement with the three crosses not in line, forming a closed space. In this way, according to the Web site of the Pinakothek (www.pinakothek .de), the emphasis is placed on the grieving Mary as a model that invites believers to contemplate the suffering of Christ. However, see Steinberg (1983|1996) for another focus point.

neural representation beyond basic features such as texture and color. I am referring to Christ's loincloth that we can easily recognize for the item of clothing it is without pausing to register anything else about it. It took a perceptive art historian to point out the obvious, grotesque penis in the "wings of excess." For hundreds of years before Leo Steinberg's (1983|1996) controversial book on *The Sexuality of Christ in*

Renaissance Art and Modern Oblivion, the giant member had been hiding in plain view.

The focus on the genitals seems so scandalously out of place that we have no choice but to ignore it or to deny it. Yet this focus might not have been intended to offend. Steinberg argues the prominent display of Christ's sex purported to highlight that Jesus was most fully human in every sense. For the miracle of the incarnation of God to be complete, the Son had to be human all the way. Renaissance artists like Lucas Cranach emphasized it by focusing on the genitals; others like Matthias Grünewald did it by portraying the suffering of Christ in ways that effectively look unbearable. This line of thought went lost in the ages that followed. Today with the controversial artist Mideo Cruz we know the mood is very different ("Philippine 'phallic' art exhibit forced to close," BBC News, August 9, 2011). If the transgression cannot be denied, it must be punished.

Taboo

In the case of transgressions that require punishment, consciousness comes at a cost. To denounce the violation, we have to invest energy. Faced with the prospect of losing time and wasting effort, we may prefer to deny that there is a problem in the first place. Our semantic system would imply a bias against explicitly recognizing what has been recognized already unconsciously or automatically—it would be an intentional blindness, inspired by loss aversion (Kahneman & Tversky, 1979), not unlike the dynamics behind some of the most infamous cases of "looking away." Classic examples are the German response in the Nazi era to the holocaust, captured with the phrase "*Davon haben wir nichts gewusst*" ("We knew nothing about that"; see Longerich, 2010), and the bystander effect in the onlookers' passiveness to the murder of Kitty Genovese (Darley & Latané, 1968; see Manning, Levine, & Collins, 2007, for a reappraisal). When suspicious patterns of data carry onerous implications, the temptation would be to apply the negative capability strategically. Then we deny what should really be obvious before it actually becomes too clear.

In *Totem and Taboo* Sigmund Freud (1913|1999) suggested an additional motivation to look away. Taboo violations would be contagious; the person who violates a taboo *becomes* taboo. The gaze must avoid contact, or we are sullied by what we see. When the taboo is strong enough and fully internalized, it will influence our gaze control even when nobody is watching us. Wishing to keep our conscience clean, we look away, and if our gaze happens to touch the wrong thing anyway, we need a healthy dose of bad faith (in Sartre's [1943|1992] sense of the concept) in order to delude ourselves into believing we never saw what we were not supposed to see. Yet, Freud (1913|1999) also decreed that taboos are inherently concerned with objects of ambivalence; they prohibit what is secretly desired, often unbeknownst to the self—themes of a sexual nature and/or involving violence onto others (particularly rivals, power figures, fathers, etc.). The taboo would simultaneously attract and repel. In the words of James Elkins (1996, p. 119), describing his observations of Christ's wings of excess in Lucas Cranach's painting (figure 7.3):

It makes me think of my vision streaming toward the image, heading right at it, about to strike its surface head-on, and then suddenly veering away like a bug sweeping past the windshield as I drive. Or else it's like magnetic lines of force, bending and curving around an object and utterly incapable of contacting it.

The bending and curving of the gaze around the taboo object constitutes evidence that it *was* seen. At some level the prohibition kicks in, counteracting the attraction and pushing the gaze trajectory away from the sensitive information. Figure 7.4, based on data that are very dear to me (Weaver, Lauwereyns, & Theeuwes, 2011), shows that such bending and curving is not merely the figment of an art historian's imagination. During a four-month stay in Jan Theeuwes's lab in Amsterdam, my former Ph.D. student Matt Weaver conducted an eye movement experiment using irrelevant word cues in a paradigm inspired by that of Sheliga, Riggio, and Rizzolatti (1994). This paradigm produces curved saccade trajectories. In Matt's version, the subjects are first given a word cue (presented for a hundred milliseconds) to the left or right of the fixation point. Critically, the word is either neutral or taboo (Weaver et al.'s article includes the most colorful list of ten Dutch words ever published in a scientific journal). Then, after a delay of zero, three hundred, or seven hundred milliseconds, an arrow instructs the target location for the saccade.

Our data replicated the curved saccade effect. Apparently, saccadic eye movements are not exactly the type of ballistic motor action with stereotyped spatial vectors they once were thought to be. Instead, the trajectories of individual saccades express a level of competition in the motor programming. Port and Wurtz (2003) have traced sequential activity in the superior colliculus that could explain the curving of saccades. This neural mechanism pertained to curved saccades that veered from one

Sequence of Events

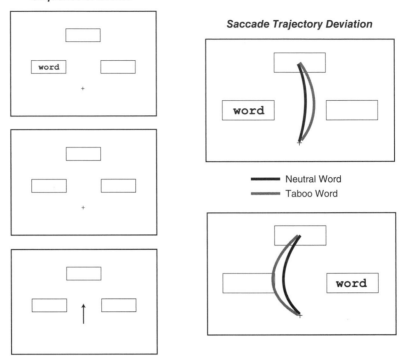

Figure 7.4
The effect of taboo words on saccade trajectories (after Weaver, Lauwereyns, & Theeuwes, 2011). The three panels on the left display the sequence of events. Subjects are asked to ignore the initial word cue (top left panel) and to make a saccade in the direction indicated by the arrow (bottom left panel). The two panels on the right show average saccade trajectories. These deviate to the right if the word cue appears on the left (top right panel) and vice versa (bottom right panel). The deviation in the trajectories is more pronounced for taboo words (gray traces) than for neutral words (black traces).

target to another. Such trajectories imply competition between different attractors. The eyes move first toward one item, then toward another. Our data, as well as those by Sheliga, Riggio, and Rizzolatti (1994), show a different type of curving, with the eyes taking a detour to avoid one item while moving to another. Still, reason allows us to assume that this kind of curving also reflects the dynamic strengths of different saccade target representations in the superior colliculus. Sometimes a curved trajectory is due to multiple activations; sometimes it is the product of differential suppression and activation.

In our study, we found that the curving happened as a function of the semantic information carried by the word cues. This was observable in two ways. First, the saccades were bent more strongly for word cues to the right than to the left. This hemifield effect suggests a role for language since the information from word cues in the right hemifield is fed straight to the left brain half, the dominant hemisphere for language processing (a fact first glimpsed by Paul Broca in the 1860s; Schiller, 1992). This laterality effect by itself is noteworthy enough, as it could imply linguistic intrusion onto the dynamics of saccade programming in the superior colliculus. However, even more interesting is Big Effect No. 2. The taboo words produced stronger bends than neutral words, pushing the eyes further away from the no-go zone. This effect was seen only in trials with a delay of seven hundred milliseconds between the word cue and the arrow. It takes some time for the taboo mechanisms to wake up and start inhibiting, but once they are in action, the gaze has to dance to their tune.

The curved saccades provide double evidence, of seeing *and* not-seeing, a complex interaction in the sensorimotor control of vision. It will be interesting to compare this kind of twisted seeing with other chimeric forms such as those of blindsight (Cowey, 2010; Weiskrantz, 2009) and subliminal perception (Custers & Aarts, 2010; Wiens, 2006). Whether due to characteristics of the observer or the information, we find evidence of disavowed seeing—visual pattern recognition denied by the observer. The pattern recognition can be quite sophisticated, the denial no less impressive in being vehement. I suspect that in all of these cases the gaze essentially functions as a mediator, an instrument that can be recruited to operate in service of consciousness.

In blindsight, the gaze shows reflexive orienting but is unable to focus on what is seen without cortex (Isa & Yoshida, 2009), and so the information remains outside of consciousness. In subliminal perception, the brief exposure duration never gives the gaze a chance to focus on what is automatically decoded by superfast mechanisms (heavily reliant on bias) in brain areas such as the amygdala. Thus, in both blindsight and subliminal perception, the lack of gaze fixation prevents the information from reaching consciousness. Conversely, in dealing with sensitive images involving taboos or moral violations, we regulate the content of consciousness by aiming the gaze away from problem zones (Van Reekum et al., 2007).

We wish to avoid processing the information consciously, and so we prevent gaze fixation. An effective way to control our thoughts is to control our eyes, though preferably not as per Jesus's advice, offered with respect to the adulterous gaze in the Sermon on the Mount ("[I]f thy right eye offend thee, pluck it out," the Gospel of Matthew, 5:29, the King James version of the Bible, Anonymous, 1611|2004). Rather than resorting to self-mutilation, we may look for ways to facilitate the strategic

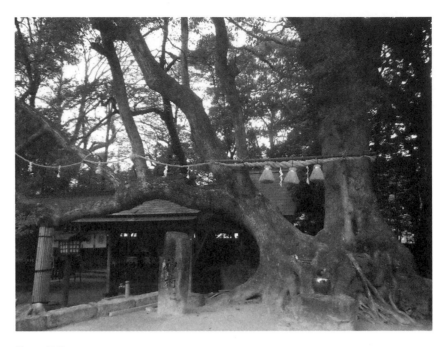

Figure 7.5
A venerable camphor tree at a Shinto shrine in Kirishima, Kagoshima prefecture, Japan, photographed on December 25, 2010 (which makes it my favorite kind of Christmas tree). Nobody knows how old the tree is, but the locals agree it has to be at least a thousand years old. The inscription in stone declares it holy, and the demarcation between sacred object and profane observer is further underscored by the *shimenawa* ("enclosing rope"), festooned with *shide* (one of multiple readings would be "four hands"; zigzagged white paper streamers).

control of the gaze. Figure 7.5 shows the Shinto approach, using visual cues (the rope and paper streamers) to signal what is sacred (the ancient tree). In this case, our gaze is allowed to make contact with the object in question. However, the contact is given boundaries. The visual cues mark the taboo. They tell us to keep an appropriate distance, to show proper respect. In other cases, the visual cues mark the limits of where we can go and what we are allowed to see. They become vivid, visible symbols of the invisible.

Vanishing Point

With visual cues that mark prohibitions we move to yet another form of not-seeing, controlled by the gaze. We can have our eyes open in ways that prevent seeing. Sometimes we stare and do not see. Here is a vivid description of the "trance stare," as given by André Weitzenhoffer (1989|2000, p. 181) in a chapter on the induction of hypnosis:

The subject seems to be staring, unblinking, possibly unseeing, at some indefinite point in space, although sometimes one can determine that his eyes are fixed on some definite object or point, usually the one he was looking at, at the onset of hypnosis. If he is facing you, you may have the impression he is staring right through you at something further away.

From Walt Disney's 1967 animation movie *The Jungle Book* we remember the cunning python Kaa's eyes beaming their psychedelic tricks onto those of the gullible Mowgli in hopes of applying the bone-crushing coils in preparation for dinner. Mowgli merely smiled, his eyes opened wide and unmoving. Weitzenhoffer (1969, 1971) was the first researcher empirically to connect the induction of hypnosis with altered eye movement characteristics in a line of work that has yet to be developed (for other gestures in this direction, see Kallio et al., 2011; Tada, Yamada, & Hariu, 1990). Again, the gaze may be a key to making the transition to an altered mind state. What we currently know about the neural mechanisms of hypnosis reinforces this proposal. Neural structures that show differential activity during hypnosis include areas such as the anterior cingulate cortex, the right inferior parietal lobule, and the thalamus—important players in what is often loosely called the "executive attentional network" (Oakley & Halligan, 2009; Rainville et al., 1997, 2002).

Somehow the trance stare and the executive attentional network go hand in hand during hypnosis, but at the moment we know next to nothing about the dynamics and the underlying mechanisms. This is not surprising given the sluggish temporal profile of fMRI data and the problem of confounding factors when studying correlations between eye movements and BOLD signals. However, the techniques are improving, and we are encouraged in hoping that the questions can be studied in the lab before too long. One interesting issue, casually raised by Weitzenhoffer in the quote above, is that with respect to the point of fixation in the trance stare. Sometimes the gaze rests on a particular object or point, usually the same as that being looked at when hypnosis sets in. Sometimes the gaze appears locked to infinity, the vanishing point, nothing of this world. In both cases, the eyes remain still. Blinks are limited. But the spatial selection of the gaze is completely different: focused on one concrete thing or on absolutely nothing.

Figure 7.6 illustrates the latter case, with the gaze of Lewis Powell, or Lewis Payne, off into the unending distance. He (one of the alleged

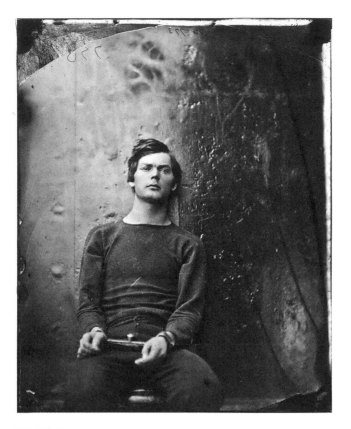

Figure 7.6
Lewis Powell, also known as Lewis Payne, photographed by Alexander Gardner in the spring or early summer of 1865. Here is what Roland Barthes wrote in relation to this photograph (1981|1999, p. 96): "I now know that there exists another *punctum* (another "stigmatum") than the "detail." This new *punctum*, which is no longer of form but of intensity, is Time, the lacerating emphasis of the *noeme* ("that-has-been"), its pure representation. In 1865, young Lewis Payne tried to assassinate Secretary of State W. H. Seward. Alexander Gardner photographed him in his cell, where he was waiting to be hanged. The photograph is handsome, as is the boy: that is the *studium*. But the *punctum* is: *he is going to die*."

conspirators in Lincoln's assassination) may be hypnotized by the prospect of his inevitable death or merely daydreaming, bored and waiting while Alexander Gardner takes the famous picture (actually one of three different portraits, all taken within the space of a few minutes, presumably, but the unmistakable stare appears only in the photograph reproduced in figure 7.6). Roland Barthes's reading of the image (given in the figure caption) does not mention the gaze, but I would venture to claim that it is the lack of convergence of Powell/Payne's eyes that set the

French philosopher going with his vicarious daydreaming. The gaze invites the somber, deeply existentialist mood.

It is the lack of convergence of the eyes that immediately gives away the not-seeing nature of this gaze. Powell/Payne is taking in the entire imaginary horizon beyond the walls of the space where he is confined. His eyes are locked onto a point vanishingly far away; the lines of sight from his two eyes are perfectly parallel. How do the eyes find their target? By which mechanisms does the trance stare manage to hold the eyes still? To what extent are these mechanisms shared with the alternative kind of stare, which is locked onto a concrete object in space? At first, the latter case would seem to be easier to understand. Somehow the target selection mechanisms pick a single object, perhaps in a way that is principally no different from other cases of voluntary gaze control. If so, areas such as the SEF, the FEF, and the LIP work with the superior colliculus to choose an object of fixation and to jointly move the eyes, their focus fully converged.

The eyes are fixed on a point; they remain still. But then the questions reemerge. When do the eyes fix on an object to process it, and when do the eyes fix on an object while the mind is focused on something else? How can gaze control serve both to see and not to see? It rings paradoxical. The most efficient way of locking out the present, the surround, is to avoid scanning and to limit the data input. We can literally close our eyes, or we can pick any point in actual space and keep our eyes fixed there. Then we daydream. We enter our personal zone of infinite thought, with words and images, old and new. In order to see a thing most fully *and* to not see a thing at all, our biology performs the same action. We hold the eyes still.

The challenge is for psychophysics and neuroscience to discover exactly how and where the fully concentrated seeing diverges from not-seeing during daydreaming or under hypnosis. We have yet to properly characterize the differences in mental states, though researchers have already begun exploring the neural correlates of daydreaming (cf. the work on the "default network," a set of neural structures active when the brain is "at rest," that is, wandering freely, unbothered by any difficult task; Mason et al., 2007). Is thought enhanced during daydreaming but reduced in hypnosis? Can we probe the cognitive features of different states? The eyes may be perfectly still and converged on a single point in all cases, but perhaps there are telltale signs of different mental states in the pupil sizes (larger during daydreaming than during hypnosis?), the likelihood of blinks (lower in hypnosis than during both daydreaming and fully concentrated vision?), and the size and frequency of microsac-cades (bigger and more frequent during fully concentrated vision than during daydreaming and hypnosis?).

More generally, we need a new look at looking at nothing. It may have specific cognitive functions. I have already alluded to the blocking out of visual noise. This would be a strategy to reduce perceptual interfer-ence on cognitive processing—a way to better focus on internal pro-cessing. However, there may be other functions. In psycholinguistic experiments, subjects are often found to fixate on empty regions where objects appeared previously. Researchers thinking about the world in terms of embodied cognition had insisted on the argument that this kind of gaze control reflects the usual mechanisms of spatial indexing and ad hoc retrieval of information from the world. But in a stimulating opinion article for *Trends in Cognitive Sciences*, Ferreira, Apel, and Henderson (2008) suggested that the looking at nothing in these cases facilitates the retrieval of relatively detailed internal representations, created earlier by the visual system. Here the gaze is used as a cue not to see but to reac-tivate a memory. In a way, this is still an argument compatible with the general framework of embodied cognition, but the actions in the world would be part and parcel of the intensive approach, oriented to meaning as it lives in neural circuits.

Truths of Stone

The orientation to meaning in the intensive approach ultimately reaches for truths that are relevant to the subject. Some of these truths require us to go beyond what is directly visible in the shapes of salient structures, bodies, things out in the world. Sometimes we need to build links *between* the visible structures to get access to things as they are—objects of thought derived from dynamics in the world. With Jean-Paul Sartre we note that building such links (tracing their trajectories) involves a construction beyond what is given externally: "The trajectory *never is*, since it is *nothing*; it vanishes immediately into purely external relations between different places; that is, in simple exteriority of indifference or spatiality" (Sartre, 1956|1992, p. 290). Alain Badiou (1988|2007, p. 181) adds, "[O]nly an interpretative intervention can declare that an event is presented in a situation; as the arrival in being of non-being, the arrival amidst the visible of the invisible." The invisible here is the underlying truth, the link between the visible structures. To see it, we must change gears, from literal seeing to virtual seeing.

The virtual seeing, similar to that of the wandering or daydreaming mind, involves covert visual processing—but not the type that Posner (1980) studied with the spatial-cueing paradigm. With the gaze fixed on an external point, the covert processing of virtual seeing does not orient to other, more peripheral external points but to information of a different kind altogether, nonexistent in the world, present in the mind thanks to memory and imagination. The neural mechanisms that enable the shift of processing away from the point of gaze fixation probably involve something more than the premotor programming that Rizzolatti (1983) postulated. The targets for virtual seeing cannot be translated to bodily coordinates when the relevant visual space is abstract—an n-dimensional manifold of possibilities and fantasies. A leap is required, a shift of perspective from a real-world plane to a fictive horizon.

Should Rizzolatti hook up with Rizzolatti to make that leap? Should we connect the premotor theory with the mirror/enactive system? When we turn the covert visual processing to internal representations, we certainly are shifting to an abstract concept of space, belonging to "the other"—not necessarily a different person, but "me" beyond here and now, an ecstatic subject in the future or past, virtually experiencing something surreal or actually possible. Terrence Deacon (1997) has suggested it would be a function of language, an orientation of covert selective processing to symbols and abstract relations, a form of seeing that focuses on semantic connections. Indeed, the seeing of truths, laws, signs, and all other types of deeper things is conventionally thought of as an act of language. With Jonathan Culler (1981|2001, p. 226) in *The Pursuit of Signs*, in the chapter on "The Turns of Metaphor," "the act of grouping distinct particulars under a common heading on the basis of perceived or imagined resemblance, which is the central act in any narrative of the origin of language, corresponds to the classical definition of the metaphor: substitution on the basis of resemblance" (see also De Man, 1979).

Does this mean that we have finally undeniably crossed the active boundaries of vision and are now roaming in the domain of language? I would rather think that the active boundaries of vision move *with* language. The metaphorical seeing of the invisible (the trajectories, the connections between things) is a form of active vision that plays out over time. Perhaps language is the tool with which we extend our visual grasp in the temporal domain. Language would be the placeholder of nothingness (what is not or no longer there; this includes memory). It gives the invisible a sustained presence. This thought comes to me via a passage from a manuscript by Leonardo da Vinci, quoted by Giorgio Agamben

(1991, p. 82, citing "Cod. Arundel, f. 131r") as *a standard for any theory of negativity*:

Among the magnitude of things that are around us, the being of nothingness holds the highest position and its grasp extends to things that have no being, and its essence resides within time, within the past and the future, and it possesses nothing of the present.

The metaphorical seeing of the invisible (the project over time) must ultimately start from the "being of nothingness." Here we stumble on the scariest, most fundamental questions—the radically ontological. For most of our story on active vision we have been naturally concerned with Merleau-Ponty's (1945|2008) phenomenology of perception, but now we must open the door to the rest of phenomenology and existentialism. For Sartre (1956|1992, p. 36), being was shaped by nothingness: "Whatever being is, it will allow this formulation: 'Being is *that*, and outside of that, *nothing*.'"

Heidegger (1927|2008, p. 279) was focused more specifically on death: "In Dasein there is always something still *outstanding*, which, as a potentiality-for-Being for Dasein itself, has not yet become 'actual'" (p. 279). What is always still outstanding: the end, death.

For Heidegger, this meant that nothingness somehow had to be incorporated in the definition of being: "Any Dasein always exists in just such a manner that its 'not-yet' *belongs* to it" (p. 287) and "Death is a way to be, which Dasein takes over as soon as it is" (p. 289).

Nothingness gives the contours of being. Shaped by death and the end, being can acquire its meaning. This project of seeing through the invisible requires time: "Within the horizon of time the projection of meaning of Being in general can be accomplished" (Heidegger, 1927|2008, p. 278). Nothingness gives the grounding, the great, massive truth of stone (made visible by Yasujirō Ozu in figure 7.7). From this negative base we can jump off, walk freely, explore, and engage in active vision. Alain Badiou (1988|2007) described this grounding in mathematical terms, with set theory. He noted that the void (apparently synonymous with nothingness, infinity, the null set, and the subtractive point of the multiple) can be added to any set, and that any two sets always have at least the void in common. This truth would be the axiom of foundation (pp. 185–187). To represent the foundational nothingness, Badiou likes to use "an old Scandinavian letter, Ø, emblem of the void, zero affected by the barring of sense" (p. 69). It is rendered beautifully in a composition with stones photographed by Ed Marshall on the glossy cover of the paperback

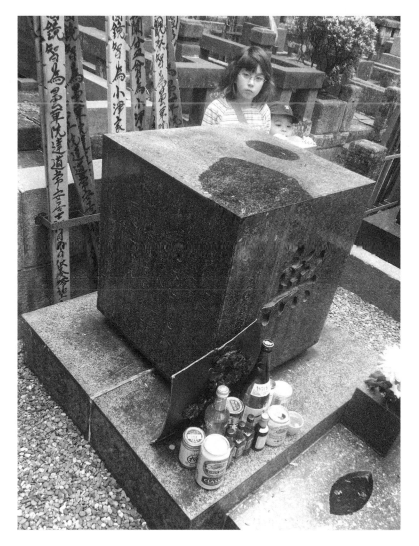

Figure 7.7
Yasujirō Ozu's grave at Engaku-ji in Kamakura, Kanagawa prefecture, Japan, photographed in April 2009. The movie director still receives his daily drinks. The massive granite block, his gravestone, bears just one character, *mu*: "nothingness," often used as a prefix to mark the absence of something. I asked the living in the picture to "look serious," and they did (at least the eldest did; the youngest had no clue what was going on, or why the stone should be interesting).

edition of *Being and Event* that I have in my hands. Our compulsive desire to turn invisible truths into stone (or rope or carp-shaped streamers) is exactly where language and vision meet. We create symbols, signs, and objects of art to embody the invisible truths that we would like to see with our own eyes.

Consciousness, the Space of Literature

Contemplating the truths of stone, we realize that they are ours for the taking. The identification of Sartre's trajectory or the naming of Badiou's event—forging the links between visible structures—is the creative task our minds relish and perform naturally. It is what we do when we tell ourselves and others what happened (what we saw), in fairy tales, bedtime stories, pillow books, travel journals, scientific articles, letters to the editor, witness reports, and sworn testimonies.

This narrative function could very well be the core feature of consciousness and returns in different guises in many, if not all, contemporary accounts.

"Consciousness is a state of mind with a self process added to it," according to Damasio (2010, p. 157), and the most elaborate of the self processes would be the autobiographical self, which tells us who we are and how we came to be that way. Consciousness would be a process that works in close cooperation with memory to write new pages in the stories of our lives. This view matches with several calls by neuroscientists to abandon the received wisdom that attention and consciousness are essentially the same thing or that attention would serve as the gatekeeper to consciousness. Instead, visual selective processing ("visual attention") can take place without consciousness, and consciousness may primarily interact with memory (e.g., Koch & Tsuchiya, 2007; Lamme, 2003). Damasio (2010) makes a further distinction between self-as-object ("the material me") and self-as-subject (the more elusive agent or observer, central to autobiographical memory). The self-as-object would be based on representations of the body.

Damasio even specifies a location for it in the brain, in the posteromedial cortices, at the "intersection of pathways associated with information from the visceral interior (interoceptive), from the musculoskeletal system (proprioceptive and kinesthetic), and from the outside world (exteroceptive)" (p. 218), a region that "was known not by an umbrella term but rather by its component parts, namely, the posterior cingulate cortex, the retrosplenial cortex, and the precuneus" (p. 219). Daniel Dennett would surely shudder at the singling out of one neural umbrella term for the substrate of consciousness. A few pages later, Damasio (2010) adds insult to injury by fully reinstating the Cartesian Theater: "Those are the cortices where images can be made and displayed—that is, where large paintings can be shown and puppet shows presented" (p. 223).

Can we move toward a position between Dennett and Damasio? From Damasio I would like to borrow the concepts of different selves at different timescales, centered on representations of the body, with distinctions between emotions and feelings. I also endorse the basic allegiance to the Spinozan parallax, insisting that mind and body are different aspects of the same thing. However, with Dennett I reject the Cartesian Theater and the notion of a fixed location for an internal viewpoint. Dennett's (1991) Center of Narrative Gravity maps onto the elusive self-as-subject. It would be a virtual abstraction in a moving pandemonium, amid complex dynamics, forming various spatiotemporal configurations across the entire brain. Perhaps the posteromedial cortices do in fact feature in these configurations, but that does not have to mean that any images are made or displayed there.

Indeed, the elusive nature of the self would follow from the variability of configurations that afford its emergence. Its gravitational force as a narrative center would follow from its grammatical position as subject, as the "I" that does something. As Marvin Minsky (1985) suggested, "I" is the name we give to whatever it is that causes everything we do. It is the thing to which we attribute agency. It is the elusive author of our actions that we load with responsibility. This also implies that for every sensation, for every thought, action, or aspect of bodily motor control, there must be neural mechanisms that support the addition of a self process (the grammatical subject "I"). It will be reasonable to expect a wide variety of neural mechanisms to play analogous roles in this addition of a self process for all the various sensations, thoughts, and actions. It is not a task for a single brain area. It does not happen on any single platform.

With consciousness, we would create a self, a home address for issues of responsibility. Daniel Wegner (2002) suggested that authorship is what it is all about in *The Illusion of Conscious Will*. Consciousness would be epiphenomenal to immediate action, unable to exert any direct influence, but crucial in developing an identity. Consciousness allows us to claim authorship for certain actions, and this sense of authorship, in turn, shapes who we are, including our implicit biases. Recent efforts in cognitive psychology show that these concepts are very tractable in elegant empirical work. My favorite example must be the study by Logan and Crump (2010) on illusions of authorship in skilled typists as a function of what is shown on the computer monitor. Interestingly, these illusions appeared to be modulated by a self-serving bias, such that subjects were more likely to take credit for corrected mistakes than to accept blame for inserted errors.

I am confident that connecting the role of consciousness with identity and the sense of authorship (or more generally: ownership) will prove to be a productive line of research. Perhaps everything will come back to the thesis of Maurice Blanchot (1955|1989) on the "space of literature." Consciousness might be that space—a virtual space where objects and events emerge as meaningful cognitive units, consistent with the etymology of poetry ("making things") and the traditional task of philosophy ("defining concepts"). Thus we find poetry and philosophy always, and usually quietly, at work in everyday life, in consciousness, where seeing connects the visible with the invisible, with memory or future, wish or fear—reality working with the imagination.

On this note, it is time to close our chapter 7. Let me bow out with this (incredibly sad, stubbornly hopeful, unbearably light) poem by Miroslav Holub (1990|1995, p. 108), translated by Ian Milner, from the 1963 collection *Where the Blood Flows*. Here, unburdened by any reductive explanation, is consciousness at its best, extreme reality working with the greatest imagination:

Reality

The small worms of pain still wriggled
    in the limpid air,
The trembling died away and
Something in us bowed low before
    the fact of the operating-table
    the fact of the window
    the fact of space
    the fact of steel
    with seven blades.

The silence was inviolable
    like the surface of a mirror.

Though we wanted to ask
Where the blood was flowing
And
Whether you were still dead,
    darling.

Coda: Esemplastic Power

Where poetry is quietly at play in everyday life, we do well to shut up and listen. When seeing connects the visible with the invisible—from memory or through anticipation, driven by wishes and fears—reality works with the imagination. This is how perception was postulated to function by the thinking poets: Wallace Stevens (1951) and Samuel Taylor Coleridge (1817|1984), to name just two who have featured in these pages. Stevens warned us against our insanity vis-à-vis the truth and urged us to incorporate the imagination. Without it, we would not achieve nobility of mind. Reality knows no values, Nature has no ethics, considers no individuals. However, perception is an act by an individual mind. It implies limited perspective, a biological body, and an internal economy of costs and benefits, preferences and aversions. The individual mind cannot help but be biased; what is inside the head ultimately determines the active boundaries of vision, what is seen and what is not.

The biases are a weakness and a blessing. The blessing is in the emergence of values, of good and bad, of ethics. To be concerned with values, to achieve nobility of mind, we need imagination "pressing back against the pressures of reality" (Stevens, 1951, p. 36), and that seems, "in the last analysis, to have something to do with our self-preservation" (same page). The crux is in how we manage our biases. The imagination would be the power through which we achieve the self-control, get to understand our wants and needs, and turn them into objects of perception and thereby into targets for action. It takes us beyond the automatic and reflexive behaviors toward the space of literature, where we can shape who we are and rewrite our biases. The imagination is the critical poetic faculty, the creative mechanism. Coleridge (1817|1984), in his *Biographia Literaria*, spoke of the "esemplastic" power of the imagination, a word he coined from Greek, meaning "to shape into one." With it we would be able to make a point, draw a line, and see a thing clearly.

Nature Has No Such Thing

The drawing of a line is a curious, imaginative gesture. With it we casually trace a perfect idea as if it were real. The infinite becomes graspable in a strange, paradoxical movement. Connecting the dots, working with finite materials, ink on paper, pixels on screens, we bring nothingness into being. It never ceased to amaze the illustrious mind of Charles Sherrington (1940|1955, p. 264):

Visual contour dominates visual space. Perceptually a contour is a line. When we hear that Nature has no such thing as a line, vision answers that all contours are lines. That every contact of fields of light or colour is sharpened and stressed into a line—a psychological line.

Nature has no such thing as a line, yet much of our primary visual cortex is devoted to detecting edges, contours, line segments. Our neural circuits are organized so as to impose the idea of lines on the structure of the visual environment. The imagination takes this process one step further, draws the line explicitly, in a creative moment that shapes the object into a structure (a "count-as-one") for vision. In this singular act, the role of the imagination in perception connects with decision making, reaching thresholds and crossing borders.

"We have to draw a line somewhere," the expression says. It means the line is not given—no physically compelling categorization, only *she says* and *he says*. The active boundaries turn from virtual (in the imagination) to actual (black on white) by a movement of the hand. Through the hand, through the sensorimotor operation of the imagination, grasping the visual, we supplement Nature with the line. We give Nature what it did not have—so now we can say, actually, Nature *does* have such a thing. This is why perception remains such an important and fascinating topic. Perception is where things emerge, made or grasped—meaningful, in our minds. From the transcendental and most abstract to the practical and mundane of everyday life, the gaining of meaning is the core question. If the question is a bit oversized, and if the approach is torturously long and hard, students of perception should take heart in the fact that few endeavors are more important.

For my part, I like to think of my life in science as one long tramping (the Kiwi word for heavy-duty hiking), taking paradoxical pleasure in the roughness of the terrain and the pain in my feet. Strange landscapes, rare moments of clarity, occasionally a magnificent flower—they are the wonders. The walk itself invents a trajectory, draws a line. Our current walk has traced one that deliberately passed through country with very different geographical features: the classics of modern philosophy and phenomenology; contemporary analytically oriented philosophy of mind and its antipode, the ("Continental") philosophy with psychoanalytic credentials; cognitive psychology and cognitive neuroscience; the more conventional hardcore neurophysiology; and—I insist, decidedly not irrelevant—literary theory and poetry. Only a book such as this one offers the space and the time to build a discourse that integrates these various perspectives.

I fully understand the risks the walk implies. The explorer's travelogue naturally must be idiosyncratic. This pushes the boundaries of the comprehensible—exactly the meaning implied by the poet Michael Palmer (2008) when he chose *Active Boundaries* as the title for his collection of essays on poetics. I will not apologize for trying to push those boundaries. I never promised this would be an easy book. My aim is not to popularize but to *do* science. For poets like Samuel Taylor Coleridge, as well as for scientists like Robert H. Wurtz, the interesting is in the difficult—again, the paradoxical pleasure. Rather than summarizing what is known, *Brain and the Gaze* extends an invitation to readers from various disciplines to explore and to take advantage of the riches in other disciplines.

The style and the approach of the present monograph reflect its main thesis on vision. The emphasis is on the active and on the dynamic range—the twilight zone, or the fuzzy area—where the seeing of things is a question, implying a degree of uncertainty. "Can you see it?" "Is this what I think it is?" Active vision works with reality and the imagination to draw the line—to draw changing lines—between what is seen and what is not. One of the greatest principles of the imagination and creative thinking remains that of *borrowing ideas*. For at least as long as we have been human—perhaps even as long as we have been hominid, primate, or mammal—we have borrowed ideas from Nature to design our tools and to shape our environments. We should be able to do more of this and to make bigger leaps in shifting from one context to another, from one perspective to another.

This book is a plea to intensify our borrowing of ideas. I will be happy if *Brain and the Gaze* inspires readers to be more promiscuous in their reading. I will be even happier if some of these readers will chart their trajectories in books as well. The topic of perception requires no defense. But in today's society, unfortunately, the genre of a book-length monograph does require a defense. The current publication culture in science (and commensurate with it, the researcher's reputation and the accolades it brings, from grants to job offers) is so desperately focused on journal articles that few researchers are willing to invest time in writing a book. This is a tragedy. It means that the knowledge and insights of any one expert are communicated in a fractionated way, distributed over dozens of brief outputs that are considered "old" within five years. Research articles give short glimpses of a particular empirical approach; review articles summarize in frantic, shallow ways, mostly limited to a single lab's line of work. It breeds researchers that know technique, but no theory. It breeds lines of research that thrive on technological invention, but not creative thought or critical insight.

So let us look up, step out into the sunlight outside the lab, look at the horizon, left and right, and apply our active vision to study active vision. Then we can come back to the lab, refreshed, reinvigorated, with a brilliant idea for a new experiment. Our current walk focused on the gaze as the chosen paradigm to study action in perception. We explored the concepts of the intensive approach, the sensorimotor system, and the neural architecture for interaction—between center and periphery, what and where, ventral and dorsal, bias and sensitivity, question and answer, hypothesis and test. We considered the intrinsic attraction of information in perception for the sake of perception. We investigated the basic paradox of vision that constructs a limited, highly selective representation of the world while conveying a sense of complete access. Vision turned out to be an enterprise that can be analyzed with concepts from economics. It also comprises important social themes. In many ways, the active boundaries of vision reflect the inherently subjective nature of the access to things as they are—bounded by the body, by degrees of freedom in movement, but also by hidden, internal factors (memory, previous experience, desire, etc.), what the poets called "the imagination" and what I have often connected with the concept of bias in an effort to reach toward Bayesian analysis (for the full story on this connection, see Lauwereyns, 2010).

The take-home message of the book is given in the title. Vision is characterized by its active boundaries—the movements of the gaze, the dynamics of internal processing. With my proposal of the intensive approach, I have specified that these active boundaries aim for meaning and that this meaning ultimately lives nowhere else than inside the subject's head. Noncontroversial though it may seem, this view departs significantly from both the classical teachings in neuroscience (still preached in textbooks) and the leading voices in contemporary philosophy of mind. Classical neuroscience tends to underestimate the active nature of vision and to overestimate the extent of internal representation. Contemporary philosophers have trouble coming to grips with the idea of internal processing and the bodily nature of the body. They tend to leave too much out there in the world and so miss the subjectivity in the subject. Both parties would benefit from reading each other.

Dynamically Coupled with the World

If nothing else, I hope this book proves its point about the benefits from reading each other. I cannot hide—I would never try to hide—that I have a vested interest and a particular vantage point, from my home turf in neuroscience, more specifically cognitive neuroscience. However, my outlook is greatly influenced, and I dare to believe *enriched*, by the ideas, opinions, and criticisms of thinkers and writers outside neuroscience. I experience this as a wonderful privilege. Perhaps the most amazing thing about the privilege is that—in principle, at the outset—it is by no means mine. It is simply there, available for anyone to enjoy. Still, in taking advantage of it and *making* it mine, I somehow have the impression that the thinkers and writers speak to me specifically, or even personally. I feel I owe them a depth of gratitude.

This is where I take my hat off to Alva Noë, the brilliant thinker and writer of *Action in Perception* (2004) and *Out of Our Heads* (2009), who inspired me to write the present book. I must confess I had not planned to write *Brain and the Gaze*. Many of the ideas were implicit in my previous book, *The Anatomy of Bias*, and there, I promised I would next address the dynamics of decision making. But things happened. In January 2010 I moved to Kyushu University, and on the plane to Japan I read Noë's (2004) *Action in Perception*. I got excited, and became irritated—a natural sequence of emotions in fine philosophical tradition. I agreed with Noë's general aim, the fundamental challenge to neuroscience, but disagreed with the externalist program and found many holes in the details. The fury with which I was taking notes shouted there was a topic that needed addressing. Ideas that were implicit begged to be made explicit.

Sometimes the appropriate response to a book is a book. Noë demanded *Brain and the Gaze*. I had to visit (in most cases *re*visit) the same sources (Merleau-Ponty, Descartes, Goethe, Dennett, Gibson, Marr, etc.) and add my own (Wurtz, Goldberg, Hikosaka, Rizzolatti, Platt, Moore, Shimojo, etc.). It quickly became clear to me that the best structure for the book would be one that built with a conceptual scheme and with materials supplied by neuroscience. But the contours—the actual shaping—would be realized by sparring with Noë and his sources. Inevitably, in choosing this structure, I have spent more time disagreeing with Noë and others than highlighting our commonalities in thought.

Here, to compensate, let me borrow a few words from Noë that I would readily have claimed authorship of if they had not been written already. The concluding lines in the last full chapter of *Out of Our Heads* (2009, p. 181) state that "we are dynamically coupled with the world, not separate from it. In so many aspects of our lives this is becoming clear. Neuroscience must come to grips with it." Indeed it must. And immediately after that (p. 183), at the beginning of the epilogue (skipping the first five, unnecessary words), "We are in the world and of it. We are patterns of active engagement with fluid boundaries and changing components. We are distributed." Noë, also in somewhat of a conciliatory mode in his epilogue, even concedes a starring role for the brain (p. 184):

> The substrate of our lives, and of our conscious experience, is the meaningful world in which we find ourselves. The broader world, and the character of our situation in it, is the raw material of a theory of conscious life. The brain plays a starring role in the story, to be sure. But the brain's job is not to "generate" consciousness. Consciousness isn't that kind of thing. It isn't a thing at all. The brain's job is to enable us to carry on as we do in relation to the world around us. Brain, body, and world—each plays a critical role in making us the kind of beings we are.

Neuroscience must come to grips with the active boundaries of vision, the sensorimotor nature of perception, and the fact that information processing is not about recreating the world inside our heads but about computing what the world does for us and what we can do for the world. This, I believe, is how far Noë and I can walk in each other's company. However, the computations happen inside our heads. Neuroscience remains the first and foremost empirical enterprise to address the information processing. We still want the level of understanding that David Marr (1982|2010) was after, though we are now ready to abandon the concept of static detailed representation. Instead, we envision the moving retina and the intensive approach in neural processing—selective and oriented toward meaning.

The Gravity of Harmony, Once More

Having abandoned the concept of static detailed representation, I renew my promise of an inquiry into the dynamics of decision making, the emergence of biases, and the creation of objects of thought. In my previous Coda, I offered as title *The Gravity of Harmony: How Neural Circuits Create Objects of Thought*. I also said it was time for me to head back to the lab and collect new data on the topic. The effort is ongoing, focused on multi-unit recording, tracking covert abstract information coding in rats as they perform spatial choice tasks (for a first output, see Takahashi et al., 2009). We are interested in the dynamics of information seeking (e.g., under which conditions are rats willing to perform operant behaviors to obtain information?) and information coding (e.g., how do rats combine bits of information to predict events?).

At the same time we are interested in the *neural* dynamics. Most of the conceptualizing in *Brain and the Gaze* and *The Anatomy of Bias* was based on what neuroscientists call "rate coding"—the traditional, rather open-ended notion that the amount of neural activity during particular time windows is critical in the correlation between brain and behavior. However, to fully abandon the static views of brain processing, we must also shift to the more dynamic analyses of neural activity (e.g., Tsuda, 2001), or as A. David Redish told me frankly during a workshop in Hokkaido, "Rate coding is dead"—a line that reminded me of Bruce Willis's memorable "Zed's dead, baby, Zed's dead" in Quentin Tarantino's 1994 movie *Pulp Fiction*. So now in my lab we look at, for example, the possibility of chaotic transitions in the spike timing of hippocampal CA1 neurons, shifting from the peak to the trough of theta oscillations.

Luckily I have a few smart colleagues and students around me who seem to understand the algorithms. Every day I realize I have much to learn. I will have my work cut out for me, just trying to catch up. The brilliant (somewhat quirky) mathematician Ichiro Tsuda is making me study general topology, and while my head is spinning from the implications for neuroscience, I try to unwind it every night by treating it to a bit of Jorge Luis Borges (I am now rereading the poems and fictions and discovering the nonfictions). I also know I need to delve further into Heidegger, Sartre, and Deleuze (via his explicator, DeLanda), possibly also Badiou. And I figure I will never be done with Descartes. Nor can there be (or would I wish there to be) relief from Dennett, Clark, Noë, the Anglo-Saxon. Thus the reading and experimenting goes on, more intensely than ever. I have no idea how long it will take me, how far I must walk, but I do think (body and mind permitting) that I will be ready one day for that next book. Writing sharpens thought, so, of course, I have to write, if for no other reason than to think. However, I already know I will want to use a different title—not *The Gravity of Harmony:*

How Neural Circuits Create Objects of Thought. "Harmony" sounds too harmonious, and the structure of the title was modeled too closely after that of *The Anatomy of Bias.* Today I think I will prefer *Being in Doubt: Intensive Biology and Virtual Consciousness.* Let me leave it at that: an empty placeholder for now, the future content wide open and yet not entirely unimaginable.

Lying in a Hammock

"Where poetry is quietly at play in everyday life, we do well to shut up and listen. When seeing connects the visible with the invisible—from memory or through anticipation, driven by wishes and fears—reality works with the imagination." These are the two sentences with which I started this Coda. But instead of duly shutting up, I moved on to talking about drawing lines, off on a tangent.

Now I should really finish, drawing another kind of line, orthogonal to the trajectory. *This is the end,* today the 24th of October 2011, a special day indeed, a thirteenth anniversary—*the* thirteenth anniversary. From today onward, this book will be in postproduction, meaning I will not let future events (publications) alter the content of the discourse. As always I eagerly look forward to what science will bring in the next few years and decades—not only neuroscience but also psychology, philosophy, poetry, and any other discipline or perspective that has something to say about consciousness, perception, how it is that we are who we are, and what it is to be or not to be. The questions are old, and always there, and always new. So, then, this is me shutting up, with a lovely, quiet humming by the contemporary Russian poet Arkadii Dragomoshchenko (2008, p. 93), invoking a strange nostalgia, not for what is lost but for what is still there after many years:

Even today I get the most pleasure from lying in a hammock with a book, gazing beyond its pages. This applies to my own writing as well. And when I write this, I see certain things, which haven't changed in forty years—for example, the big old linden tree, or sunshine under my eyelids.

Bibliography

Adamük, E. (1870). Über die Innervation der Augenbewegungen [On the innervation of eye movements]. *Centralblatt für die medicinische Wissenschaften, 8,* 65–67.

Addyman, C., & Mareschal, D. (2010). The perceptual origins of the abstract same/different concept in human infants. *Animal Cognition, 13,* 817–833.

Agamben, G. (1991). *Language and Death: The Place of Negativity* (Pinkus, K. E., & Hardt, M., Trans.). Minneapolis, MN: University of Minnesota Press.

Agamben, G. (2009). *What Is an Apparatus? And Other Essays* (Kishik, D., & Pedatella, S., Trans.). Stanford, CA: Stanford University Press.

Aguilonius, F. (1613). *Opticorum Libri Sex Philosophis juxta ac Mathematicis utiles* [Six Books of Optics Useful for Philosophers and Mathematicians Alike]. Antwerp, Belgium: Plantin Press.

Alighieri, D. (1995). *The Divine Comedy: Inferno; Purgatorio; Paradiso* (Mandelbaum, A., Trans.). New York: Alfred A. Knopf (Everyman's Library). (Original work written between 1308 and 1321.)

Allport, D. A. (1987). Selection-for-action: Some behavioral and neurophysiological considerations of attention and action. In H. Heuer & A. F. Sanders (Eds.), *Perspectives on Perception and Action* (pp. 395–419). Hillsdale, NJ: Lawrence Erlbaum Associates.

Amodio, D. M., & Frith, C. D. (2006). Meeting of minds: The medial frontal cortex and social cognition. *Nature Reviews. Neuroscience, 7,* 268–277.

Anderson, E., Siegel, E. H., Bliss-Moreau, E., & Barrett, L. F. (2011). The visual impact of gossip. *Science, 332,* 1446–1448.

Andersson, R., Ferreira, F., & Henderson, J. M. (2011). I see what you're saying: The integration of complex speech and scenes during language comprehension. *Acta Psychologica, 137,* 208–216.

Anonymous. (2004). *The Bible, King James Version, Book 42: Luke.* Project Gutenberg, EBook #7999 [http://www.gutenberg.org]. (Accessed 1 July 2011.) (Translation first published 1611.)

Antes, J. R. (1974). The time course of picture viewing. *Journal of Experimental Psychology, 103,* 62–70.

Awh, E., & Jonides, J. (2001). Overlapping mechanisms of attention and spatial working memory. *Trends in Cognitive Sciences, 5,* 119–126.

Baccus, S. A., Ölveczky, B. P., Manu, M., & Meister, M. (2008). A retinal circuit that computes object motion. *Journal of Neuroscience, 28,* 6807–6817.

Bachelard, G. [1958] (1994). *The Poetics of Space* (Jolas, M., Trans.). Boston, MA: Beacon Press.

Bach-y-Rita, P. (1972). *Brain Mechanisms in Sensory Substitution.* New York: Academic Press.

Badiou, A. [1982] (2009). *Theory of the Subject* (Bosteels, B., Trans.). London: Continuum.

Badiou, A. [1988] (2007). *Being and Event* (Feltham, O., Trans.). London: Continuum.

Bahrami, B., Olson, K., Latham, P. E., Roepstorff, A., Rees, G., & Frith, C. D. (2010). Optimally interacting minds. *Science, 329,* 1081–1085.

Ballard, D., Hayhoe, M. M., Pook, P., & Rao, R. (1997). Deictic codes for the embodiment of cognition. *Behavioral and Brain Sciences, 20,* 723–767.

Barbur, J. (2004). Learning from the pupil: Studies of basic mechanisms and clinical applications. In L. Chlupa & J. Werner (Eds.), *The Visual Neurosciences* (Vol. 1, pp. 641–656). Cambridge, MA: MIT Press.

Baron-Cohen, S. (1995). *Mindblindness.* Cambridge, MA: MIT Press.

Barthes, R. [1981] (1999). *Camera Lucida: Reflections on Photography* (Howard, R., Trans.). New York: Hill and Wang.

Baudelaire, C. [1857] (2010). E. K. Kaplan (Ed.), *Les Fleurs du Mal.* Newark, DE: European Masterpieces.

Bays, P. M., & Husain, M. (2007). Spatial remapping of the visual world across saccades. *Neuroreport, 18,* 1207–1213.

Bays, P. M., & Husain, M. (2008). Dynamic shifts of limited working memory resources in human vision. *Science, 321,* 851–854.

Berkes, P., Orban, G., Lengyel, M., & Fiser, J. (2011). Spontaneous cortical activity reveals hallmarks of an optimal internal model of the environment. *Science, 331,* 83–87.

Berlyne, D. E. (1966). Curiosity and exploration. *Science, 153,* 25–33.

Berman, R. A., Heiser, L. M., Dunn, C. A., Saunders, R. C., & Colby, C. L. (2007). Dynamic circuitry for updating spatial representations. III. From neurons to behavior. *Journal of Neurophysiology, 98,* 105–121.

Berry, D. C. (1987). The problem of implicit knowledge. *Expert Systems: International Journal of Knowledge Engineering and Neural Networks, 4,* 144–151.

Berry, D. C., & Broadbent, D. E. (1984). On the relationship between task performance and associated verbalisable knowledge. *Quarterly Journal of Experimental Psychology, 36A,* 209–231.

Bezdudnaya, T., Cano, M., Bereshpolova, Y., Stoelzel, C. R., Alonso, J. M., & Swadlow, H. A. (2006). Thalamic burst mode and inattention in the awake LGNd. *Neuron, 49,* 421–432.

Bisley, J. W., & Goldberg, M. E. (2003). Neuronal activity in the lateral intraparietal area and spatial attention. *Science, 299,* 81–86.

Blake, R., & Logothetis, N. K. (2001). Visual competition. *Nature Reviews. Neuroscience, 3,* 1–11.

Blanchot, M. [1955] (1989). *The Space of Literature* (Smock, A., Trans.). Lincoln, NE: University of Nebraska Press.

Bloom, H. [1975] (2003). *A Map of Misreading.* New York: Oxford University Press.

Borges, J. L. (1998). *Collected Fictions* (Hurley, A., Trans.). New York: Viking Penguin.

Borges, J. L. (1999). A. Coleman (Ed.), *Selected Poems.* New York: Viking Penguin.

Bouton, M. E. (2007). *Learning and Behavior: A Contemporary Synthesis.* Sunderland, MA: Sinauer.

Brenner, S. (1974). The genetics of *Caenorhabditis elegans. Genetics, 77,* 71–94.

Brentano, F. [1874] (1995). *Psychology from an Empirical Standpoint* (Rancurello, A. C., Terrell, D. B., & McAlister, L. L., Trans.; Kraus , E., & McAlister, L. L., Eds.). London: Routledge.

Bridge, H., & Cumming, B. G. (2008). Representation of binocular surfaces by cortical neurons. *Current Opinion in Neurobiology, 18*, 425–430.

Bridgeman, B., Van der Heijden, A. H. C., & Velichkovsky, B. (1994). Visual stability and saccadic eye movements. *Behavioral and Brain Sciences, 17*, 247–258.

Briggman, K. L., Helmstaedter, M., & Denk, W. (2011). Wiring specificity in the direction-selectivity of the retina. *Nature, 471*, 183–188.

Broadbent, D. E. [1958] (1961). *Perception and Communication.* London: The Scientific Book Guild.

Bromberg-Martin, E. S., & Hikosaka, O. (2009). Midbrain dopamine neurons signal preference for information about upcoming rewards. *Neuron, 63*, 119–126.

Bromberg-Martin, E. S., & Hikosaka, O. (2011). Lateral habenula neurons signal errors in the prediction of reward information. *Nature Neuroscience, 14*, 1209–1216.

Brooks, B. A., Yates, J. T., & Coleman, R. D. (1980). Perception of images moving at saccadic velocities during saccades and during fixation. *Experimental Brain Research, 40*, 71–78.

Browning, C. R., & Matthäus, J. (2004). *The Origins of the Final Solution: The Evolution of Nazi Jewish Policy, September 1939–March 1942.* Jerusalem, Israel: Yad Vashem.

Brozzoli, C., Gentile, G., Petkova, V. I., & Ehrsson, H. H. (2011). fMRI adaptation reveals a cortical mechanism for the coding of space near the hand. *Journal of Neuroscience, 31*, 9023–9031.

Burr, D. C., Morrone, M. C., & Ross, J. (1994). Selective suppression of the magnocellular visual pathway during saccadic eye movements. *Nature, 371*, 511–513.

Bushnell, E. W., & Boudreau, J. P. (1993). Motor development and the mind: The potential role of motor abilities as a determinant of aspects of perceptual development. *Child Development, 64*, 1005–1021.

Buswell, G. T. (1920). *An Experimental Study of the Eye–Voice Span in Reading.* Chicago: University of Chicago Press.

Buswell, G. T. (1935). *How People Look at Pictures: A Study of the Psychology of Perception in Art.* Chicago: University of Chicago Press.

Büttner-Ennever, J. A. (Ed.). (2006). *Neuroanatomy of the Oculomotor System (Progress in Brain Research, Volume 151).* Amsterdam, The Netherlands: Elsevier.

Cajal, S. R. (1893). La rétine des vertébrés [The retina of vertebrates]. *La Cellule, 9*, 17–257.

Carpenter, R. H. S. (1999). A neural mechanism that randomises behaviour. *Journal of Consciousness Studies, 6*, 13–22.

Cavanagh, P., Hunt, A. R., Afraz, A., & Rolfs, M. (2010). Visual stability based on remapping of attention pointers. *Trends in Cognitive Sciences, 14*, 147–153.

Cecala, A. L., & Freedman, E. G. (2009). Head-unrestrained gaze adaptation in the rhesus macaque. *Journal of Neurophysiology, 101*, 164–183.

Cerf, M., Thiruvengadam, N., Mormann, F., Kraskov, A., Quiroga, R. Q., Koch, C., et al. (2010). On-line, voluntary control of human temporal lobe neurons. *Nature, 467*, 1104–1108.

Cheal, M., & Lyon, D. R. (1991). Central and peripheral precuing of forced-choice discrimination. *Quarterly Journal of Experimental Psychology, 43A*, 859–880.

Cheal, M., Lyon, D. R., & Gottlob, L. R. (1994). A framework for understanding the allocation of attention in location-precued discrimination. *Quarterly Journal of Experimental Psychology, 47A*, 699–739.

Chun, M. M., & Jiang, Y. (1998). Contextual cueing: Implicit learning and memory of visual context guides spatial attention. *Cognitive Psychology, 36*, 28–71.

Chun, M. M., & Phelps, E. A. (1999). Memory deficits for implicit contextual information in amnesic subjects with hippocampal damage. *Nature Neuroscience*, *2*, 844–847.

Churchland, A. K., Kiani, R., & Shadlen, M. N. (2008). Decision-making with multiple alternatives. *Nature Neuroscience*, *11*, 693–702.

Clark, A. (1997). *Being There: Putting Brain, Body and World Together Again*. Cambridge, MA: MIT Press.

Clark, A. (2003). *Natural-Born Cyborgs: Minds, Technologies, and the Future of Human Intelligence*. New York: Oxford University Press.

Clark, A. (2008). *Supersizing the Mind: Embodiment, Action, and Cognitive Extension*. New York: Oxford University Press.

Cohen, M. R., & Maunsell, J. H. (2010). A neuronal population measure of attention predicts performance on individual trials. *Journal of Neuroscience*, *30*, 15241–15253.

Coleridge, S. T. [1817] (1984). J. Engell & W. J. Bate (Eds.), *The Collected Works of Samuel Taylor Coleridge: Biographia Literaria or Biographical Sketches of My Literary Life and Opinions*. Princeton, NJ: Princeton University Press.

Coleridge, S. T. (2001). J. C. C. Mays (Ed.), *The Collected Works of Samuel Taylor Coleridge: Poetical Works I*. Princeton, NJ: Princeton University Press.

Conradie, C. J., Johl, R., Beukes, M., Fischer, O., & Ljungberg, C. (Eds.). (2010). *Signergy*. Amsterdam, The Netherlands: John Benjamins.

Conway, B. R., Chatterjee, S., Field, G. D., Horwitz, G. D., Johnson, E. N., Koida, K., et al. (2010). Advances in color science: From retina to behavior. *Journal of Neuroscience*, *30*, 14955–14963.

Corneil, B. D., Munoz, D. P., Chapman, B. B., Admans, T., & Cushing, S. L. (2008). Neuromuscular consequences of reflexive covert orienting. *Nature Neuroscience*, *11*, 13–15.

Courchesne, E., Hillyard, S. A., & Galambos, R. (1975). Stimulus novelty, task relevance and the visual evoked potential in man. *Electroencephalography and Clinical Neurophysiology*, *39*, 131–143.

Cowey, A. (2010). The blindsight saga. *Experimental Brain Research*, *200*, 3–24.

Cox, D., Meyers, E., & Sinha, P. (2004). Contextually evoked object-specific responses in human visual cortex. *Science*, *304*, 115–117.

Crick, F. (1984). Function of the thalamic reticular complex: The searchlight hypothesis. *Proceedings of the National Academy of Sciences of the United States of America*, *81*, 4586–4590.

Crick, F. [1994] (1995). *The Astonishing Hypothesis: The Scientific Search for the Soul*. New York: Touchstone.

Crist, R. E., Kapadia, M., Westheimer, G., & Gilbert, C. D. (1997). Perceptual learning of spatial localization: Specificity for orientation, position and context. *Journal of Neurophysiology*, *78*, 2889–2894.

Culler, J. [1981] (2001). *The Pursuit of Signs: Semiotics, Literature, Deconstruction*. London: Routledge Classics.

Custers, R., & Aarts, H. (2010). The unconscious will: How the pursuit of goals operates outside of conscious awareness. *Science*, *329*, 47–50.

Damasio, A. (2010). *Self Comes to Mind: Constructing the Conscious Brain*. New York: Pantheon Books.

Darley, J. M., & Latané, B. (1968). Bystander intervention in emergencies: Diffusion of responsibility. *Journal of Personality and Social Psychology*, *8*, 377–383.

Darwin, C. [1859] (1866). *On the Origin of Species by Means of Natural Selection, or the Preservation of Favoured Races in the Struggle for Life*. London: John Murray.

Darwin, C. [1872] (1965). *The Expression of the Emotions in Man and Animals*. Chicago: University of Chicago Press.

Daw, N. D., O'Doherty, J. P., Dayan, P., Seymour, B., & Dolan, R. J. (2006). Cortical substrates for exploratory decisions in humans. *Nature, 441*, 876–879.

Dawkins, R. [1996] (1997). *Climbing Mount Improbable*. New York: W. W. Norton & Company.

Deacon, T. W. (1997). *The Symbolic Species: The Co-evolution of Language and the Brain*. New York: W. W. Norton & Company.

Deaner, R. O., & Platt, M. L. (2003). Reflexive social attention in monkeys and humans. *Current Biology, 13*, 1609–1613.

Deaner, R. O., Khera, A. V., & Platt, M. L. (2005). Monkeys pay per view: Adaptive valuation of social images by rhesus monkeys. *Current Biology, 15*, 546–548.

De Cuypere, L. (2008). *Limiting the Iconic: From the Metatheoretical Foundations to the Creative Possibilities of Iconicity in Language*. Amsterdam, The Netherlands: John Benjamins.

De Graef, P., Christiaens, D., & d'Ydewalle, G. (1990). Perceptual effects of scene context on object identification. *Psychological Research, 52*, 317–329.

DeLanda, M. [2002] (2004). *Intensive Science and Virtual Philosophy*. New York: Continuum.

Deleuze, G. [1968] (1994). *Difference and Repetition* (Patton, P., Trans.). New York: Columbia University Press.

De Man, P. (1979). *Allegories of Reading: Figural Language in Rousseau, Nietzsche, Rilke, and Proust*. New Haven, CT: Yale University Press.

Demb, J. B., Haarsma, L., Freed, M. A., & Sterling, P. (1999). Functional circuitry of the retinal ganglion cell's nonlinear receptive field. *Journal of Neuroscience, 19*, 9756–9767.

Demos, K. E., Kelley, W. M., Ryan, S. L., Davis, F. C., & Whalen, P. J. (2008). Human amygdala sensitivity to the pupil size of others. *Cerebral Cortex, 18*, 2729–2734.

Dennett, D. C. (1987). *The Intentional Stance*. Cambridge, MA: MIT Press.

Dennett, D. C. (1991). *Consciousness Explained*. Boston, MA: Little, Brown and Company.

Descartes, R. [1637] (2006). *A Discourse on the Method of Correctly Conducting One's Reason and Seeking Truth in the Sciences* (Maclean, I., Trans.). Oxford: Oxford University Press.

Descartes, R. [1641] (1996). *Meditations on First Philosophy: With Selections from the Objections and Replies* (Cottingham, J., Trans., Ed.). Cambridge, UK: Cambridge University Press.

Desimone, R., Albright, T. D., Gross, C. G., & Bruce, C. (1984). Stimulus-selective properties of inferior temporal neurons in the macaque. *Journal of Neuroscience, 4*, 2051–2062.

Deubel, H., & Schneider, W. X. (1996). Saccade target selection and object recognition: Evidence for a common attentional mechanism. *Vision Research, 14*, 1827–1837.

De Weerd, P., Gattass, R., Desimone, R., & Ungerleider, L. G. (1995). Responses of cells in monkey visual cortex during perceptual filling-in of an artificial scotoma. *Nature, 377*, 731–734.

Dickinson, A. (1980). *Contemporary Animal Learning Theory*. Cambridge, UK: Cambridge University Press.

Dinsmoor, J. A. (2001). Stimuli inevitably generated by behavior that avoids electric shock are inherently reinforcing. *Journal of the Experimental Analysis of Behavior, 75*, 311–333.

Dixson, A. F. (2009). *Sexual Selection and the Origins of Human Mating Systems*. Oxford: Oxford University Press.

Dixson, B. J., Grimshaw, G. M., Linklater, W. L., & Dixson, A. F. (2011). Eye-tracking of men's preferences for waist-to-hip ratio and breast size of women. *Archives of Sexual Behavior, 40*, 43–50.

Dolar, M. (1996). At first sight. In R. Salecl & S. Žižek (Eds.), *Gaze and Voice as Love Objects* (pp. 129–153). Durham, NC: Duke University Press.

Donders, F. C. (1869). Over de snelheid van psychische processen [On the speed of mental processes]. *Nederlands Archief voor Genees- en Natuurkunde, 4,* 117–145.

Donders, F. C. (1969). On the speed of mental processes (W. G. Koster, Trans.). In W. G. Koster (Ed.), *Attention and Performance II, Acta Psychologica, 30,* 412–431.

Downing, C. J. (1988). Expectancy and visual-spatial attention: Effects on perceptual quality. *Journal of Experimental Psychology. Human Perception and Performance, 14,* 188–202.

Dragomoshchenko, A. (2008). *Dust* (Pavlov, E., Epstein, T., Avagyan, S., & Lucic, A., Trans.). Champaign, IL: Dalkey Archive Press.

Driver, J., Davis, G., Ricciardelli, P., Kidd, P., Maxwell, E., & Baron-Cohen, S. (1999). Gaze perception triggers reflexive visuospatial orienting. *Visual Cognition, 6,* 509–540.

Duhamel, J. R., Colby, C. L., & Goldberg, M. E. (1992). The updating of the representation of visual space in parietal cortex by intended eye movements. *Science, 255,* 90–92.

Duhamel, J. R., Colby, C. L., & Goldberg, M. E. (1998). Ventral intraparietal area of the macaque: Congruent visual and somatic response properties. *Journal of Neurophysiology, 79,* 126–136.

Dundes, A. (Ed.). [1981] (1992). *The Evil Eye: A Casebook.* Madison, WI: University of Wisconsin Press.

Egner, T., Monti, J. M., & Summerfield, C. (2010). Expectation and surprise determine neural population responses in the ventral visual stream. *Journal of Neuroscience, 30,* 16601–16608.

Einhäuser, W., Martin, K. A., & König, P. (2004). Are switches in perception of the Necker cube related to eye position? *European Journal of Neuroscience, 20,* 2811–2820.

Einhäuser, W., Moeller, G. U., Schumann, F., Conradt, J., Vockeroth, J., Bartl, K., et al. (2009). Eye–head coordination during free exploration in human and cat. *Annals of the New York Academy of Sciences, 1164,* 353–366.

Einstein, A. (1954). C. Seelig (Ed.), *Ideas and Opinions* (Bargmann, B., Trans.). New York: Wings Books.

Elkins, J. (1996). *The Object Stares Back: On the Nature of Seeing.* New York: Simon & Schuster.

Elston, M. A. [1987] (1990). Women and anti-vivisection in Victorian England, 1870–1900. In N. A. Rupke (Ed.), *Vivisection in Historical Perspective* (pp. 259–294). London: Routledge.

Emery, N. J., Lorincz, E. N., Perrett, D. I., Oram, M. W., & Baker, C. I. (1997). Gaze following and joint attention in rhesus monkeys (*Macaca mulatta*). *Journal of Comparative Psychology, 111,* 286–293.

Enroth-Cugell, C., & Robson, J. G. (1966). The contrast sensitivity of retinal ganglion cells of the cat. *Journal of Physiology, 187,* 517–552.

Érdi, P. (1996). The brain as a hermeneutic device. *Bio Systems, 38,* 179–189.

Eriksen, C. W., & Collins, J. F. (1969). Temporal course of selective attention. *Journal of Experimental Psychology, 80,* 254–261.

Euler, T., Detwiler, P. B., & Denk, W. (2002). Directionally selective calcium signals in dendrites of starburst amacrine cells. *Nature, 418,* 845–852.

Fanselow, E. E., Sameshima, K., Baccala, L. A., & Nicolelis, M. A. (2001). Thalamic bursting in rats during different awake behavioral states. *Proceedings of the National Academy of Sciences of the United States of America, 98,* 15330–15335.

Farkas, I., Helbing, D., & Vicsek, T. (2002). Mexican waves in an excitable medium. *Nature, 419,* 131–132.

Faverey, H. [1994] (2004). *Against the Forgetting: Selected Poems* (Jones, F. R., Trans.). New York: New Directions Publishing.

Ferreira, F., & Henderson, J. M. (1990). Use of verb information in syntactic parsing: Evidence from eye movements and word-by-word self-paced reading. *Journal of Experimental Psychology. Learning, Memory, and Cognition, 16*, 555–568.

Ferreira, F., Apel, J., & Henderson, J. M. (2008). Taking a new look at looking at nothing. *Trends in Cognitive Sciences, 12*, 405–410.

Ferrier, D. (1876). *The Functions of the Brain.* New York: G. P. Putnam's Sons.

Fetz, E. E. (1969). Operant conditioning of cortical unit activity. *Science, 163*, 955–958.

Fias, W., Dupont, P., Reynvoet, B., & Orban, G. A. (2002). The quantitative nature of the task differentiates between ventral and dorsal stream. *Journal of Cognitive Neuroscience, 14*, 646–658.

Findlay, J. M. (2003). *Active Vision: The Psychology of Looking and Seeing.* Oxford: Oxford University Press.

Findlay, J. M. (2009). Saccadic eye movement programming: Sensory and attentional factors. *Psychological Research, 73*, 127–135.

Fogassi, L., Ferrari, P. F., Gesierich, B., Rozzi, S., Chersi, F., & Rizzolatti, G. (2005). Parietal lobe: From action organization to intention understanding. *Science, 308*, 662–667.

Frazier, L., & Rayner, K. (1982). Making and correcting errors during sentence comprehension: Eye movements in the analysis of structurally ambiguous sentences. *Cognitive Psychology, 14*, 178–210.

Freud, S. [1913] (1999). *Totem and Taboo* (Strachey, J., Trans.). London: Routledge.

Fried, S. I., Münch, T. A., & Werblin, F. S. (2002). Mechanisms and circuitry underlying directional selectivity in the retina. *Nature, 420*, 411–414.

Friedman, A. (1979). Framing pictures: The role of knowledge in automatized encoding and memory for gist. *Journal of Experimental Psychology. General, 108*, 316–355.

Friesen, C. K., & Kingstone, A. (1998). The eyes have it! Reflexive orienting is triggered by nonpredictive gaze. *Psychonomic Bulletin & Review, 5*, 490–495.

Fritsch, G., & Hitzig, E. [1870] (2009). Electric excitability of the cerebrum [Über die elektrische Erregbarkeit des Grosshirns] (Crump, T., & Lama, S., Trans.). *Epilepsy & Behavior, 15*, 123–130.

Gallese, V., & Goldman, A. (1998). Mirror neurons and the simulation theory of mind-reading. *Trends in Cognitive Sciences, 2*, 493–501.

Gallese, V., Fadiga, L., Fogassi, L., & Rizzolatti, G. (1996). Action recognition in the premotor cortex. *Brain, 119*, 593–609.

Gattass, R., Gross, C. G., & Sandell, J. H. (1981). Visual topography of V2 in the macaque. *Journal of Comparative Neurology, 201*, 519–539.

Gattass, R., Sousa, A. P., & Gross, C. G. (1988). Visuotopic organization and extent of V3 and V4 of the macaque. *Journal of Neuroscience, 8*, 1831–1845.

Gauthier, I., Hayward, W. G., Tarr, M. J., Anderson, A. W., Skudlarski, P., & Gore, J. C. (2002). BOLD activity during mental rotation and viewpoint-dependent object recognition. *Neuron, 34*, 161–171.

Gauthier, I., Skudlarski, P., Gore, J. C., & Anderson, A. W. (2000). Expertise for cars and birds recruits brain areas involved in face recognition. *Nature Neuroscience, 3*, 191–197.

Gerlach, K. D., Spreng, R. N., Gilmore, A. W., & Schacter, D. L. (2011). Solving future problems: Default network and executive activity associated with goal-directed mental simulations. *NeuroImage, 55*, 1816–1824.

Gibboni, R. R., III, Zimmerman, P. E., & Gothard, K. M. (2009). Individual differences in scanpaths correspond with serotonin transporter genotype and behavioral phenotype in rhesus monkeys (*Macaca mulatta*). *Frontiers in Behavioral Neuroscience, 3*, 50.

Gibson, J. J. [1979] (1986). *The Ecological Approach to Visual Perception*. Hillsdale, NJ: Lawrence Erlbaum Associates.

Gigerenzer, G. (2002). *Reckoning with Risk: Learning to Live with Uncertainty*. London: Allen Lane, Penguin Press.

Gilbert, C. D., Sigman, M., & Crist, R. E. (2001). The neural basis of perceptual learning. *Neuron, 31*, 681–697.

Gilbert, T. D., & Wilson, T. D. (2007). Prospection: Experiencing the future. *Science, 317*, 1351–1354.

Girard, R. (2008). R. Doran (Ed.), *Mimesis and Theory: Essays on Literature and Criticism, 1953–2005*. Stanford, CA: Stanford University Press.

Glimcher, P. W. (2003). *Decisions, Uncertainty, and the Brain: The Science of Neuroeconomics*. Cambridge, MA: MIT Press.

Goethe, J. W. [1810] (2006). *Theory of Colours* (Eastlake, C. L., Trans.). Mineola, NY: Dover Publications Inc.

Goldberg, M. E., & Wurtz, R. H. (1972a). Activity of superior colliculus in behaving monkey. I. Visual receptive fields of single neurons. *Journal of Neurophysiology, 35*, 542–559.

Goldberg, M. E., & Wurtz, R. H. (1972b). Activity of superior colliculus in behaving monkey. II. Effect of attention on neuronal responses. *Journal of Neurophysiology, 35*, 560–574.

Gollisch, T., & Meister, M. (2010). Eye smarter than scientists believed: Neural computations in circuits of the retina. *Neuron, 65*, 150–164.

Goodale, M. A., & Milner, A. D. (1992). Separate visual pathways for perception and action. *Trends in Neurosciences, 15*, 20–25.

Goodale, M. A., Milner, A. D., Jakobson, L. S., & Carey, D. P. (1991). A neurological dissociation between perceiving objects and grasping them. *Nature, 349*, 154–156.

Gottlieb, J., Kusunoki, M., & Goldberg, M. E. (1998). The representation of visual salience in monkey parietal cortex. *Nature, 391*, 481–484.

Grabenhorst, F., & Rolls, E. T. (2011). Value, pleasure and choice in the ventral prefrontal cortex. *Trends in Cognitive Sciences, 15*, 56–67.

Graziano, M. S., Yap, G. S., & Gross, C. G. (1994). Coding of visual space by premotor neurons. *Science, 266*, 1054–1057.

Green, D. M., & Swets, J. A. [1966] (1988). *Signal Detection Theory and Psychophysics*. Los Altos, CA: Peninsula Publishing.

Gregory, R. L. (1966). *Eye and Brain: The Psychology of Seeing*. London: World University Library.

Greimel, E., Schulte-Rüther, M., Fink, G. R., Piefke, M., Herpertz-Dahlmann, B., & Konrad, K. (2010). Development of neural correlates of empathy from childhood to early adulthood: An fMRI study in boys and adult men. *Journal of Neural Transmission, 117*, 781–791.

Grimes, J. (1996). On the failure to detect changes in scenes across saccades. In K. Akins (Ed.), *Perception (Vancouver Studies in Cognitive Science), 2* (pp. 89–110). New York: Oxford University Press.

Grimes, W. N., Zhang, J., Graydon, C. W., Kachar, B., & Diamond, J. S. (2010). Retinal parallel processors: More than 100 independent microcircuits operate within a single interneuron. *Neuron, 65*, 873–885.

Gross, C. G. (2009). Early steps toward animal rights. *Science, 324*, 466–467.

Grüsser, O.-J. (1994). Early concepts on efference copy and reafference. *Behavioral and Brain Sciences, 17*, 262–265.

Guo, C. C., & Raymond, J. L. (2010). Motor learning reduces eye movement variability through reweighting of sensory inputs. *Journal of Neuroscience, 30*, 16241–16248.

Guthrie, B. L., Porter, J. D., & Sparks, D. L. (1983). Corollary discharge provides accurate eye position information to the oculomotor system. *Science, 221*, 1193–1195.

Han, X., Xian, S. X., & Moore, T. (2009). Dynamic sensitivity of area V4 neurons during saccade preparation. *Proceedings of the National Academy of Sciences of the United States of America, 106*, 13046–13051.

Hanes, D. P., & Schall, J. D. (1996). Neural control of voluntary movement initiation. *Science, 274*, 427–430.

Hannula, D. E., & Ranganath, C. (2009). The eyes have it: Hippocampal activity predicts expression of memory in eye movements. *Neuron, 63*, 592–599.

Hannula, D. E., Ryan, J. D., Tranel, D., & Cohen, N. J. (2007). Rapid onset relational memory effects are evident in eye movement behavior, but not in hippocampal amnesia. *Journal of Cognitive Neuroscience, 19*, 1690–1705.

Hansen, D. W., & Ji, Q. (2010). In the eye of the beholder: A survey of models for eye and gaze. *IEEE Transactions on Pattern Analysis and Machine Intelligence, 32*, 478–500.

Hare, B., Brown, M., Williamson, C., & Tomasello, M. (2002). The domestication of social cognition in dogs. *Science, 298*, 1634–1636.

Hare, B., Call, J., Agnetta, B., & Tomasello, M. (2000). Chimpanzees know what conspecifics do and do not see. *Animal Behaviour, 59*, 771–785.

Harper, G. M. [1928] (1969). *Spirit of Delight*. Freeport, NY: Books for Libraries Press.

Harris, L. T., & Fiske, S. T. (2006). Dehumanizing the lowest of the low. *Psychological Science, 17*, 847–853.

Hart, A. (1986). *Knowledge Acquisition for Expert Systems*. London: Kogan Page.

Hayhoe, M., Bensinger, D. G., & Ballard, D. H. (1998). Task constraints in visual working memory. *Vision Research, 38*, 125–137.

Hebb, D. O. (1946). Emotion in man and animal: An analysis of the intuitive processes of recognition. *Psychological Review, 53*, 88–106.

Heidegger, M. [1962] (2008). *Being and Time* (Macquarrie, J., & Robinson, E., Trans.). New York: HarperPerennial.

Henderson, J. M. (1993). Visual attention and saccadic eye movements. In G. d'Ydewalle & J. Van Rensbergen (Eds.), *Perception and Cognition: Advances in Eye Movement Research* (pp. 37–50). Amsterdam, The Netherlands: North-Holland.

Henderson, J. M. (2003). Human gaze control during real-world scene perception. *Trends in Cognitive Sciences, 7*, 498–504.

Henderson, J. M., & Hollingworth, A. (2003). Eye movements and visual memory: Detecting changes to saccade targets in scenes. *Perception & Psychophysics, 65*, 58–71.

Henderson, J. M., Weeks, P. A., Jr., & Hollingworth, A. (1999). The effects of semantic consistency on eye movements during complex scene viewing. *Journal of Experimental Psychology. Human Perception and Performance, 25*, 210–228.

Herbert, Z. (2007). *The Collected Poems 1956–1998* (Valles, A., Trans.). New York: HarperCollins.

Herrmann, E., Call, J., Hernández-Lloreda, M. V., Hare, B., & Tomasello, M. (2007). Humans have evolved specialized skills of social cognition: The cultural intelligence hypothesis. *Science, 317*, 1360–1366.

Hess, E. H., & Polt, J. M. (1960). Pupil size as related to interest value of visual stimuli. *Science, 132*, 349–350.

Hess, E. H., & Polt, J. M. (1964). Pupil size in relation to mental activity during simple problem-solving. *Science, 140*, 1190–1192.

Hikosaka, O., & Sakamoto, M. (1987). Dynamic characteristics of saccadic eye movements in the albino rat. *Neuroscience Research*, *4*, 304–308.

Hockney, D. (2001). *Secret Knowledge: Rediscovering the Lost Techniques of the Old Masters*. London: Thames & Hudson.

Hollingworth, A., & Henderson, J. M. (2002). Accurate visual memory for previously attended objects in natural scenes. *Journal of Experimental Psychology. Human Perception and Performance*, *28*, 113–136.

Hollingworth, A., Schrock, G., & Henderson, J. M. (2001). Change detection in the flicker paradigm: The role of fixation position within the scene. *Memory & Cognition*, *29*, 296–304.

Holmes, R. (2008). *The Age of Wonder: How the Romantic Generation Discovered the Beauty and Terror of Science*. London: HarperPress.

Holub, M. [1990] (1995). *Poems: Before & After* (Milner, I., Milner, J., Osers, E., & Theiner, G., Trans.). Newcastle upon Tyne, UK: Bloodaxe Books.

Howard, I. P. (1996). Alhazen's neglected discoveries of visual phenomena. *Perception*, *25*, 1203–1217.

Huang, X., & Paradiso, M. A. (2008). V1 response timing and surface filling-in. *Journal of Neurophysiology*, *100*, 39–47.

Hubel, D. H., & Wiesel, T. N. (1959). Receptive fields of single neurones in the cat's striate cortex. *Journal of Physiology*, *148*, 574–591.

Huddleston, W. E., & DeYoe, E. A. (2008). The representation of spatial attention in human parietal cortex dynamically modulates with performance. *Cerebral Cortex*, *18*, 1272–1280.

Hung, C. P., Kreiman, G., Poggio, T., & DiCarlo, J. J. (2005). Fast readout of object identity from macaque inferior temporal cortex. *Science*, *310*, 863–866.

Hurley, S. (1998). *Consciousness in Action*. Cambridge, MA: MIT Press.

Hurley, S. (2008). The shared circuits model (SCM): How control, mirroring, and simulation can enable imitation, deliberation, and mindreading. *Behavioral and Brain Sciences*, *31*, 1–22.

Iacoboni, M. [2008] (2009). *Mirroring People: The Science of Empathy and How We Connect with Others*. New York: Picador.

Isa, T., & Yoshida, M. (2009). Saccade control after V1 lesion revisited. *Current Opinion in Neurobiology*, *19*, 608–614.

Ishihara, T., Iino, Y., Mohri, A., Mori, I., Gengyo-Ando, K., Mitani, S., et al. (2002). HEN-1, a secretory protein with an LDL receptor motif, regulates sensory integration and learning in *Caenorhabditis elegans*. *Cell*, *109*, 639–649.

Ito, M., Tamura, H., Fujita, I., & Tanaka, K. (1995). Size and position invariance of neuronal responses in monkey inferotemporal cortex. *Journal of Neurophysiology*, *73*, 218–226.

Jakobson, R. (1960). Linguistics and poetics. In T. A. Sebeok (Ed.), *Style in Language* (pp. 350–377). Cambridge, MA: MIT Press.

James, W. [1890] (1950a). *The Principles of Psychology. Volume 1*. New York: Dover Publications Inc.

James, W. [1890] (1950b). *The Principles of Psychology. Volume 2*. New York: Dover Publications Inc.

Jenkins, I. (1973). Art for art's sake. In P. P. Wiener (Ed.), *Dictionary of the History of Ideas: Studies of Selected Pivotal Ideas* (Vol. 1, pp. 108–111). New York: Charles Scribner's Sons.

Johansson, R. S., Westling, G., Bäckström, A., & Flanagan, J. R. (2001). Eye–hand coordination in object manipulation. *Journal of Neuroscience*, *21*, 6917–6932.

Johnson, A., & Redish, A. D. (2007). Neural assemblies in CA3 transiently encode paths forward of the animal at a decision point. *Journal of Neuroscience*, *27*, 12176–12189.

Jones, A., Wilkinson, H. J., & Braden, I. (1961). Information deprivation as a motivational variable. *Journal of Experimental Psychology*, *62*, 126–137.

Jonides, J. (1981). Voluntary versus automatic control over the mind's eye's movement. In J. B. Long & A. D. Baddeley (Eds.), *Attention and Performance IX* (pp. 187–203). Hillsdale, NJ: Lawrence Erlbaum Associates.

Kahneman, D. (1973). *Attention and Effort*. Englewood Cliffs, NJ: Prentice-Hall.

Kahneman, D., & Tversky, A. (1979). Prospect theory: An analysis of decision under risk. *Econometrica*, *47*, 263–291.

Kallio, S., Hyönä, J., Revonsuo, A., Sikka, P., & Nummenmaa, L. (2011). The existence of a hypnotic state revealed by eye movements. *PLoS ONE*, *6*, e26374.

Kandel, E. R., Schwartz, J. H., & Jessel, T. H. (2000). *Principles of Neural Science*. New York: McGraw-Hill.

Kang, M. J., Rangel, A., Camus, M., & Camerer, C. F. (2011). Hypothetical and real choice differentially activate common valuation areas. *Journal of Neuroscience*, *31*, 461–468.

Kant, I. [1781] (2007). *Critique of Pure Reason* (Weigelt, M., Trans.). London: Penguin Books.

Kanwisher, N., & Yovel, G. (2009). Face perception. In G. G. Berntson & J. T. Cacioppo (Eds.), *Handbook of Neuroscience for the Behavioral Sciences* (Vol. 2, pp. 841–858). Hoboken, NJ: John Wiley & Sons.

Kanwisher, N., McDermott, J., & Chun, M. M. (1997). The fusiform face area: A module in human extrastriate cortex specialized for face perception. *Journal of Neuroscience*, *17*, 4302–4311.

Keats, J. (2002). G. F. Scott (Ed.), *Selected Letters of John Keats* (Revised Edition). Cambridge, MA: Harvard University Press.

Keats, J. [1978] (2003). *Complete Poems* (Stillinger, J., Ed.). Cambridge, MA: The Belknap Press, Harvard University Press.

Kim, J. H., Auerbach, J. M., Rodríguez-Gómez, J. A., Velasco, I., Gavin, D., Lumelsky, N., et al. (2002). Dopamine neurons derived from embryonic stem cells function in an animal model of Parkinson's disease. *Nature*, *418*, 50–56.

Ko, H.-K., Poletti, M., & Rucci, M. (2010). Microsaccades precisely relocate gaze in a high visual acuity task. *Nature Neuroscience*, *13*, 1549–1553.

Kobayashi, S., Schultz, W., & Sakagami, M. (2010). Operant conditioning of primate prefrontal neurons. *Journal of Neurophysiology*, *103*, 1843–1855.

Koch, C., & Tsuchiya, N. (2007). Attention and consciousness: Two distinct brain processes. *Trends in Cognitive Sciences*, *11*, 16–22.

Kohler, E., Keysers, C., Umiltà, M. A., Fogassi, L., Gallese, V., & Rizzolatti, G. (2002). Hearing sounds, understanding actions: Action representation in mirror neurons. *Science*, *297*, 846–848.

Komatsu, H., Kinoshita, M., & Murakami, I. (2000). Neural response in the retinotopic representation of the blind spot in the macaque V1 to stimuli for perceptual filling-in. *Journal of Neuroscience*, *20*, 9310–9319.

Kornmüller, A. E. (1931). Eine experimentelle Anästhesie der äusseren Augenmuskeln am Menschen und ihre Auswirkungen. [Experimental anesthesia of the outer eye muscles in humans and its effects.] *Journal für Psychologie und Neurologie*, *41*, 354–366.

Kovács, Á. M., Téglás, E., & Endress, A. D. (2010). The social sense: Susceptibility to others' beliefs in human infants and adults. *Science*, *330*, 1830–1834.

Krajbich, I., Armel, C., & Rangel, A. (2010). Visual fixations and the computation and comparison of value in simple choice. *Nature Neuroscience*, *13*, 1292–1298.

Kravitz, D. J., Saleem, K. S., Baker, C. I., & Mishkin, M. (2011). A new neural framework for visuospatial processing. *Nature Reviews. Neuroscience*, *12*, 217–230.

Kreiman, G., Koch, C., & Fried, I. (2000). Imagery neurons in the human brain. *Nature*, *408*, 357–361.

LaBerge, D. (1995). *Attentional Processing: The Brain's Art of Mindfulness*. Cambridge, MA: Harvard University Press.

LaBerge, D., & Buchsbaum, M. S. (1990). Positron emission tomographic measurements of pulvinar activity during an attention task. *Journal of Neuroscience*, *10*, 613–619.

Lacan, J. [1966] (2004). *Écrits: A Selection* (Sheridan, A., Trans.). London: Routledge.

Lamme, V. A. F. (2003). Why visual attention and awareness are different. *Trends in Cognitive Sciences*, *7*, 12–18.

Langston, R. F., Ainge, J. A., Couey, J. J., Canto, C. B., Bjerknes, T. L., Witter, M. P., et al. (2011). Development of the spatial representation system in the rat. *Science*, *328*, 1576–1580.

Langton, S. R. H., & Bruce, V. (1999). Reflexive visual orienting in response to the social attention of others. *Visual Cognition*, *6*, 541–568.

Lauwereyns, J. (1998). Exogenous/endogenous control of space-based/object-based attention: Four types of visual selection? *European Journal of Cognitive Psychology*, *10*, 41–74.

Lauwereyns, J. (2010). *The Anatomy of Bias: How Neural Circuits Weigh the Options*. Cambridge, MA: MIT Press.

Lauwereyns, J., & d'Ydewalle, G. (1996). Knowledge acquisition in poetry criticism: The expert's eye movements as an information tool. *International Journal of Human–Computer Studies*, *45*, 1–18.

Lauwereyns, J., Takikawa, Y., Kawagoe, R., Kobayashi, S., Koizumi, M., Coe, B., et al. (2002a). Feature-based anticipation of cues that predict reward in monkey caudate nucleus. *Neuron*, *33*, 463–473.

Lauwereyns, J., Watanabe, K., Coe, B., & Hikosaka, O. (2002b). A neural correlate of response bias in monkey caudate nucleus. *Nature*, *418*, 413–417.

Lavie, N., Ro, T., & Russell, C. (2003). The role of perceptual load in processing distractor faces. *Psychological Science*, *14*, 510–515.

Lederer, R. [1987] (2006). *Anguished English: An Anthology of Accidental Assaults upon the English Language*. Layton, UT: Wyrick & Company.

Le Gros Clark, W. E. (1932). The structure and connections of the thalamus. *Brain*, *55*, 406–470.

Lenggenhager, B., Tadi, T., Metzinger, T., & Blanke, O. (2007). Video ergo sum: Manipulating bodily self-consciousness. *Science*, *317*, 1096–1099.

Leslie, A. M. (1994). Pretending and believing: Issues in the theory of ToMM. *Cognition*, *50*, 211–238.

Lettvin, J. Y., Maturana, H. R., McCulloch, W. S., & Pitts, W. H. (1959). What the frog's eye tells the frog's brain. [IRE]. *Proceedings of the Institute of Radio Engineers*, *47*, 1940–1951.

Levin, D. T., & Simons, D. J. (1997). Failure to detect changes to attended objects in motion pictures. *Psychonomic Bulletin & Review*, *4*, 501–506.

Lévinas, E. [1972] (2003). *Humanism of the Other* (Poller, N., Trans.). Chicago: University of Illinois.

Li, N., & DiCarlo, J. J. (2008). Unsupervised natural experience rapidly alters invariant object representation in visual cortex. *Science*, *321*, 1502–1507.

Li, N., & DiCarlo, J. J. (2010). Unsupervised natural visual experience rapidly reshapes size-invariant object representation in inferior temporal cortex. *Neuron*, *67*, 1062–1075.

Li, Y., Van Hooser, S. D., Mazurek, M., White, L. E., & Fitzpatrick, D. (2008). Experience with moving visual stimuli drives the early development of cortical direction selectivity. *Nature, 456*, 952–956.

Lim, S.-L., O'Doherty, J. P., & Rangel, A. (2011). The decision value computations in the vmPFC and striatum use a relative value code that is guided by visual attention. *Journal of Neuroscience, 31*, 13214–13223.

Livingstone, M. [2002] (2008). *Vision and Art: The Biology of Seeing*. New York: ABRAMS.

Lloyd, J., & Mitchinson, J. (2006). *The Book of General Ignorance*. London: Faber and Faber Limited.

Locke, J. [1689] (1975). P. H. Nidditch (Ed.), *An Essay Concerning Human Understanding*. Oxford: Oxford University Press.

Loftus, G. R., & Mackworth, N. H. (1978). Cognitive determinants of fixation location during picture viewing. *Journal of Experimental Psychology. Human Perception and Performance, 4*, 565–572.

Logan, G. D., & Crump, M. J. (2010). Cognitive illusions of authorship reveal hierarchical error detection in skilled typists. *Science, 330*, 683–686.

Logothetis, N. K., & Sheinberg, D. L. (1996). Visual object recognition. *Annual Review of Neuroscience, 19*, 577–621.

Longerich, P. (2010). *Holocaust: The Nazi Persecution and Murder of the Jews*. Oxford: Oxford University Press.

Lynd-Balta, E., & Haber, S. N. (1994). The organization of midbrain projections to the striatum in the primate: Sensorimotor-related striatum versus ventral striatum. *Neuroscience, 59*, 625–640.

Mack, A., & Rock, I. (1998). *Inattentional Blindness*. Cambridge, MA: MIT Press.

Mackworth, N. H., & Morandi, A. J. (1967). The gaze selects informative details within pictures. *Perception & Psychophysics, 2*, 547–552.

Manning, R., Levine, M., & Collins, A. (2007). The Kitty Genovese murder and the social psychology of helping: The parable of the 38 witnesses. *American Psychologist, 62*, 555–562.

Mansouri, F. A., Tanaka, K., & Buckley, M. J. (2009). Conflict-induced behavioural adjustment: A clue to the executive functions of the prefrontal cortex. *Nature Reviews. Neuroscience, 10*, 141–152.

Markram, H. (2006). The Blue Brain Project. *Nature Reviews. Neuroscience, 7*, 153–160.

Marr, D. [1982] (2010). *Vision: A Computational Investigation into the Human Representation and Processing of Visual Information*. Cambridge, MA: MIT Press.

Masland, R. H. (2001). The fundamental plan of the retina. *Nature Neuroscience, 4*, 877–886.

Mason, M. F., Norton, M. I., Van Horn, J. D., Wegner, D. M., Grafton, S. T., & Macrae, C. N. (2007). Wandering minds: The default network and stimulus-independent thought. *Science, 315*, 393–395.

Matin, E. (1974). Saccadic suppression: A review and an analysis. *Psychological Bulletin, 81*, 899–917.

Matin, L., Picoult, E., Stevens, J. K., Edwards, M. W., Jr., Young, D., & MacArthur, R. (1982). Oculoparalytic illusion: Visual-field dependent spatial mislocalizations by humans partially paralyzed with curare. *Science, 216*, 198–201.

Matsumoto, M., & Hikosaka, O. (2009). Two types of dopamine neuron distinctly convey positive and negative motivational signals. *Nature, 459*, 837–841.

Matsumoto, M., & Komatsu, H. (2005). Neural responses in the macaque V1 to bar stimuli with various lengths presented on the blind spot. *Journal of Neurophysiology, 93*, 2374–2387.

Maturana, H. R., Lettvin, J. Y., McCulloch, W. S., & Pitts, W. H. (1960). Anatomy and physiology of vision in the frog (*Rana pipiens*). *Journal of General Physiology*, *43*, 129–175.

Mazer, J. A., & Gallant, J. L. (2003). Goal-related activity in V4 during free viewing visual search: Evidence for a ventral stream visual salience map. *Neuron*, *40*, 1241–1250.

McAlonan, K., Cavanaugh, J., & Wurtz, R. H. (2008). Guarding the gateway to cortex with attention in visual thalamus. *Nature*, *456*, 391–394.

Mehta, R., & Zhu, R. (2009). Blue or red? Exploring the effects of color on cognitive task performances. *Science*, *323*, 1226–1229.

Melcher, D. (2007). Predictive remapping of visual features precedes saccadic eye movements. *Nature Neuroscience*, *10*, 903–907.

Merleau-Ponty, M. [1945] (2008). *Phenomenology of Perception* (Smith, C., Trans.). New York: Routledge Classics.

Merriam, E. P., Genovese, C. R., & Colby, C. L. (2003). Spatial updating in human parietal cortex. *Neuron*, *39*, 361–373.

Messinger, A., Squire, L. R., Zola, S. M., & Albright, T. D. (2005). Neural correlates of knowledge: Stable representation of stimulus associations across variations in behavioral performance. *Neuron*, *48*, 359–371.

Metzinger, T. (2004). *Being No One: The Self-Model Theory of Subjectivity*. Cambridge, MA: MIT Press.

Mevorach, C., Hodsoll, J., Allen, H., Shalev, L., & Humphreys, G. (2010). Ignoring the elephant in the room: A neural circuit to downregulate salience. *Journal of Neuroscience*, *30*, 6072–6079.

Miller, G. (2000). *The Mating Mind: How Sexual Choice Shaped the Evolution of Human Nature*. New York: Doubleday, Random House, Inc.

Minsky, M. (1985). *The Society of Mind*. New York: Simon & Schuster.

Mitchell, J. F., Stoner, G. R., & Reynolds, J. H. (2004). Object-based attention determines dominance in binocular rivalry. *Nature*, *429*, 410–413.

Mitroff, S. R., Simons, D. J., & Levin, D. T. (2004). Nothing compares 2 views: Change blindness can occur despite preserved access to the changed information. *Perception & Psychophysics*, *66*, 1268–1281.

Moore, T., & Armstrong, K. M. (2003). Selective gating of visual signals by microstimulation of frontal cortex. *Nature*, *421*, 370–373.

Moore, T., & Fallah, M. (2001). Control of eye movements and spatial attention. *Proceedings of the National Academy of Sciences of the United States of America*, *98*, 1273–1276.

Moore, T., Armstrong, K. M., & Fallah, M. (2003). Visuomotor origins of covert spatial attention. *Neuron*, *40*, 671–683.

Moriguchi, Y., Ohnishi, T., Decety, J., Hirakata, M., Maeda, M., Matsuda, H., et al. (2009). The human mirror neuron system in a population with deficient self-awareness: An fMRI study in alexithymia. *Human Brain Mapping*, *30*, 2063–2076.

Mulvey, L. [1989] (2009). *Visual and Other Pleasures*. New York: Palgrave Macmillan.

Münch, T. A., da Silveira, R. A., Siegert, S., Viney, T. J., Awatramani, G. B., & Roska, B. (2009). Approach sensitivity in the retina processed by a multifunctional neural circuit. *Nature Neuroscience*, *12*, 1308–1316.

Nakamura, K., & Colby, C. L. (2002). Updating of the visual representation in monkey striate and extrastriate cortex during saccades. *Proceedings of the National Academy of Sciences of the United States of America*, *99*, 4026–4031.

Nardo, D., Santangelo, V., & Macaluso, E. (2011). Stimulus-driven orienting of visuo-spatial attention in complex dynamic environments. *Neuron*, *69*, 1015–1028.

Necker, L. A. (1832). Observations on some remarkable optical phaenomena seen in Switzerland; and on an optical phaenomenon which occurs on viewing a figure of a crystal or geometrical solid. *London & Edinburgh Philosophical Magazine and Journal of Science*, *1*, 329–337.

Neisser, U. (1967). *Cognitive Psychology*. New York: Appleton-Century-Crofts.

Neisser, U., & Becklen, R. (1975). Selective looking: Attending to visually specified events. *Cognitive Psychology*, *7*, 480–494.

Nelissen, K., Luppino, G., Vanduffel, W., Rizzolatti, G., & Orban, G. A. (2005). Observing others: Multiple action representation in the frontal lobe. *Science*, *310*, 332–336.

Niedenthal, P. M., Mermillod, M., Maringer, M., & Hess, U. (2010). The Simulation of Smiles (SIMS) model: Embodied simulation and the meaning of facial expression. *Behavioral and Brain Sciences*, *33*, 417–433.

Nobre, A. C., Rao, A., & Chelazzi, L. (2006). Selective attention to specific features within objects: Behavioral and electrophysiological evidence. *Journal of Cognitive Neuroscience*, *18*, 539–561.

Noë, A. (2004). *Action in Perception*. Cambridge, MA: MIT Press.

Noë, A. (2009). *Out of Our Heads: Why You Are Not Your Brain and Other Lessons from the Biology of Consciousness*. New York: Hill and Wang.

Noudoost, B., & Moore, T. (2011). Control of visual cortical signals by prefrontal dopamine. *Nature*, *474*, 372–375.

Oakley, D. A., & Halligan, P. W. (2009). Hypnotic suggestion and cognitive neuroscience. *Trends in Cognitive Sciences*, *13*, 264–270.

O'Connor, D. H., Fukui, M. M., Pinsk, M. A., & Kastner, S. (2002). Attention modulates responses in the human lateral geniculate nucleus. *Nature Neuroscience*, *5*, 1203–1209.

O'Doherty, J., Kringelbach, M. L., Rolls, E. T., Hornak, J., & Andrews, C. (2001). Abstract reward and punishment representations in the human orbitofrontal cortex. *Nature Neuroscience*, *4*, 95–102.

Öhman, A., & Mineka, S. (2001). Fears, phobias, and preparedness: Toward an evolved module of fear and fear learning. *Psychological Review*, *108*, 483–522.

O'Keefe, J., & Nadel, L. (1978). *The Hippocampus as a Cognitive Map*. Oxford: Oxford University Press.

Olson, C. (1967). R. Creely (Ed.), *Selected Writings of Charles Olson*. New York: New Directions Books.

Olson, C. R., & Gettner, S. N. (1995). Object-centered direction selectivity in the macaque supplementary eye field. *Science*, *269*, 985–988.

Ölveczky, B. P., Baccus, S. A., & Meister, M. (2003). Segregation of object and background motion in the retina. *Nature*, *423*, 401–408.

Oomura, Y., Yoshimatsu, H., & Aou, S. (1983). Medial preoptic and hypothalamic neuronal activity during sexual behavior of the male monkey. *Brain Research*, *266*, 340–343.

Palmer, M. (2008). *Active Boundaries: Selected Essays and Talks*. New York: New Directions Books.

Palmer, M. (2011). *Thread*. New York: New Directions Books.

Palmer, S. E. (1999). *Vision Science: Photons to Phenomenology*. Cambridge, MA: MIT Press.

Peelen, M. V., Fei-Fei, L., & Kastner, S. (2009). Neural mechanisms of rapid natural scene categorization in human visual cortex. *Nature*, *460*, 94–97.

Perloff, M. [1991] (1994). *Radical Artifice: Writing Poetry in the Age of Media*. Chicago: University of Chicago Press.

Perner, J., Mauer, M. C., & Hildenbrand, M. (2011). Identity: Key to children's understanding of belief. *Science*, *333*, 474–477.

Petersen, S. E., Robinson, D. L., & Keys, W. (1985). Pulvinar nuclei of the behaving rhesus monkey: Visual responses and their modulation. *Journal of Neurophysiology*, *54*, 867–886.

Petrusca, D., Grivich, M. I., Sher, A., Field, G. D., Gauthier, J. L., Greschner, M., et al. (2007). Identification and characterization of a Y-like primate retinal ganglion cell type. *Journal of Neuroscience*, *27*, 11019–11027.

Platt, M. L. (2002). Neural correlates of decisions. *Current Opinion in Neurobiology, 12,* 141–148.

Platt, M. L., & Glimcher, P. W. (1999). Neural correlates of decision variables in parietal cortex. *Nature, 400,* 233–238.

Poe, E. A. [1850] (2009). *The Poetic Principle.* Baltimore, MD: The Edgar Allen Poe Society of Baltimore.

Polk, T. A., Drake, R. M., Jonides, J. J., Smith, M. R., & Smith, E. E. (2008). Attention enhances the neural processing of relevant features and suppresses the processing of irrelevant features in humans: A functional magnetic resonance imaging study of the Stroop task. *Journal of Neuroscience, 28,* 13786–13792.

Popper, K. [1935] (2002). *The Logic of Scientific Discovery.* London: Routledge.

Port, N. L., & Wurtz, R. H. (2003). Sequential activity of simultaneously recorded neurons in the superior colliculus during curved saccades. *Journal of Neurophysiology, 90,* 1887–1903.

Porter, G., Troscianko, T., & Gilchrist, I. D. (2007). Effort during visual search and counting: Insights from pupillometry. *Quarterly Journal of Experimental Psychology, 60,* 211–229.

Posner, M. I. (1980). Orienting of attention. *Quarterly Journal of Experimental Psychology, 32,* 3–25.

Posner, M. I., & Keele, S. W. (1968). On the genesis of abstract ideas. *Journal of Experimental Psychology, 77,* 353–363.

Posner, M. I., & Mitchell, R. F. (1967). Chronometric analysis of classification. *Psychological Review, 74,* 392–409.

Powers, R. (1995). *Galatea 2.2.* New York: Farrar, Straus and Giroux.

Powers, R. (1999). Eyes wide open. *The New York Times,* April 18.

Powers, R. (2006). *The Echo Maker.* New York: Farrar, Straus and Giroux.

Rainville, P., Duncan, G. H., Price, D. D., Carrier, B., & Bushnell, M. C. (1997). Pain affect in human anterior cingulate but not somatosensory cortex. *Science, 277,* 968–971.

Rainville, P., Hofbauer, R. K., Bushnell, M. C., Duncan, G. H., & Price, D. D. (2002). Hypnosis modulates activity in brain structures involved in the regulation of consciousness. *Journal of Cognitive Neuroscience, 14,* 887–901.

Ratcliff, R., & Smith, P. (2004). A comparison of sequential sampling models for two-choice reaction time. *Psychological Review, 111,* 333–367.

Rayner, K., Li, X., Williams, C. C., Cave, K. R., & Well, A. D. (2007). Eye movements during information processing tasks: Individual differences and cultural effects. *Vision Research, 47,* 2714–2726.

Redgrave, P., & Gurney, K. (2006). The short-latency dopamine signal: A role in discovering novel actions? *Nature Reviews. Neuroscience, 7,* 967–975.

Rensink, R. A., O'Regan, J. K., & Clark, J. J. (1997). To see or not to see: The need for attention to perceive changes in scenes. *Psychological Science, 8,* 368–373.

Rilke, R. M. (1995). *Ahead of All Parting: The Selected Poetry and Prose of Rainer Maria Rilke* (Mitchell, S., Trans.). New York: The Modern Library.

Rizzini, L., Favory, J. J., Cloix, C., Faggionato, D., O'Hara, A., Kaiserli, E., et al. (2011). Perception of UV-B by the Arabidopsis UVR8 protein. *Science, 332,* 103–106.

Rizzolatti, G. (1983). Mechanisms of selective attention in mammals. In J. P. Ewert, R. R. Capranica, & D. J. Ingle (Eds.), *Advances in Vertebrate Neuroethology* (pp. 261–297). London: Plenum Press.

Rizzolatti, G., & Arbib, M. A. (1998). Language within our grasp. *Trends in Neurosciences, 21,* 188–194.

Rizzolatti, G., Fadiga, L., Gallese, V., & Fogassi, L. (1996). Premotor cortex and the recognition of motor actions. *Brain Research. Cognitive Brain Research, 3,* 131–141.

Ro, T., Russell, C., & Lavie, N. (2001). Changing faces: A detection advantage in the flicker paradigm. *Psychological Science, 12*, 94–99.

Robinson, D. A. (1972). Eye movements evoked by collicular stimulation in the alert monkey. *Vision Research, 12*, 1795–1808.

Robinson, D. A., & Fuchs, A. F. (1969). Eye movements evoked by stimulation of the frontal eye fields. *Journal of Neurophysiology, 32*, 637–648.

Robinson, D. L., & Kertzman, C. (1995). Covert orienting of attention in macaques III. Contributions of the superior colliculus. *Journal of Neurophysiology, 74*, 713–721.

Robinson, D. L., Petersen, S. E., & Keys, W. (1986). Saccade-related and visual activities in the pulvinar nuclei of the behaving rhesus monkey. *Experimental Brain Research, 62*, 625–634.

Rolfs, M., Jonikaitis, D., Deubel, H., & Cavanagh, P. (2011). Predictive remapping of attention across eye movements. *Nature Neuroscience, 14*, 252–256.

Rolls, E. T. (2008). *Memory, Attention, and Decision-Making: A Unifying Computational Neuroscience Approach*. Oxford: Oxford University Press.

Rosenbluth, D., & Allman, J. M. (2002). The effect of gaze angle and fixation distance on the responses of neurons in V1, V2, and V4. *Neuron, 33*, 143–149.

Ross, J., & Ma-Wyatt, A. (2004). Saccades actively maintain perceptual continuity. *Nature Neuroscience, 7*, 65–69.

Ryan, J. D., Althoff, R. R., Whitlow, S., & Cohen, N. J. (2000). Amnesia is a deficit in relational memory. *Psychological Science, 11*, 454–461.

Saalmann, Y. B., & Kastner, S. (2011). Cognitive and perceptual functions of the visual thalamus. *Neuron, 71*, 209–223.

Sakai, K., Hikosaka, O., Miyauchi, S., Takino, R., Sasaki, Y., & Pütz, B. (1998). Transition of brain activation from frontal to parietal areas in visuomotor sequence learning. *Journal of Neuroscience, 18*, 1827–1840.

Salecl, R., & Žižek, S. (1996). Introduction. In R. Salecl & S. Žižek (Eds.), *Gaze and Voice as Love Objects* (pp. 1–4). Durham, NC: Duke University Press.

Sanders, G., Sinclair, K., & Walsh, T. (2007). Testing predictions from the hunter–gatherer hypothesis. II. Sex differences in the visual processing of near and far space. *Evolutionary Psychology, 5*, 666–679.

Sartre, J.-P. [1943] (1992). *Being and Nothingness: A Phenomenological Essay on Ontology* (Barnes, H. E., Trans.). New York: Washington Square Press.

Schafer, R. J., & Moore, T. (2011). Selective attention from voluntary control of neurons in prefrontal cortex. *Science, 332*, 1568–1571.

Schell, A., Rieck, K., Schell, K., Hammerschmidt, K., & Fischer, J. (2011). Adult but not juvenile Barbary macaques spontaneously recognize group members from pictures. *Animal Cognition, 14*, 503–509.

Scheumann, M., & Call, J. (2004). The use of experimenter-given cues by South African fur seals (*Arctocephalus pusillus*). *Animal Cognition, 7*, 224–230.

Schiller, F. (1992). *Paul Broca: Founder of French Anthropology, Explorer of the Brain*. Oxford: Oxford University Press.

Schmidt, J., Scheid, C., Kotrschal, K., Bugnyar, T., & Schloegl, C. (2011). Gaze direction — A cue for hidden food in rooks (*Corvus frugilegus*)? *Animal Cognition, 88*, 88–93.

Schmuckler, M. A., & Jewell, D. T. (2007). Infants' visual–proprioceptive intermodal perception with imperfect contingency information. *Developmental Psychobiology, 49*, 387–398.

Schneider, K. A., Richter, M. C., & Kastner, S. (2004). Retinotopic organization and functional subdivisions of the human lateral geniculate nucleus: A high-resolution functional magnetic resonance imaging study. *Journal of Neuroscience, 24*, 8975–8985.

Schoups, A., Vogels, R., Qian, N., & Orban, G. (2001). Practising orientation identification improves orientation coding in V1 neurons. *Nature, 412*, 549–553.

Schultes, R. E., Hofman, A., & Rätsch, C. (2001). *Plants of the Gods: Their Sacred, Healing, and Hallucinogenic Powers*. Rochester, VT: Healing Arts Press.

Schultz, W. (1998). Predictive reward signal of dopamine neurons. *Journal of Neurophysiology, 80*, 1–27.

Schultz, W., Dayan, P., & Montague, P. R. (1997). A neural substrate of prediction and reward. *Science, 275*, 1593–1599.

Schwartz, G., Harris, R., Shrom, D., & Berry, M. J., II. (2007). Detection and prediction of periodic patterns by the retina. *Nature Neuroscience, 10*, 552–554.

Sergent, J., Ohta, S., & MacDonald, B. (1992). Functional neuroanatomy of face and object processing: A positron emission study. *Brain, 115*, 15–36.

Sheliga, B. M., Riggio, L., & Rizzolatti, G. (1994). Orienting of attention and eye movements. *Experimental Brain Research, 98*, 507–522.

Shepherd, S. V., Klein, J. T., Deaner, R. O., & Platt, M. L. (2009). Mirroring of attention by neurons in macaque parietal cortex. *Proceedings of the National Academy of Sciences of the United States of America, 106*, 9489–9494.

Sherrington, C. (1906). *The Integrative Action of the Nervous System*. New York: Charles Scribner's Sons.

Sherrington, C. [1940] (1955). *Man on His Nature*. Middlesex, UK: Penguin Books.

Sheth, S. A., Abuelem, T., Gale, J. T., & Eskandar, E. N. (2011). Basal ganglia neurons dynamically facilitate exploration during associative learning. *Journal of Neuroscience, 31*, 4878–4885.

Shimojo, S., Kamitani, Y., & Nishida, S. (2001). Afterimages of perceptually filled-in surface. *Science, 293*, 1677–1680.

Shimojo, S., Simion, C., Shimojo, E., & Scheier, C. (2003). Gaze bias both reflects and influences preference. *Nature Neuroscience, 6*, 1317–1322.

Shinkai, Y., Yamamoto, Y., Fujiwara, M., Tabata, T., Murayama, T., Hirotsu, T., et al. (2011). Behavioral choice between conflicting alternatives is regulated by a receptor guanylyl cyclase, GCY-28, and a receptor tyrosine kinase, SCD-2, in AIA interneurons of *Caenorhabditis elegans*. *Journal of Neuroscience, 31*, 3007–3015.

Siebeck, R., & Frey, R. (1953). Die Wirkungen muskelerschlaffender Mittel auf die Augenmuskeln [The effects of muscle relaxants on the eye muscles]. *Anaesthesia, 2*, 138–141.

Silverman, I., & Eals, M. (1992). Sex differences in spatial abilities: Evolutionary theory and data. In J. Barkow, L. Cosmides, & J. Tooby (Eds.), *The Adapted Mind: Evolutionary Psychology and the Generation of Culture* (pp. 533–549). New York: Oxford University Press.

Silverman, M., & Mack, A. (2006). Change blindness and priming: When it does and does not occur. *Consciousness and Cognition, 15*, 409–422.

Simons, D. J., & Chabris, C. F. (1999). Gorillas in our midst: Sustained inattentional blindness for dynamic events. *Perception, 28*, 1059–1074.

Simons, D. J., & Rensink, R. A. (2005). Change blindness: Past, present, and future. *Trends in Cognitive Sciences, 9*, 16–20.

Singer, T., Seymour, B., O'Doherty, J. P., Stephan, K. E., Dolan, R. J., & Frith, C. D. (2006). Empathic neural responses are modulated by the perceived fairness of others. *Nature, 439*, 466–469.

Singer, W. (1977). Control of thalamic transmission by corticofugal and ascending reticular pathways in the visual system. *Physiological Reviews, 57*, 386–420.

Smith, A. M. (2001). *Alhacen's Theory of Visual Perception. Volume 1: Introduction and Latin Text*. Philadelphia: American Philosophical Society.

Sokolov, E. N. (1963). *Perception and the Conditioned Reflex* (Waydenfeld, S. W., Trans.). New York: The Macmillan Company.

Sokolov, E. N., Spinks, J. A., Näätänen, R., & Lyytinen, H. (2002). *The Orienting Response in Information Processing*. Mahwah, NJ: Lawrence Erlbaum Associates.

Sommer, M. A., & Wurtz, R. H. (2002). A pathway in primate brain for internal monitoring of movements. *Science, 296*, 1480–1482.

Sommer, M. A., & Wurtz, R. H. (2006). Influence of the thalamus on spatial visual processing in frontal cortex. *Nature, 444*, 374–377.

Sperry, R. W. (1950). Neural basis of the spontaneous optokinetic response produced by visual inversion. *Journal of Comparative and Physiological Psychology, 43*, 482–489.

Spinoza. [1677] (2001). *Ethics* (White, W. H., Trans.). Hertfordshire, UK: Wordsworth Editions.

Staub, A. (2011). Word recognition and syntactic attachment in reading: Evidence for a staged architecture. *Journal of Experimental Psychology. General, 140*, 407–433.

Stein, G. (2008). J. Retallack (Ed.), *Selections*. Berkeley, CA: University of California Press.

Steinberg, L. [1983] (1996). *The Sexuality of Christ in Renaissance Art and Modern Oblivion*. Chicago: University of Chicago Press.

Sternberg, S. (1969a). The discovery of processing stages: Extensions of Donders' method. In W.G. Koster (Ed.), *Attention and performance II, Acta Psychologica, 30*, 276–315.

Sternberg, S. (1969b). Memory scanning: Mental processes revealed by reaction-time experiments. *American Scientist, 57*, 421–457.

Stevens, J. K., Emerson, R. C., Gerstein, G. L., Kallos, T., Neufeld, G. R., Nichols, C. W., et al. (1976). Paralysis of the awake human: Visual perceptions. *Vision Research, 16*, 93–98.

Stevens, W. (1951). *The Necessary Angel: Essays on Reality and the Imagination*. New York: Vintage Books.

Stevens, W. [1954] (1984). *Collected Poems*. London: Faber and Faber Limited.

Supèr, H., & Romeo, A. (2011). Rebound spiking as a neural mechanism for surface filling-in. *Journal of Cognitive Neuroscience, 23*, 491–501.

Supèr, H., Spekreijse, H., & Lamme, V. A. F. (2001). A neural correlate of working memory in monkey primary visual cortex. *Science, 293*, 120–124.

Tada, T., Yamada, F., & Hariu, T. (1990). Changes of eye-blink activities during hypnotic state. *Perceptual and Motor Skills, 71*, 832–834.

Takahashi, M., Lauwereyns, J., Sakurai, Y., & Tsukada, M. (2009). A code for spatial alternation during fixation in rat hippocampal CA1 neurons. *Journal of Neurophysiology, 102*, 556–567.

Takeuchi, T., Puntous, T., Tuladhar, A., Yoshimoto, S., & Shirama, A. (2011). Estimation of mental effort in learning visual search by measuring pupil response. *PLoS ONE, 6*, e21973.

Taylor, J. G. (2001). *The Race for Consciousness*. Cambridge, MA: MIT Press.

Thakral, P. P. (2011). The neural substrates associated with inattentional blindness. *Consciousness and Cognition, 20*, 1768–1775.

Theeuwes, J. (1991). Exogenous and endogenous control of attention: The effect of visual onsets and offsets. *Perception & Psychophysics, 51*, 279–290.

Theeuwes, J., Kramer, A. F., Hahn, S., Irwin, D. E., & Zelinsky, G. J. (1999). Influence of attentional capture on oculomotor control. *Journal of Experimental Psychology. Human Perception and Performance, 25*, 1595–1608.

Theyel, B. B., Llano, D. A., & Sherman, S. M. (2010). The corticothalamocortical circuit drives higher-order cortex in the mouse. *Nature Neuroscience, 13*, 84–88.

Thiele, A., Henning, P., Kubischik, M., & Hoffmann, K. P. (2002). Neural mechanisms of saccadic suppression. *Science, 295*, 2460–2462.

Tomasello, M., Call, J., & Hare, B. (1998). Five primate species follow the visual gaze of conspecifics. *Animal Behaviour*, *55*, 1063–1069.

Tomasello, M., Hare, B., & Agnetta, B. (1999). Chimpanzees, *Pan troglodytes*, follow gaze direction geometrically. *Animal Behaviour*, *58*, 769–777.

Torralba, A., Oliva, A., Castelhano, M. S., & Henderson, J. M. (2006). Contextual guidance of eye movements and attention in real-world scenes: The role of global features in object search. *Psychological Review*, *113*, 766–786.

Treisman, A. (1969). Strategies and models of selective attention. *Psychological Review*, *76*, 282–299.

Treisman, A., & Gelade, G. (1980). A feature-integration theory of attention. *Cognitive Psychology*, *12*, 97–136.

Treisman, A., & Sato, S. (1990). Conjunction search revisited. *Journal of Experimental Psychology. Human Perception and Performance*, *8*, 194–214.

Tremblay, L., & Schultz, W. (1999). Relative reward preference in primate orbitofrontal cortex. *Nature*, *398*, 704–708.

Tsuda, I. (2001). Toward an interpretation of dynamic neural activity in terms of chaotic dynamical systems. *Behavioral and Brain Sciences*, *24*, 793–810.

Tsutsui, K.-I., Sakata, H., Naganuma, T., & Taira, M. (2002). Neural correlates for perception of 3D surface orientation from texture gradient. *Science*, *298*, 409–412.

Umeno, M. M., & Goldberg, M. E. (1997). Spatial processing in the monkey frontal eye field. I. Predictive visual responses. *Journal of Neurophysiology*, *78*, 1373–1383.

Umiltà, M. A., Kohler, E., Gallese, V., Fogassi, L., Fadiga, L., Keysers, C., et al. (2001). I know what you are doing: A neurophysiological study. *Neuron*, *31*, 155–165.

Ungerleider, L. G., & Mishkin, M. (1982). Two cortical visual systems. In D. J. Ingle, M. A. Goodale, & R. J. W. Mansfield (Eds.), *Analysis of Visual Behavior* (pp. 549–586). Cambridge, MA: MIT Press.

Van der Heijden, A. H. C. (2004). *Attention in Vision: Perception, Communication, and Action*. Hove, UK: Psychology Press.

Van der Meer, M. A., Johnson, A., Schmitzer-Torbert, N. C., & Redish, A. D. (2010). Triple dissociation of information processing in dorsal striatum, ventral striatum, and hippocampus on a learned spatial decision task. *Neuron*, *67*, 25–32.

Van Reekum, C. M., Johnstone, T., Urry, H. L., Thurrow, M. E., Schaefer, H. S., Alexander, A. L., et al. (2007). Gaze fixations predict brain activation during the voluntary regulation of picture-induced negative affect. *NeuroImage*, *36*, 1041–1055.

Vick, S. J., & Anderson, J. R. (2000). Learning and limits of use of eye gaze by capuchin monkeys (*Cebus apella*) in an object-choice task. *Journal of Comparative Psychology*, *114*, 200–207.

Vieth, G. A. U. (1818). Über die Richtung der Augen [On the direction of the eyes]. *Annalen der Physik*, *28*, 233–253.

Vogels, R., & Orban, G. A. (1996). Coding of stimulus invariances by inferior temporal neurons. *Progress in Brain Research*, *112*, 195–211.

von Helmholtz, H. [1910] (2000). J. P. C. Southall (Ed.), *Helmholtz's Treatise on Physiological Optics*. Bristol, UK: Thoemmes Press.

von Holst, E., & Mittelstädt, H. (1950). Das Reafferenzprinzip: Wechselwirkungen zwischen Zentralnervensystem und Peripherie [The reafference principle: Interactions between the central nervous system and the periphery]. *Naturwissenschaften*, *37*, 464–476.

Vroman, L. (1965). A resemblance between the clotting of blood plasma and the breakdown of cytoplasm. *Nature*, *204*, 496–497.

Vroman, L. (2011). *Daar* [There]. Amsterdam, The Netherlands: Querido.

Wagner, D. D., Dal Cin, S., Sargent, J. D., Kelley, W. M., & Heatherton, T. F. (2011). Spontaneous action representation in smokers when watching movie characters smoke. *Journal of Neuroscience, 31*, 894–898.

Waldrop, K. (2009). *Transcendental Studies: A Trilogy*. Berkeley, CA: University of California Press.

Wallace, D. F. (2003). *Everything and More: A Compact History of Infinity*. New York: W. W. Norton & Company.

Wallis, J. D., Anderson, K. C., & Miller, E. K. (2001). Single neurons in prefrontal cortex encode abstract rules. *Nature, 411*, 953–956.

Wang, Y., Ramsey, R., & Hamilton, A. F. de C. (2011). The control of mimicry by eye contact is mediated by medial prefrontal cortex. *Journal of Neuroscience, 31*, 12001–12010.

Weaver, M. D., & Lauwereyns, J. (2011). Attentional capture and hold: The oculomotor correlates of the change detection advantage for faces. *Psychological Research, 75*, 10–23.

Weaver, M. D., Lauwereyns, J., & Theeuwes, J. (2011). The effect of semantic information on saccade trajectory deviations. *Vision Research, 51*, 1124–1128.

Weaver, M. D., Phillips, J., & Lauwereyns, J. (2010). Semantic influences from a brief peripheral cue depend on task set. *Quarterly Journal of Experimental Psychology, 63*, 1249–1255.

Wegner, D. M. (2002). *The Illusion of Conscious Will*. Cambridge, MA: MIT Press.

Wei, W., Hamby, A. M., Zhou, K., & Keller, M. B. (2011). Development of asymmetric inhibition underlying direction selectivity in the retina. *Nature, 469*, 402–406.

Weiskrantz, L. (2009). Is blindsight just degraded normal vision? *Experimental Brain Research, 192*, 413–416.

Weitzenhoffer, A. M. (1969). Hypnosis and eye movements. I. Preliminary report on a possible slow eye movement correlate of hypnosis. *American Journal of Clinical Hypnosis, 11*, 221–227.

Weitzenhoffer, A. M. (1971). Ocular changes associated with passive hypnotic behavior. *American Journal of Clinical Hypnosis, 14*, 102–121.

Weitzenhoffer, A. M. [1989] (2000). *The Practice of Hypnotism*. New York: John Wiley & Sons.

West, R. (1932). Curare in man. *Proceedings of the Royal Society of Medicine, 25*, 1107–1116.

Whalen, P. J., Kagan, J., Cook, R. G., Davis, F. C., Kim, H., Polis, S., et al. (2004). Human amygdala responsivity to masked fearful eye whites. *Nature, 306*, 261.

Wiens, S. (2006). Subliminal emotion perception in brain imaging: Findings, issues, and recommendations. *Progress in Brain Research, 156*, 105–121.

Williams, M. A., Baker, C. I., Op de Beeck, H. P., Shim, W. M., Dang, S., Triantafyllou, C., et al. (2008). Feedback of visual information to foveal retinotopic cortex. *Nature Neuroscience, 11*, 1439–1445.

Wills, T. J., Cacucci, F., Burgess, N., & O'Keefe, J. (2011). Development of the hippocampal cognitive map in preweanling rats. *Science, 328*, 1573–1576.

Winawer, J., Witthoft, N., Frank, M. C., Wu, L., Wade, A. R., & Boroditsky, L. (2007). Russian blues reveal effects of language on color discrimination. *Proceedings of the National Academy of Sciences of the United States of America, 104*, 7780–7785.

Wittgenstein, L. [1953] (2003). *Philosophical Investigations* (Anscombe, G. E. M., Trans.). Oxford: Blackwell Publishing.

Wolpert, D. M., Ghahramani, Z., & Jordan, M. I. (1995). An internal model for sensorimotor integration. *Science, 269*, 1880–1882.

Wróbel, A., Ghazaryan, A., Bekisz, M., Bogdan, W., & Kamiński, J. (2007). Two streams of attention-dependent beta activity in the striate recipient zone of cat's lateral posterior-pulvinar complex. *Journal of Neuroscience, 27*, 2230–2240.

Wunderlich, K., Schneider, K. A., & Kastner, S. (2005). Neural correlates of binocular rivalry in the human lateral geniculate nucleus. *Nature Neuroscience, 8*, 1595–1602.

Wurtz, R. H. (1969). Visual receptive fields of striate cortex neurons in awake monkeys. *Journal of Neurophysiology, 32*, 727–742.

Wurtz, R. H. (2008). Neuronal mechanisms of visual stability. *Vision Research, 48*, 2070–2089.

Wurtz, R. H., & Goldberg, M. E. (1972a). Activity of superior colliculus in behaving monkey. III. Cells discharging before eye movements. *Journal of Neurophysiology, 35*, 575–586.

Wurtz, R. H., & Goldberg, M. E. (1972b). Activity of superior colliculus in behaving monkey. IV. Effects of lesions on eye movements. *Journal of Neurophysiology, 35*, 587–596.

Wurtz, R. H., & Goldberg, M. E. (Eds.). (1989). *The Neurobiology of Saccadic Eye Movements*. Amsterdam, The Netherlands: Elsevier.

Wurtz, R. H., McAlonan, K., Cavanaugh, J., & Berman, R. A. (2011). Thalamic pathways for active vision. *Trends in Cognitive Sciences, 15*, 177–184.

Yantis, S., & Jonides, J. (1990). Abrupt visual onsets and selective attention: Voluntary versus automatic allocation. *Journal of Experimental Psychology. Human Perception and Performance, 16*, 121–134.

Yarbus, A. L. [1965] (1967). *Eye Movements and Vision* (Haigh, B., Trans.). New York: Plenum Press.

Yonehara, K., Balint, K., Noda, M., Nagel, G., Bamberg, E., & Roska, B. (2011). Spatially asymmetric reorganization of inhibition establishes a motion-sensitive circuit. *Nature, 469*, 407–410.

Yorzinski, J. L., & Platt, M. L. (2010). Same-sex gaze attraction influences mate-choice copying in humans. *PLoS ONE, 5*, e9115.

Yu, C., Ballard, D., & Aslin, R. (2005). The role of embodied intention in early lexical acquisition. *Cognitive Science, 29*, 961–1005.

Zeki, S. (2000). *Inner Vision: An Exploration of Art and the Brain*. Oxford: Oxford University Press.

Zhou, H., & Desimone, R. (2011). Feature-based attention in the frontal eye field and area V4 during visual search. *Neuron, 70*, 1205–1217.

Žižek, S. [2006] (2009). *The Parallax View*. Cambridge, MA: MIT Press.

Index